Handbook of Aging and Diseases of Aging

Handbook of Aging and Diseases of Aging

Editor: Oliver Fincher

AMERICAN
MEDICAL PUBLISHERS
www.americanmedicalpublishers.com

AMERICAN
MEDICAL PUBLISHERS
www.americanmedicalpublishers.com

Cataloging-in-Publication Data

Handbook of aging and diseases of aging / edited by Oliver Fincher.
p. cm.
Includes bibliographical references and index.
ISBN 978-1-63927-580-9
1. Geriatrics. 2. Older people--Diseases. 3. Aging.
4. Older people--Health and hygiene. 5. Gerontology. I. Fincher, Oliver.
RC952 .H363 2023
618.97--dc23

American Medical Publishers,
41 Flatbush Avenue,
1st Floor, New York,
NY 11217, USA

ISBN 978-1-63927-580-9 (Hardback)

Contents

Preface

Aging refers to the process of growing older. It primarily applies to humans, fungi and certain other animals. Contrarily, there are certain simple animals, bacteria and perennial plants that are virtually immortal. It is a biological process. Usually, it is linked to the dynamic changes in the physiological, behavioral, biological, social, environmental and psychological processes. There are numerous symptoms of aging, which develop and start to show up with time. These symptoms include wrinkles, hair graying, high frailty, decline in female fertility, muscle loss, hearing loss, increased likelihood of osteoarthritis and menopause in females. There are various diseases associated with aging such as cataract, atherosclerosis, Alzheimer's disease, cardiovascular disease, hypertension, cancer, type-2 diabetes, arthritis and osteoporosis. The occurrence of these diseases develops exponentially with age. This book unravels the recent studies on aging and the diseases associated with it. It presents researches and studies performed by experts across the globe. Those in search of information to further their knowledge will be greatly assisted by this book.

This book is a comprehensive compilation of works of different researchers from varied parts of the world. It includes valuable experiences of the researchers with the sole objective of providing the readers (learners) with a proper knowledge of the concerned field. This book will be beneficial in evoking inspiration and enhancing the knowledge of the interested readers.

In the end, I would like to extend my heartiest thanks to the authors who worked with great determination on their chapters. I also appreciate the publisher's support in the course of the book. I would also like to deeply acknowledge my family who stood by me as a source of inspiration during the project.

Editor

1

Depression, Loneliness, Social Support, Activities of Daily Living, and Life Satisfaction in Older Adults at High-Risk of Dementia

Sunghee Kim, Kwisoon Choe and Kyoungsook Lee *

Department of Nursing, Chung-Ang University, Dongjak-gu, Seoul 06974, Korea; sung1024@cau.ac.kr (S.K.); kwisoonchoe@cau.ac.kr (K.C.)

* Correspondence: kyoungsooklee0628@gmail.com

Abstract: As the number of older adults with dementia increases, early diagnosis and intervention are crucially important. The purpose of this study was to conduct dementia screening on older adults to determine whether there are differences in depression, loneliness, social support, daily activities of living, and life satisfaction between older adults at high-risk for dementia compared with low-risk older adults. We hypothesized a negative relationship between high-risk older adults and these factors. This study also hypothesized a moderating effect for social support on the relationship between daily living activities and life satisfaction. This study used a cross-sectional design with survey data. Participants were recruited at 15 public community health centers in South Korea. A total of 609 older adults (male 208, female 401) living in the community were screened for early dementia, and 113 participants (18.9%) were assigned to the high-risk group. As hypothesized, participants in the high-risk group showed significantly more negative results in terms of activities of daily living, depression, loneliness, social support, and life satisfaction compared with participants in the low-risk group. The findings of this study provide a theoretical basis for the importance of early screening for dementia and policies for effective dementia prevention.

Keywords: dementia; depression; loneliness; activities of daily living; social support; life satisfaction

---

1. Introduction

The rapid increase in the elderly population worldwide has been accompanied by a concomitant increase in the incidence and prevalence of dementia within this population. In 2019, the Korean Center for Dementia reported that the number of older adults with dementia over the age of 65 years was approximately 750,000 in South Korea [1]. Dementia is a disease that leads directly to a deterioration in the quality of life of older adults [2] and places severe physical, psychological, and economic burdens on both persons with dementia and their family care givers [3]. Given the increased incidence and prevalence of dementia, and the devastating effects of the disease, it is of paramount importance that dementia be detected early and that intervention is made as soon as possible to slow the progress of the disease for the patient's and their family care givers' quality of life.

Early screening for cognitive impairment in older adults is pivotal, particularly once older adults or their family members notice a decline in memory or difficulty performing daily activities such as paying bills, shopping, or managing medications [4]. The dementia evaluation test generally consists of a series of assessments including patient history, physical examination, functional assessment, cognitive testing, laboratory studies, and imaging studies. An initial screening test is performed for patients with suspected dementia before these are conducted.

Above all, identifying the risk factors for dementia is as essential for delaying or preventing dementia [5] as early screening. In the literature review, depression, loneliness, and poor social support were shown to be the main risk factors. Depression is generally known as a risk factor for dementia [6–9]. Depression at any age, specifically late-life depression, was associated with dementia such as Alzheimer's disease [6], and may be a response to cognitive impairment in older persons [7]. Loneliness and poor social networks were also known the major risk factor of dementia among older adults [5,10–14]. Loneliness induced by low social participation and infrequent social contact was related to the occurrence of dementia [5]. For example, loneliness increased the risk of dementia among people aged 65 years and older in China [11]. Poor social networks and social support resulted in poor social engagement, and poor social engagement increased the risk of dementia [14]. Frequency of social contacts for all types of dementia was a significant protective factor [6]. In addition, social support through community engagement and marriage is known to be a protective factor against the risk of dementia [13,14]. In particular, social support from family members such as children reduced the risk of dementia, whereas negative social support increased the risk [15].

In addition, older adults with dementia have difficulty performing daily activities, so-called activities of daily living (ADL), across the stage of dementia [16]. ADL disability can predict the occurrence and degree of dementia [17]. Furthermore, ADL is closely related to life satisfaction of older adults with dementia [18]. Life satisfaction is a protective factor for dementia [19], and ADL affects life satisfaction among older adults regardless of dementia [20].

To confirm the risk factors of dementia and the usefulness of the early screening test for dementia among older adults, the research question in this study was, "does the high-risk group who was detected by early screening for dementia show any differences in variables known as risk factors for dementia when comparing with those of low-risk group?" and "is there a difference in daily living activities and life satisfaction between the high-risk and low-risk groups classified by the early screening test?". The third research question was, "Does social support have a moderating effect on the relationship between ADL and life satisfaction?". According to the conceptual model of quality of life [21], social functioning moderates the relationship between physical functioning and life satisfaction. The authors wanted to confirm whether this model applies to the group of dementia.

The purpose of this study was to identify whether there are differences in depression, loneliness, social support, daily activities of living, and life satisfaction between older adults at high-risk for dementia compared with low-risk older adults by means of an early screening test for dementia in community. Furthermore, the authors sought to identify the moderating effect of social support on the relationship between ADL and life satisfaction of older adults in both groups.

2. Materials and Methods

2.1. Research Design

This study used a cross-sectional design with survey data.

2.2. Participants

Participants were recruited at 15 public health centers in South Korea. Public health centers are medical facilities operated by the government to promote health and prevent people's diseases in the community. Public health centers in South Korea recommend that people in their 60s receive an early screening test for dementia, so the authors recruited those aged 60 and over who visit public health centers in their community via convenience sampling. The inclusion criteria were: older adults aged 60 years or older, willingness to take a test for early dementia screening, living in the community, and able to communicate without cognitive impairment. Older adults were not eligible if they could not communicate with discernible cognitive impairment, could not read or understand the questionnaires of this study, and did not voluntarily agree to participate in this study.

2.3. Instruments

2.3.1. Mini-Mental State Examination for Dementia Screening (MMSE-DS)

The Korean version of the MMSE-DS [22] was used to identify cognitive impairment in participants. The high risk for dementia was determined according to the standardized criteria (Table 1) of the previous study [22], which verified the reliability and validity of MMSE-DS. Therefore, we did not verify the reliability and validity of the scale separately in this study. This scale is commonly used as a screening test for dementia in public health centers in South Korea. MMSE-DS is composed of items that investigate orientation (time, place), memory (memory registration and recall), attention and calculation capabilities, language skills, understanding, and judgment.

Table 1. Mini-Mental State Examination for Dementia Screening (MMSE-DS) criteria.

Age	Sex	Educational Year			
		0–3	4–6	7–12	13 and Over
60–69	Male	20	24	25	26
	Female	19	23	25	26
70–74	Male	21	23	25	26
	Female	18	21	25	26
75–79	Male	20	22	25	25
	Female	17	21	24	26
80 and over	Male	18	22	24	25
	Female	16	20	24	27

If the score is lower than that given in the table above, refer it to the diagnostic test.

2.3.2. Geriatric Depression Scale Short Form-Korea

The Geriatric Depression Scale Short Form-Korea (GDSSF-K) was used to assess depression. The GDSSF-K was standardized by Kee [23]. It comprises 15 items with a "yes" or "no" response resulting in a total possible score of 15 points. The higher the score, the higher the degree of depression. This scale is a shortened form of the 30-item Geriatric Depression Scale (GDS) developed by Yesavage et al. [24].

2.3.3. UCLA Loneliness Scale

The revised UCLA (University of California, Los Angeles) Loneliness Scale [25] was used to measure loneliness. This is a 4-point Likert-type scale, consisting of 20 items, and the range of total score is 20–80. The higher the score, the greater the degree of loneliness experienced.

2.3.4. Instrumental Activities of Daily Living Scale

The Korean version of the Instrumental Activities of Daily Living Scale [26] was used to evaluate everyday functions such as shopping, food preparation, housekeeping, laundry, transportation, responsibility for own medications, and handling finances. This 15-item scale was developed based on Lawton's Instrumental Activities of Daily Living Scale [27] and rated on a 4-point Likert-type scale. The range of total score is between 15 and 60.

2.3.5. Lubben Social Network Scale

Social support was measured using the Lubben Social Network Scale [28]. The scale measures the degree of social support received from the older person's family network, network of friends, caregivers, and living arrangements. It consists of 10 items rated on a 6-point Likert-type scale from 0 to 5; a score of 20 or less shows a limited social network.

2.3.6. Life Satisfaction Scale

The Life Satisfaction Scale was developed by Yoon [29] based on the Memorial University of Newfoundland of Scale for Happiness [30]. It consists of a total of 20 items rated on a 4-point Likert-type scale ranging from 0 to 3 points. The higher the score, the higher the level of life satisfaction.

2.4. Data Collection and Ethical Considerations

This study was conducted in accordance with the Declaration of Helsinki, and the protocol was approved by the institutional review board of Chung-Ang University (1041078-201410-HR-151-01). The authors recruited nursing and social welfare college students on a part-time basis. We trained them on the purpose of the study and how to collect the data using the questionnaire. After obtaining cooperation from the public health centers for data collection, trained college students explained the aims of the research to older persons who came for dementia screening. Participants who volunteered for this study were asked to complete a consent form and a questionnaire. The questionnaire took an average of approximately 20 min to complete, and it did not need break time in answering the questionnaires. When participants asked for help filling out the questionnaire, nursing students, social welfare students, and health center staff trained in this study helped them. After removing 11 questionnaires due to missing data, a total of 609 questionnaires were used in the data analysis.

2.5. Data Analysis

The data were analyzed using SPSS Statistics 23.0 (IBM Corp., Armonk, NY, USA) [31]. We analyzed the general characteristics of the participants in terms of frequencies, percentages, means, and standard deviations. As a result of the Kolmogorov-Smirnov and Shapiro-Wilk tests, the Mann–Whitney U test was used to compare differences between the two groups because the dependent variable was not normally distributed. The correlations between variables were analyzed using Spearman's correlation analysis. Next, the authors used the standard method of determining whether a moderating effect exists, which entails adding a (linear) interaction term in a multiple regression model [32]. The four demographic variables (i.e., sex, age, education level, and marital status), ADL, and social support were added into the model step by step sequentially. In the first model, sex, age, education level, and marital status were entered. In the second model, ADL was added into the first model, and social support was added in the third model. Finally, the interaction term (ADL and social support) was added in the fourth model to test the moderating effect of social support. All statistical tests were set at the 0.05 significance level. Internal consistency reliability was assessed using Cronbach's alpha.

3. Results

3.1. General Characteristics

A total of 609 older persons living in the community (208 males, 401 females) were screened for early dementia. Based on MMSE-DS scoring criteria, 113 people (18.9%) were assigned to a high-risk group for dementia. There were no statistically significant differences in other general characteristics except marital status (Table 2). There were more single participants (widowed, separated, divorced, unmarried) in the high-risk group.

3.2. Scale Characteristics

Based on the entire study sample (N = 609), the mean score for the Geriatric Depression Scale Short Form-Korea (GDSSF-K) was 4.57 (SD = 4.03). The mean score for the UCLA Loneliness Scale was 38.35 (SD = 10.60), the mean score for the Instrumental Activities of Daily Living Scale (IADL) was 52.71 (SD = 9.76), and the mean score for the Lubben Social Network Scale was 25.49 (SD = 10.09). The mean score for the Life Satisfaction Scale was 44.77 (SD = 8.03). The Cronbach's alpha reliability for the GDSSF-K was 0.97, for the UCLA Loneliness Scale it was 0.92, and for IADL, it was 0.97. For the

Lubben Social Network Scale, it was found to be 0.86. The Cronbach's alpha of the Life Satisfaction Scale was 0.90.

Table 2. Demographic characteristics.

Demographic Characteristics		High-Risk Group (n = 113) N (%)	Low-Risk Group (n = 496) N (%)	Chi-Square	
				χ^2	p
Sex	Male	45 (39.8%)	163 (32.9%)	1.98	0.159
	Female	68 (60.2%)	333 (67.1%)		
Marital status	Single	70 (61.9%)	236 (47.6%)	7.60	0.006
	Married	43 (38.1%)	260 (52.4%)		
Age (years)	60–69	13 (11.5%)	59 (11.9%)	1.93	0.588
	70–74	28 (24.8%)	144 (29.0%)		
	75–79	32 (28.3%)	149 (30.1%)		
	80 and over	40 (35.4%)	144 (29.0%)		
Education level	None	40 (35.4%)	216 (43.5%)	8.40	0.078
	Elementary school	45 (39.8%)	177 (35.7%)		
	Middle school	20 (17.7%)	49 (9.9%)		
	High school	5 (4.4%)	39 (7.9%)		
	Bachelor's and higher	3 (2.7%)	15 (3.0%)		

3.3. Depression, Loneliness, ADL, Social Support, and Life Satisfaction between the Two Groups

There were differences in depression, loneliness, ADL, social support, and life satisfaction between the groups. The mean depression and loneliness scores of the high-risk group were higher than those of the low-risk group, while the mean scores of ADL, social support, and life satisfaction were lower than those of the low-risk group. This study's effect size was small according to r, a common effect size statistic for the Mann–Whitney test (Table 3).

Table 3. Univariate analyses in both group (N = 609).

	Group	N	Mean Rank	U	Z	p	r
Depression	High-risk	113	347.60	23,210.000	−2.872	0.004	0.12
	Low-risk	496	295.29				
Loneliness	High-risk	113	364.68	20,828.000	−4.162	<0.001	0.17
	Low-risk	492	288.83				
Activities of Daily Living (ADL)	High-risk	113	266.45	23,668.000	−2.656	0.008	0.11
	Low-risk	496	313.78				
Social support	High-risk	113	253.46	22,199.500	−3.398	0.001	0.14
	Low-risk	494	315.56				
Life satisfaction	High-risk	112	247.25	21,364.500	−3.742	<0.001	0.15
	Low-risk	493	315.66				

3.4. Correlations between Variables

Positive correlations were found between depression and loneliness (r = 0.536, $p < 0.01$) and between ADLs, social support, and life satisfaction. However, negative correlations were found between two negative emotions (depression and loneliness) and positive variables (ADL, social support, and life satisfaction; Table 4).

3.5. Moderating Effect of Social Support on the Relationship between ADL and Life Satisfaction

As hypothesized, social support moderated the relationship between daily life activities and life satisfaction in both groups. The interaction effect of social support on the relationship between ADL and life satisfaction was statistically significant ($\beta = 0.108$, $p = 0.006$). The explanatory power was 27.2%

in model 4. Therefore, social support has a moderating role in the relationship between ADL and life satisfaction. In both the high-risk and low-risk groups for dementia, ADL influenced life satisfaction, and the higher the social support, the higher the life satisfaction (Table 5).

Table 4. Spearman's correlation between variables (N = 609).

Variables	1	2	3	4	5
1. Depression	1				
2. Loneliness	0.536 **	1			
3. Activities of Daily Living (ADL)	−0.298 **	−0.297 **	1		
4. Social support	−0.325 **	−0.564 **	0.255 **	1	
5. Life satisfaction	−0.693 **	−0.632 **	0.301 **	0.438 **	1

** $p < 0.01$.

Table 5. Moderating effect of social support on the relationship between ADL and life satisfaction (N = 609).

Variables	Model 1		Model 2		Model 3		Model 4	
	β	p-Value	β	p-Value	β	p-Value	β	p-Value
Sex	0.004	0.934	0.028	0.540	0.005	0.901	<0.001	0.997
Age	−0.048	0.263	0.017	0.689	0.021	0.580	0.024	0.526
Education level	0.092	0.047	0.075	0.093	0.097	0.018	0.093	0.022
Marital status	−0.118	0.040	−0.111	0.046	−0.107	0.035	−0.105	0.037
Activities of Daily Living (ADL)			0.278	<0.001	0.176	<0.001	0.222	<0.001
Social support					0.390	<0.001	0.393	<0.001
ADL × Social support							0.108	0.006
F	0.873	0.457	45.577	<0.001	39.180	<0.001	32.667	<0.001
R^2	0.053		0.124		0.263		0.272	
Adjusted R^2	0.043		0.114		0.253		0.261	
ΔR^2	0.053	<0.001	0.071	<0.001	0.139	<0.001	0.009	0.006

4. Discussion

This study screened older adults living in local communities for their dementia risk using the validated Korean version of the Mini-Mental State Examination for Dementia Screening (MMSE-DS) [22]. Based on the results of this test, 113 (18.9%) participants were identified as the high-risk group, and the MMSE-DS score was lower in older adults without a spouse than the counterpart. This finding is consistent with that of a previous study [33] that older adults living alone exhibited lower MMSE-DS scores than those who did not live alone.

In this study, older adults at high risk for dementia showed significantly more negative results than those of the low-risk group. In other words, the older adults in the high-risk group experienced higher levels of depression and loneliness, and lower levels of daily living activities, social support, and life satisfaction than their low-risk counterparts.

The finding that older adults in the high-risk group had higher depression scores than those in the low-risk is consistent with previous findings that depression increases the risk of dementia [8,9]. Depression in older adults manifests in physical symptoms such as loss of appetite and sleep disturbance, and psychological aspects such as cognitive decline and lack of motivation. Depression and dementia influence each other in diagnosis and treatment [34]. To prevent dementia in older adults, staff working at facilities for older adults in the community should provide them with interventions aimed at relieving depression. Staff working with older adults must learn to recognize depressive symptoms such as loss of appetite, lessened speech, decreased activity, and sleep disturbances for early detection of dementia.

In this study, the high-risk group had a higher loneliness score than the low-risk group. Loneliness occurs when individuals cannot satisfy their needs in meaningful social relationships [35]. Several factors, such as deterioration in health, changes to the family structure, loss of roles, and reduced contact with family and friends can induce loneliness. Feelings of loneliness may signal early dementia [36]. Although lowered cognitive functioning may not exacerbate loneliness [37], we need to pay attention to loneliness among older adults and attempt to alleviate their loneliness to prevent dementia.

The results of this study show that older adults in the high-risk group had lower ADL scores than those in the low-risk group. The problems of daily activities in older adults with dementia deteriorates approximately three times faster than in older adults who do not have dementia [38]. Previous studies [39–41] reported that a low ADL score effectively predicts the onset of cognitive disorders such as Alzheimer's disease. Even though the ability to perform daily activities gradually decreases due to aging, we should continuously observe older adults' ability to perform daily activities since a decline in daily activities may reflect a decline in cognitive function.

Older adults in the high-risk group showed smaller social support network size and satisfaction than their counterparts in this study. Low social participation, infrequent social contacts, and loneliness are significantly associated with dementia [5]. In addition, this study's results are consistent with other studies that report that social isolation is a more significant risk factor for dementia than physical inactivity, hypertension, diabetes, and obesity [42]. Conversely, Social contact is a significant protective factor for dementia [6]. Thus, it needs to promote social ties and reduce social isolation and disengagement for dementia prevention [14].

Moreover, the finding of this study revealed that social support has a moderating role between daily living activities and life satisfaction in both high-risk and low-risk groups in this study. This finding shows that the conceptual model of quality of life [21] can be applied to older adults with dementia as well as older adults with stroke. This result confirms once again that the importance of social support for older adults cannot be overemphasized.

It will be possible to increase older adults' life satisfaction by enhancing their social networks, such as participation in social activities. In the results of a study on older adults in Spain [43], perceived social support was a predictor of life satisfaction. Social support is critical for improving patients' health outcomes. Social support is a protective factor of dementia [6,13–15] even in daily life activities as well as positive effects against negative emotions such as loneliness or depression.

In this study, more older adults in the high-risk group were without spouses (widowed, separated, divorced, unmarried) than those in the low-risk group. Among other social factors, community engagement was protective for women, while for men, being married was associated with a lower incidence of dementia [13]. More research is needed to understand the relationship between dementia and marriage, but social support from a spouse may be buffering against dementia. Older adults living alone are at risk for early and late dementia [44]. Establishing meaningful social support from interpersonal relationships is a valuable preventive intervention to enhance life satisfaction and reduce the risk of dementia among older adults. In addition to family relations, there is a need to prepare various social supports in the form of relationships that seniors care for older adults with early dementia or young adults take care of older adults by residing in an intimate living space.

Life satisfaction is an essential concept in dementia research [45,46]. In this study, the high-risk group had a lower life satisfaction score than the low-risk group. Low life satisfaction alone did not directly affect dementia but may lead to an increased death risk after five years [47]. We should constantly seek ways to increase the life satisfaction of older adults to prevent dementia.

This study has several limitations. Participants were limited to a small sample of older adults living in a particular region of South Korea, therefore limiting the generalizability of our findings. Given that chronic physical illnesses such as diabetes, cancer, and metabolic disorders affect participants' cognitive function, the authors should have considered these variables in this study, but not. The authors also should have checked for depression because depression can affect cognitive function but may not. These variables need to be considered in future studies on dementia. In addition, we did not take into account the male to female ratio in this study. Thus, it is necessary to consider the male to female ratio in future research. In this study, the ratio of the high-risk group and the low-risk group could not be predicted because both groups were classified according to the MMSE-DS criteria among the participants participating in the early dementia screening test. In the future, research is needed to equalize the ratio of the high-risk group and the low-risk group and compare the two groups' variables. Another limitation derives from the study's cross-sectional design which means that while we observed a relationship between social structure and life satisfaction, causality was not established.

5. Conclusions

The most important finding is that depression, loneliness, social support, ADL, and life satisfaction showed negative results in the high-risk group of dementia. Social support has a moderating role between ADL and life satisfaction in both dementia high-risk and low-risk groups. This study's findings also provide a theoretical basis for the importance of early screening for dementia and implications for caregivers and medical personnel.

For early detection of dementia, it is necessary to carefully assess older adults' psychological changes, such as depression and loneliness, provide psychosocial interventions for their psychological well-being, and promote social support from their social networks. It is also necessary to actively provide opportunities for older adults to belong to families and communities and make it as convenient as possible to access such resources.

Furthermore, people should be continuously informed of the importance of early dementia screening so that older adults can receive regular early dementia screening. Above all, it is necessary to support a continuous dementia prevention program for older adults in high-risk groups and evaluate the program's effectiveness. It is also necessary to identify differences according to the type of social support sources such as friends, co-workers, or family members separately in future studies and the types of social support services (e.g., face-to-face services and online services).

Author Contributions: Conceptualization, S.K. and K.C.; methodology, S.K. and K.C.; formal analysis, K.C.: writing—original draft preparation, S.K., K.L., and K.C.; writing—review and editing, K.L.; All authors have read and agreed to the published version of the manuscript.

Acknowledgments: The authors are most grateful to the participants for their participation in this study.

References

1. Korean Center for Dementia. Korean Dementia Observatory. 2019. Available online: https://www.nid.or.kr/info/dataroom_view.aspx?bid=209 (accessed on 11 June 2020).
2. Suvosree, B.; Asmus, V.; Marie-Louise, H.H.; Frans, B.W.; Gunhild, W. Generic and disease-specific measures of quality of life in patients with mild Alzheimer's disease. *Dement. Geriatr. Cogn. Disord.* **2010**, *30*, 327–333.
3. World Health Organization. Dementia: A Public Health Priority. Available online: https://apps.who.int/iris/bitstream/handle/10665/75263/9789241564458_jsessionid=E2450FBE77E063FF93E43388200F2D93?sequence=1 (accessed on 6 July 2020).
4. Panegyres, P.K.; Berry, R.; Burchell, J. Early dementia screening. *Diagnostics* **2016**, *6*, 6. [CrossRef]
5. Kuiper, J.S.; Zuidersma, M.; Voshaar, R.C.O.; Zuidema, S.U.; van den Heuvel, E.R.; Stolk, R.P.; Smidt, N. Social relationships and risk of dementia: A systematic review and meta-analysis of longitudinal cohort studies. *Ageing Res. Rev.* **2015**, *2*, 39–57. [CrossRef]
6. Brzezińska, A.; Bourke, J.; Rivera-Hernández, R.; Tsolaki, M.; Woźniak, J.; Kaźmierski, J. Depression in Dementia or Dementia in Depression? Systematic Review of Studies and Hypotheses. *Curr. Alzheimer Res.* **2020**, *17*, 16–28. [CrossRef]
7. Bellou, V.; Belbasis, L.; Tzoulaki, I.; Middleton, L.T.; Ioannidis, J.P.; Evangelou, E. Systematic evaluation of the associations between environmental risk factors and dementia: An umbrella review of systematic reviews and meta-analyses. *Alzheimer's Dement.* **2017**, *13*, 406–418. [CrossRef]
8. Kaup, A.R.; Byers, A.L.; Falvey, C.; Simonsick, E.M.; Satterfield, S.; Ayonayon, H.N.; Yaffe, K. Trajectories of depressive symptoms in older adults and risk of dementia. *JAMA Psychiatry* **2016**, *73*, 525–531. [CrossRef]

9. Köhler, S.; van Boxtel, M.; Jolles, J.; Verhey, F. Depressive symptoms and risk for dementia: A 9-year follow-up of the Maastricht Aging Study. *Am. J. Geriatr. Psychiatry* **2011**, *19*, 902–905. [CrossRef]
10. Balouch, S.; Rifaat, E.; Chen, H.L.; Tabet, N. Social networks and loneliness in people with Alzheimer's dementia. *Int. J. Geriatr. Psychiatry* **2019**, *34*, 666–673. [CrossRef]
11. Zhou, Z.; Wang, P.; Fang, Y. Loneliness and the risk of dementia among older Chinese adults: Gender differences. *Aging Ment. Health* **2018**, *22*, 519–525. [CrossRef] [PubMed]
12. Sutin, A.R.; Stephan, Y.; Luchetti, M.; Terracciano, A. Loneliness and risk of dementia. *J. Gerontol. Ser. B* **2020**, *75*, 1414–1422. [CrossRef] [PubMed]
13. Murata, C.; Saito, T.; Saito, M.; Kondo, K. The association between social support and incident dementia: A 10-year follow-up study in Japan. *Int. J. Environ. Res. Public Health* **2019**, *16*, 239. [CrossRef]
14. Penninkilampi, R.; Casey, A.N.; Singh, M.F.; Brodaty, H. The association between social engagement, loneliness, and risk of dementia: A systematic review and meta-analysis. *J. Alzheimer's Dis.* **2018**, *66*, 1619–1633. [CrossRef]
15. Khondoker, M.; Rafnsson, S.B.; Morris, S.; Orrell, M.; Steptoe, A. Positive and negative experiences of social support and risk of dementia in later life: An investigation using the English Longitudinal Study of Ageing. *J. Alzheimer's Dis.* **2017**, *58*, 99–108. [CrossRef]
16. Giebel, C.M.; Sutcliffe, C.; Challis, D. Activities of daily living and quality of life across different stages of dementia: A UK study. *Aging Ment. Health* **2015**, *19*, 63–71. [CrossRef]
17. Fauth, E.B.; Schwartz, S.; Tschanz, J.T.; Østbye, T.; Corcoran, C.; Norton, M.C. Baseline disability in activities of daily living predicts dementia risk even after controlling for baseline global cognitive ability and depressive symptoms. *Int. J. Geriatr. Psychiatry* **2013**, *28*, 597–606. [CrossRef]
18. Ng, S.T.; Tey, N.P.; Asadullah, M.N. What matters for life satisfaction among the oldest-old? Evidence from China. *PLoS ONE* **2017**, *12*, e0171799. [CrossRef]
19. Rawtaer, I.; Gao, Q.; Nyunt, M.S.; Feng, L.; Chong, M.S.; Lim, W.S.; Lee, T.S.; Yap, P.; Yap, K.B.; Ng, T.P. Psychosocial risk and protective factors and incident mild cognitive impairment and dementia in community dwelling elderly: Findings from the Singapore Longitudinal Ageing Study. *J. Alzheimer's Dis.* **2017**, *57*, 603–611. [CrossRef]
20. Palmer, K.; Di Iulio, F.; Varsi, A.E.; Gianni, W.; Sancesario, G.; Caltagirone, C.; Spalletta, G. Neuropsychiatric predictors of progression from amnestic mild cognitive impairment to Alzheimer's disease: The role of depression and apathy. *J. Alzheimer's Dis.* **2010**, *20*, 175–183. [CrossRef] [PubMed]
21. Chan, S.H.; Pan, Y.; Xu, Y.; Yeung, K.C. Life satisfaction of 511 elderly Chinese stroke survivors: Moderating roles of social functioning and depression in a quality of life model. *Clin. Rehabil.* **2020**. [CrossRef]
22. Kim, T.H.; Jhoo, J.H.; Park, J.H.; Kim, J.L.; Ryu, S.H.; Moon, S.W.; Choo, I.H.; Lee, D.W.; Yoon, J.C.; Do, Y.J.; et al. Korean version of mini mental status examination for dementia screening and its' short form. *Psychiatry Investig.* **2010**, *7*, 102–108. [CrossRef]
23. Kee, B.S. A preliminary study for the standardization of geriatric depression scale short form-Korea version. *J. Korean Neuropsychiatr. Assoc.* **1996**, *35*, 298–307.
24. Yesavage, J.A.; Brink, T.L.; Rose, T.L.; Adey, M. Development and validation of a Geriatric Depression Screening Scale: A preliminary report. *J. Psychiatr. Res.* **1983**, *17*, 37–49. [CrossRef]
25. Russell, D.; Peplau, L.A.; Cutrona, C.E. The revised UCLA Loneliness Scale: Concurrent and discriminant validity evidence. *J. Pers. Soc. Psychol.* **1980**, *39*, 472–480. [CrossRef]
26. Song, M. Construction of a Functional Status Prediction Model for the Elderly. Ph.D. Thesis, Seoul National University, Seoul, Korea, 1990.
27. Lawton, M.P.; Brody, E.M. Assessment of older people: Self-maintaining and instrumental activities of daily living. *Gerontologist* **1996**, *9*, 179–186. [CrossRef]
28. Lubben, J.E. Assessing social networks among elderly populations. *Fam. Community Health* **1998**, *11*, 42–52. [CrossRef]
29. Yoon, G. Successful aging and quality of life. In Proceedings of the Korean Psychological Association Conference Proceeding, Seoul, Korea, May 1995; pp. 45–75.
30. Kozma, A.; Stones, M.J. The measurement of happiness: Development of the Memorial University of Newfoundland Scale of Happiness (MUNSH). *J. Gerontol.* **1980**, *35*, 906–912. [CrossRef]
31. Field, A. *Discovering Statistics Using IBM SPSS Statistics*, 5th ed.; SAGE Publications: Thousand Oaks, CA, USA, 2017.

32. Aiken, L.S.; West, S.G. *Multiple Regression: Testing and Interpreting Interactions*, 1st ed.; SAGE Publications: Thousand Oaks, CA, USA, 1991.
33. Kim, H.; Lee, S.; Ku, B.D.; Ham, S.G.; Park, W.S. Associated factors for cognitive impairment in the rural highly elderly. *Brain Behav.* **2019**, *9*, e01203. [CrossRef]
34. Bennett, S.; Thomas, A.J. Depression and dementia: Cause, consequence or coincidence? *Maturitas* **2014**, *79*, 184–190. [CrossRef]
35. Teguo, M.T.; Simo-Tabue, N.; Stoykova, R.; Meillon, C.; Cogne, M.; Amiéva, H.; Dartigues, J.F. Feelings of loneliness and living alone as predictors of mortality in the elderly: The PAQUID study. *Psychosom. Med.* **2016**, *78*, 904–909. [CrossRef]
36. Holwerda, T.J.; Deeg, D.J.; Beekman, A.T.; van Tilburg, T.G.; Stek, M.L.; Jonker, C.; Schoevers, R.A. Feelings of loneliness, but not social isolation, predict dementia onset: Results from the Amsterdam Study of the Elderly (AMSTEL). *J. Neurol. Neurosurg. Psychiatry* **2014**, *85*, 135–142. [CrossRef]
37. Donovan, N.J.; Wu, Q.; Rentz, D.M.; Sperling, R.A.; Marshall, G.A.; Glymour, M.M. Loneliness, depression and cognitive function in older US adults. *Int. J. Geriatr. Psychiatry* **2017**, *32*, 564–573. [CrossRef]
38. Lee, H.J. Changes in cognitive function and functional disability in older adults. Comparison of groups converted and not converted to dementia among cognitively normal older adults. *Korean J. Soc. Welf. Stud.* **2013**, *44*, 323–355.
39. Roehr, S.; Riedel-Heller, S.G.; Kaduszkiewicz, H.; Wagner, M.; Fuchs, A.; van der Leeden, C.; Wolfsgruber, S. Is function in instrumental activities of daily living a useful feature in predicting Alzheimer's disease dementia in subjective cognitive decline? *Int. J. Geriatr. Psychiatry* **2019**, *34*, 193–203. [CrossRef]
40. Mao, H.F.; Chang, L.H.; Tsai, A.Y.J.; Huang, W.N.W.; Tang, L.Y.; Lee, H.J.; Shyu, Y.I.L. Diagnostic accuracy of Instrumental Activities of Daily Living for dementia in community-dwelling older adults. *Age Ageing* **2018**, *47*, 551–557. [CrossRef]
41. Cornelis, E.; Gorus, E.; Beyer, I.; Bautmans, I.; De Vriendt, P. Early diagnosis of mild cognitive impairment and mild dementia through basic and instrumental activities of daily living: Development of a new evaluation tool. *PLoS Med.* **2017**, *14*, e1002250. [CrossRef]
42. Desai, R.; John, A.; Stott, J.; Charlesworth, G. Living alone and risk of dementia: A systematic review and meta-analysis. *Ageing Res. Rev.* **2020**, *62*, 101122. [CrossRef]
43. Dumitrache, C.G.; Rubio, L.; Rubio-Herrera, R. Perceived health status and life satisfaction in old age, and the moderating role of social support. *Aging Ment. Health* **2017**, *21*, 751–757. [CrossRef]
44. Sundström, A.; Westerlund, O.; Kotyrlo, E. Marital status and risk of dementia: A nationwide population-based prospective study from Sweden. *BMJ Open* **2016**, *6*, e008565. [CrossRef]
45. Moniz-Cook, E.; Manthorpe, J. *Early Psychosocial Interventions in Dementia Evidence-Based Practice*; Jessica Kingsley: London, UK; Philadelphia, PA, USA, 2009.
46. Rabins, P.V.; Black, B.S. Measuring quality of life in dementia: Purposes, goals, challenges and progress. *Int. Psychogeriatr.* **2007**, *19*, 401–407. [CrossRef]
47. Peitsch, L.; Tyas, S.L.; Menec, V.H.; St John, P.D. General life satisfaction predicts dementia in community living older adults: A prospective cohort study. *Int. Psychogeriatr.* **2016**, *28*, 1101. [CrossRef]

2

Amino Acid Levels as Potential Biomarker of Elderly Patients with Dementia

Edyta Socha [1], Piotr Kośliński [1], Marcin Koba [1,*], Katarzyna Mądra-Gackowska [2], Kornelia Kędziora-Kornatowska [2], Marcin Gackowski [1] and Emilia Daghir-Wojtkowiak [3]

1 Department of Toxicology and Bromatology, Faculty of Pharmacy, Collegium Medicum of Nicolaus Copernicus University, 85-067 Bydgoszcz, Poland; edyta.siminska@gmail.com (E.S.); piotr.koslinski@cm.umk.pl (P.K.); marcin.gackowski@cm.umk.pl (M.G.)

2 Department of Geriatrics, Faculty of Health Sciences, Collegium Medicum of Nicolaus Copernicus University, 85-067 Bydgoszcz, Poland; katarzyna.madra@cm.umk.pl (K.M.-G.); kasiakor@interia.pl (K.K.-K.)

3 Department of Biopharmaceutics and Pharmacodynamics, Medical University of Gdańsk, 80-210 Gdańsk, Poland; emilia.daghir@gmail.com

* Correspondence: kobamar@cm.umk.pl

Abstract: Dementia is a clinical syndrome characterized by cognitive impairment, in which there is disturbance of multiple higher cortical functions. The primary risk factor of dementia is old age, and due to significant changes in the worldwide demographic structure, the prevalence of cognitive impairment is increasing dramatically with aging populations in most countries. Alzheimer's disease is the predominant and leading cause of dementia. The aim of this study was to evaluate the modifications of amino acids that characterize the initial stages of dementia to help our understanding of the complex and multifactorial pathogenesis of neurodegenerative disorders. A total of 123 participants were divided into two groups: healthy elderly subjects and patients with mild or moderate dementia. The results of this study indicate that the serum levels of three amino acids were changed significantly in patients with dementia, in relation to the subjects without dementia. In particular, we observed differences in concentrations for serine, arginine and isoleucine (all of them were significantly increased in patients with dementia, compared with the control group). Our results suggest that the metabolisms of some amino acids seem be changed in patients with dementia. We conclude that amino acid profiling might be helpful for the better understanding of biochemical and metabolic changes related to the pathogenesis and progression of dementia. However, considering the multifactorial, heterogenous and complex nature of this disease, validation with a greater study sample in further research is required.

Keywords: neurodegenerative diseases; mild dementia; moderate dementia; amino acids; arginine; serine; isoleucine

---

1. Introduction

Dementia is a clinical syndrome characterized by cognitive impairment, in which we observe the disturbance of multiple higher cortical functions, including thinking, memory, orientation, calculation, comprehension, language, learning capability and judgment [1]. The primary risk factor of dementia is old age, and due to significant changes in the worldwide demographic structure, the prevalence of cognitive impairment is increasing dramatically with aging populations in most countries. Currently, neurodegenerative disorders are one of the greatest global challenges for medical and social care, due to an aging society and the rapidly increasing costs of dementia [2].

Dementia occurs in cerebrovascular disease, Parkinson's disease and in other conditions affecting the brain, but indisputably, Alzheimer's disease (AD) is the predominant and leading cause of dementia [1]. Based on the most recent available data, AD is estimated to be responsible for up to 80% of dementia cases. Therefore, the authors of this paper mainly refer to AD as a leading cause of dementia [3].

Research to date has tended to focus on the amyloid cascade hypothesis in the development of AD. However, increasing recent evidence suggests that this hypothesis indicating the role of amyloid-β (Aβ) protein aggregation in AD pathogenesis does not encapsulate the heterogenous and complex symptomology of AD [4,5]. Growing clinical evidence shows that AD-associated cognitive impairment is the outcome of an especially complex pathogenesis. In addition to the well-defined and known amyloid plaques and neurofibrillary tangles, the pathology of AD includes inflammation, considerable DNA damage, substantial neuronal loss, the initiation of apoptotic pathways, chronic oxidative stress, alteration of the energy metabolism, and extensive mitochondrial malfunction. Long-term failures to find effective anti-Tau or anti-amyloid therapy have led to the hypothesis that specific proteins are only confluent lesions and not the sole and ultimate causes of AD. Numerous recent papers present evidence pointing to severe metabolic dysfunction as a leading cause of AD. Current data show the causative relationship between obesity and AD [6,7]. Furthermore, numerous studies reported significant improvement in the cognitive, functional, and cellular statuses of AD patients who were treated with conventional medicines, used in treating atherosclerosis, diabetes, and other metabolic disorders [6,8,9]. Hence, the current vision of AD pathogenesis must reach beyond the confirmed regular information and look for alternative research approaches in order to develop novel diagnosis, preventive, and therapeutic methods. It is very important to quest for better understanding of the biochemical changes at different stages of the disease, which are an integral part of the complex and multifactorial pathogenesis of dementia.

It is essential to advance the understanding of early disease mechanisms and to identify early biomarkers and novel therapeutic targets. Currently available diagnostic biomarkers are limited to the measurements of the Aβ, tau, and p-tau levels in plasma and cerebrospinal fluid (CSF) that represent rather limited, hypothesis-driven biomarker development [4,6]. Furthermore, neuroimaging is very expensive and available only at specialized sites. Most health care systems in the world cannot afford using Positron Emission Tomography (PET) as a routine diagnostic tool for screenings of the very high number of patients from the risk group (elderly subjects in an aging society). The limitations in the routine use of CSF biomarkers include the lumbar puncture, which is invasive, time-consuming, and complicated for many clinics [10].

Taking into account the current state of dementia diagnostics, it is important to identify a putative biomarker. In recent years, there has been an increasing interest in such research, with the use of various easy-to-collect biological materials such as serum (e.g., our study) or saliva. It is interesting to note that several recent studies indicated the antioxidant properties of saliva are limited in patients with dementia, and salivary redox biomarkers may be used for differentiating the various stages of dementia. Despite the very interesting and promising results, there are some important limitations, such as factors affecting the quantity and quality of saliva (e.g., drugs, periodontal diseases, oral mucosa disorders, age, various systemic diseases, xenobiotics, dental materials, dental treatment, physical exercise, and diet). Unfortunately, a perfect dementia biomarker or diagnostics method still does not exist, and it is important to conduct new research and strive to improve and develop the diagnostics area [11,12]. Several recent studies have identified changes in the plasma amino acid (AA) profile in the material of patients with AD and other advanced stages of neurodegenerative diseases [13–20], but there is still insufficient data for this aspect that takes into account the earlier stages of dementia. Amino acids play essential roles in the regulation and control of pivotal functions of human organisms, including the central nervous system (CNS), where AAs act as regulators of the energy metabolism, neurotransmitters, and neuromodulators. Neurotransmission is a key function of AAs in the CNS. Neurotransmission amino acids are compounds that are synthesized and stored in neurons. They are released when the nerve impulse is conducted. Alterations in plasma amino acid profiles in neurodegenerative diseases may be influenced by neurodegeneration, received treatment, mitochondrial disfunction, or malabsorption in the gastroenteric tract [15,20].

Furthermore, amino acids are involved in energy production and nitrogenous waste production and elimination as well. The human body needs amino acids in large amounts for the synthesis of body proteins and other important nitrogen-containing compounds, such as peptide hormones, creatine, and some neurotransmitters. Hence, amino acids are a large and important part of the human diet. Processing these essential amino acids for energy requires the disposal of nitrogenous waste material, a process which occurs primarily in the liver and small intestine during the urea cycle. Disturbed amino acid and nitrogen metabolism is associated with neurological disorders and, in some cases, dementia. When neurons cannot catabolize glucose effectively, they may become reliant upon amino acid oxidation during energy production. If the mechanism used to metabolize amino acids becomes dysregulated, or if neuronal amino acids become depleted, the neurons may die. This might contribute to disease progression. In addition to these main functions, amino acids and their metabolic derivatives are involved in cell signaling and in many different metabolic pathways [4].

The aim of this study was to evaluate the modifications of amino acids that characterize the initial stages of dementia to help our understanding of the complex and multifactorial pathogenesis of dementia.

2. Materials and Methods

2.1. Subjects and Serum Samples

A total of 123 participants were recruited from the Department of Geriatrics, Collegium Medicum in Bydgoszcz, Nicolaus Copernicus University in Toruń. They were divided into two groups: 50 healthy elderly subjects with no dementia diagnosed (23 males, 27 females; mean age ± SD: 77.09 ± 7.08 years) and 73 patients with mild or moderate dementia (17 males, 56 females; mean age ± SD: 81.89 ± 6.38 years). Table 1 reports the clinical and demographic characteristics of the two groups of participants.

Table 1. Demographic and clinical characteristics of the study groups.

	Control Group (n = 50)	Case Group (n = 73)	p-Value
Mean age ± SD, years	77.09 ± 7.08	81.89 ± 6.38	
Gender, n (%)			$P = 0.014$
Male	23 (46)	17 (23.3)	
Female	27 (54)	56 (76.7)	
Mean BMI ± SD	28.01 ± 5.37	25.79 ± 6.34	
Drugs, n (%)			$P = 0.664$
Painkillers	16 (32)	22 (30.1)	
Duretics	15 (30)	13 (17.8)	
Anti-coagulants	13 (26)	18 (24.7)	
Anticancer medications	0 (0)	1 (1.4)	
Mineral supplements	1 (2)	1 (1.4)	
Thyroid medications	5 (10)	10 (13.7)	
Folic acid	2 (4)	6 (8.2)	
Vitamin D3	5 (10)	13 (17.8)	
Smoking, n (%)			$P = 0.862$
Non-smoker	39 (78)	55 (75.3)	
Former smoker	4 (8)	6 (8.2)	
Occasional smoker	0 (0)	0 (0)	
Active smoker	0 (0)	2 (2.7)	
Passive smoker	0 (0)	0 (0)	
Medical history, n (%)			$P = 0.284$
Hypertension	35 (70)	52 (71)	
Diabetes	7 (14)	26 (35)	

Table 1. *Cont.*

	Control Group (n = 50)	Case Group (n = 73)	p-Value
Kidney disease	2 (4)	0 (0)	
Liver disease	0 (0)	1 (1.4)	
Thyroid disease	7 (14)	13 (17.8)	
Cancer	4 (8)	10 (13.7)	

Investigators classified patients into two groups in accordance with the current clinical standard: a group of elderly patients without dementia and a group of elderly patients with dementia (from mild dementia to moderate dementia). Participants of the study were chosen from older adults, who were referred to a comprehensive geriatric assessment by a general practitioner, mainly because of persistent symptoms of memory loss reported over a six-month span. Patients were included in the study prior to a clinical diagnosis of the cause of dementia. They were admitted to the geriatric clinic for a comprehensive geriatric assessment to evaluate their cognitive status. Patients with causes of reversible dementia were excluded. Patients had laboratory tests ordered to rule out reversible causes of dementia (e.g., B12 deficiency or hypothyroidism). The International Statistical Classification of Diseases and Related Health Problems (ICD-10) criteria were adopted for the clinical diagnosis of dementia. Furthermore, diagnosis of dementia was based on a review of the patient's medical history and symptoms via a physical examination and a brain scan, such as a CT or MRI scan. A mini-mental state examination (MMSE) and a clock-drawing test (CDR) were used to diagnose the severity of dementia. The mean score on the MMSE for healthy elderly subjects with no dementia diagnosed was 27 points. For patients with mild dementia, it was 21 points, and for patients with moderate dementia, it was 16 points.

The assignment to the groups was documented in a survey that was previously reviewed and approved by the ethics committee. This study was conducted with all approved international guidelines for human research and was in accordance with the Declaration of Helsinki. The ethics committee of Nicolaus Copernicus University in Toruń and Collegium Medicum in Bydgoszcz approved this study (consent number: KB 173/2018). Written, informed consent was required from the participants. An informed consent form, an investigator survey form, and a patient survey form were also reviewed and approved by the ethics committee.

Antecubital whole-blood samples were drawn from a peripheral vein in the morning hours (always between 6 and 7 a.m.). Overnight fasting and 15 min of rest before the blood test were obligatory. The needle was inserted into the vein, and the blood was withdrawn to vacuum tubes (the test's 5 mL tube contained a clot activator and serum gel separator, and it had no anticoagulant). Blood collected in the tube was kept for 30 min. Serum from the blood after clotting was separated out and, after appropriate preparation and centrifuging, was frozen at −80 °C until analysis was performed.

2.2. *Chemicals and Materials*

A system consisting of an AccQ Fluor reagent kit (Waters, En Yvelines Cedex, France, amino acid standards (Waters), internal standard α-aminobutyric acid (Sigma Aldrich, Saint Louis, MO, USA), acetonitrile and methanol (Sigma Aldrich), and deionized water purified with Direct–QUV (Millipore, Molsheim, France) was used for all aqueous solutions.

2.3. *Instrumentation*

A Shimadzu high-performance liquid chromatography (HPLC) system, combined with a Diode-Array Detection (DAD) detector and an RF-20A XS fluorescence detector (Shimadzu, Kyoto, Japan) were used.

2.4. Chromatographic Method

Chromatographic analysis, which was aimed at measuring the amino acid concentrations in the samples, was carried out using high-performance liquid chromatography (HPLC) with fluorescence detection, using an AccQ Tag column (Waters). The final parameters of the chromatographic system consisted of a 150 mm × 3.9 mm chromatographic column by AccQ Tag (Waters), a fluorescence detection excitation/emission of 250/395, mobile phase A conducted with an AccQ Tag Eluent A (Buffer), mobile phase B conducted with acetonitrile, mobile phase C conducted with water and a gradient elution, a flow of 1 mL/min, an injection volume of 5 µL, and an analysis time of 35 min.

2.5. Data Modelling

In prior analysis, the data were cantered and standardized. To check the presence of outliers or extreme values, we visualized the AA distributions as density plots and quantile–quantile plots. The normal distribution of the AA data was checked using the Shapiro–Wilk test. To check whether the distribution of each AA differed between investigated groups, we performed either a Kruskal–Wallis test (for non-normal distribution) or a *t*-test (for normally distributed data). To check the presence of linear correlations between the amino acids, a Pearson correlation coefficient was calculated for each amino acid against each other. The relationship between the categorical variables and the disease status was checked using the Fisher test.

2.5.1. Random Forest Algorithm

The random forest (RF) model was used to evaluate the impact of amino acids on classification between groups. The RF algorithm is a machine learning-based algorithm constructed from decision trees trained using bootstrap aggregation, where each new tree is fit from a bootstrap sample of the training observations. The out-of-bag (OOB) error is the average error for each, calculated using predictions from the trees that not contained in their respective bootstrap samples. The model was built for 22 variables, which we hypothesized would have an impact on classification between both groups.

2.5.2. Missing Values and Unbalance in the Data Structure

As the data (50 controls and 73 cases) had missing values and were unbalanced, we first imputed the missing values. The imputation technique was specified via the impute function, relative to a feature class. Next, we split the data into training and test sets (7:3) with further application of the random over-sampling examples (ROSE) algorithm to balance it [21].

2.5.3. Model Development and Variable Importance

The RF model was fitted using the training data, with the setting for the optimal number of trees and variables giving the lowest error rate on the training set. After training the RF model, we assessed the variable importance to address the question of which variables were the most important in building the model and had a significant impact on the outcome. The variable importance was calculated based on the Gini index by calculating each feature's importance as the sum over the number of splits across all tress that included the feature, proportional to the number of samples it split.

2.5.4. Model Performance

The model performance was checked on the validation set using such metrics as accuracy, sensitivity, specificity, and area under the curve (AUC). The variables based on the Gini index were further included in the logistic regression model. The inference on their impact was based on the calculation of the odds ratio (OR), a 95% confidence interval and the *p*-value.

All analyses were conducted in R (7. R Core Team, 2014), and figures were produced using the package ggplot2.

3. Results

Comparison: Elderly subjects with no dementia as the control group (n = 50) versus elderly patients with dementia (n = 73).

In Figure 1, we present a visualization of the raw data for each AA (asparagine (ASP), serine (SER), glutamine (GLU), glycine (GLY), histidine (HIS), arginine (ARG), threonine (THR), alanine (ALA), proline (PRO), tyrosine (TYR), valine (VAL), methionine (MET), lysine (LYS), isoleucine (ILE), leucine (LEU), and phenylalanine (PHE)) for the two groups. To maintain the same scale for each AA and for data analysis purposes, we centered and standardized the raw values. In Figure 2, we present a visualization of the centered and standardized data for each AA for the two groups. From a visual inspection, we might observe a slight difference in the ARG mean between both groups. Not all amino acid concentrations were normally distributed. Under such a scenario, we calculated the average and SD for each distribution, but only for those AAs with normal distributions (Figure 3, Table 2).

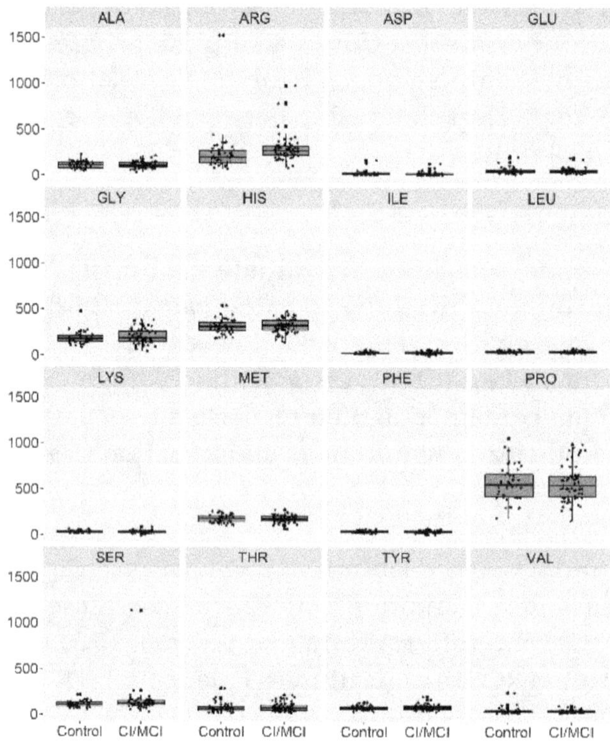

Figure 1. Visualization of the raw data for 16 amino acids in patients with no cognitive impairment or with Mild Cognitive Impairment (MCI) (depicted as 0) and with mild or moderate dementia (depicted as 1).

Table 2. The mean (±SD) for each metabolite signal distribution.

Compound Name	Mean (± SD)
ALA	0.27 (± 0.30)
GLY	0.75 (± 0.35)
HIS	1.24 (± 0.23)
LEU	−0.56 (± 0.22)
MET	0.71 (± 0.22)
PRO	1.74 (± 0.30)
TYR	−0.04 (± 0.27)

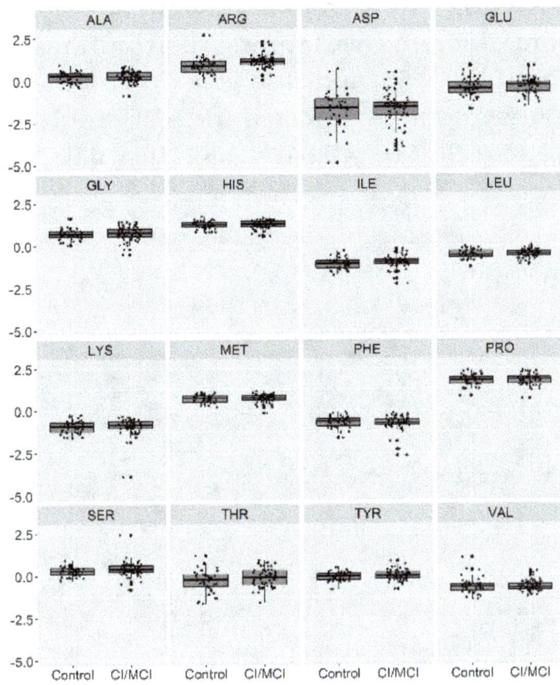

Figure 2. Visualization of the centered and standardized data for 16 amino acids in patients with no CI or with MCI (depicted as 0) and with mild or moderate dementia (depicted as 1).

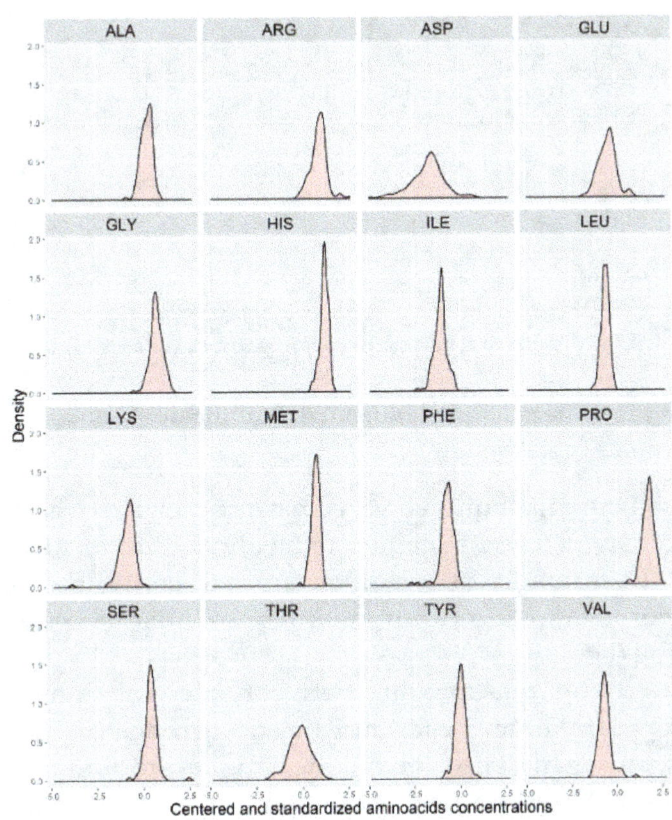

Figure 3. Distribution of the centered and standardized amino acids in a group of 123 individuals (with no separation between the two groups).

To investigate whether AA distributions were homogeneous and whether the AA concentration data originated from two or more different overlapping distributions (e.g., groups), we provided the distribution of each AA in the control ($n = 50$) and case ($n = 73$) groups (Figure 4). As shown in Figure 4, separation between the two groups might be expected for ARG. At $\alpha = 0.05$, the distribution between both groups significantly differed for SER ($p = 0.042$), ARG ($p = 0.0003$), and ILE ($p = 0.035$).

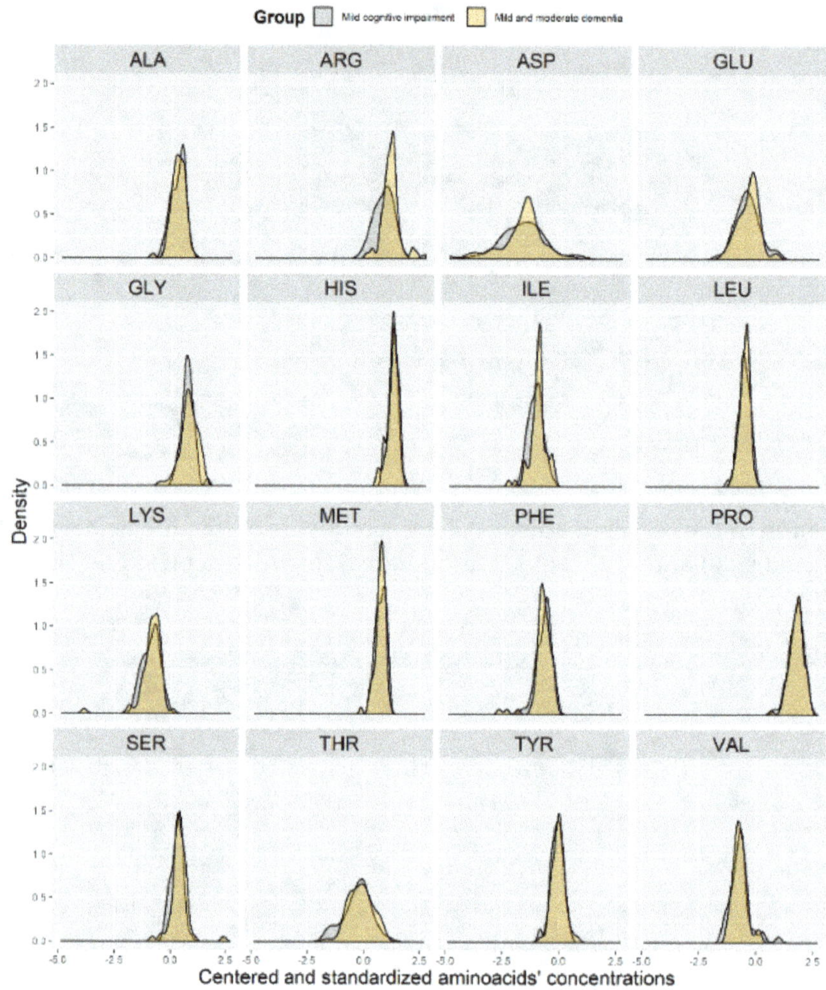

Figure 4. Distribution of the centered and standardized amino acid concentrations between the two groups (controls (grey) versus cases (yellow)).

Additionally, we checked the distribution of AA concentrations between sexes (Figure 5). As shown in Figure 5, the distribution between sexes seemed to be almost identical.

The authors analyzed the influence of age on amino acid concentrations to check whether there was any trend (e.g., higher or lower concentration with age). Neither a positive nor a negative trend with age was observed in the data.

We further investigated the relationship between alcohol consumption, smoking status, concomitant diseases, drugs intake, and diet and the occurrence of cognitive impairment (using the Fisher exact test). No relationship between alcohol intake, smoking status, and drug intake and cognitive impairment was found. Only the relationship with diabetes ($p = 0.009$) was found to be significant at $\alpha = 0.05$.

However, we found a significant difference between the presence of mild-to-moderate dementia and the frequency of meat consumption (3 or 4 times per week, $p = 0.007$), tea drinking (5 or 6 times per week, $p = 0.0008$), fish consumption (2–3 times per month, $p = 0.044$), and sweets intake (5–6 times per week, $p = 0.044$). The visual representation of the above-mentioned significant differences is presented in Figure 6. However, these results should be interpreted with caution as the investigated group was small, and a large disproportion between the compared groups was present.

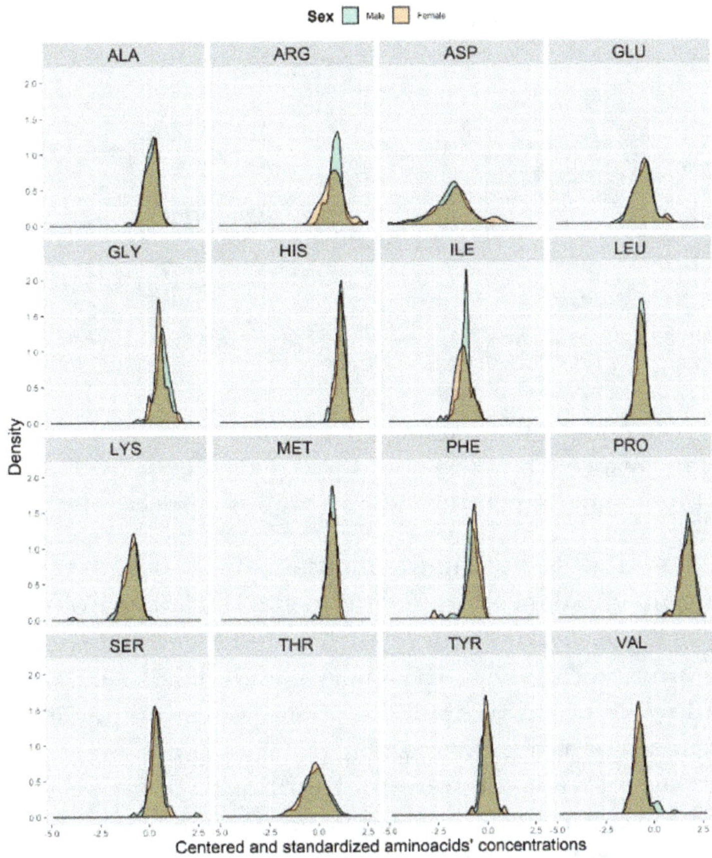

Figure 5. Histograms of the centered and standardized amino acid concentrations between males (blue) and females (pink).

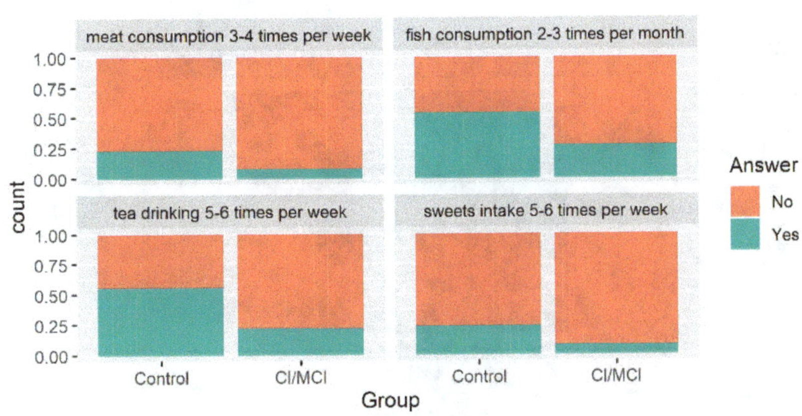

Figure 6. Distribution of patients' groups with regard to their classification (x-axis) and the proportions for categorical variables which appeared to be significant ($\alpha = 0.05$) in Fisher's test.

The random forest model was built for 22 variables, which we hypothesized had an impact on the splitting between both groups. The OOB error rate was the lowest with 150 trees (Figure 7). The optimal number of variables was set at three.

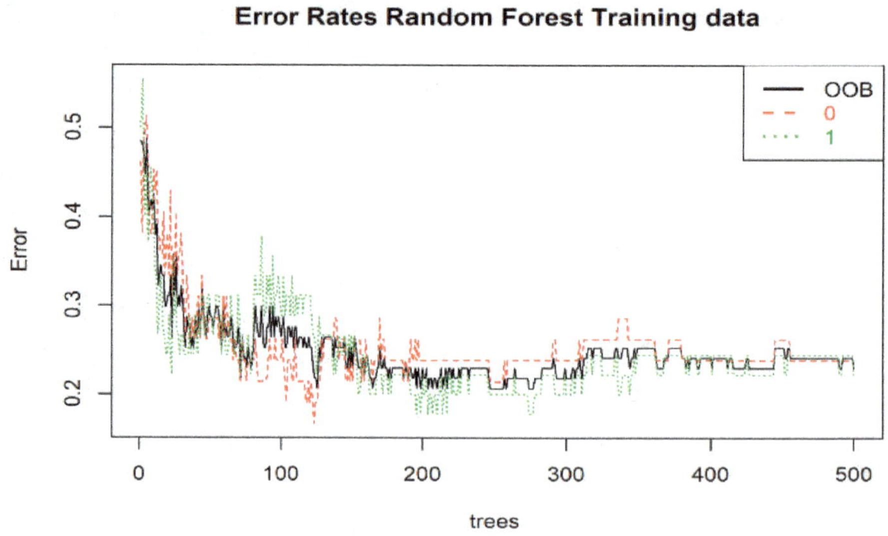

Figure 7. Error rate for the random forest training set. On the x- and y-axis, one can observe the number of trees and the error rate, respectively. The out-of-bag (OOB) score for the model is presented as a black solid line; 0 and 1 represent the control and case groups, respectively.

The missing values were imputed using the medians or modes, depending on the variable type. The available data were highly unbalanced (referring to classification problems where we had unequal instances for different classes). As a consequence, an unbalanced dataset would bias the prediction model towards the more common class. We artificially balanced the samples according to a smoothed bootstrap approach and allowed for aiding both the phases of estimation and accuracy evaluation of a binary classifier in the presence of a rare class [21].

In order to select the most relevant variables contributing to patient classification, after developing the RF model, we assessed the contribution of each variable to the classification between both groups. The RF algorithm selected the top four variables (Figure 8).

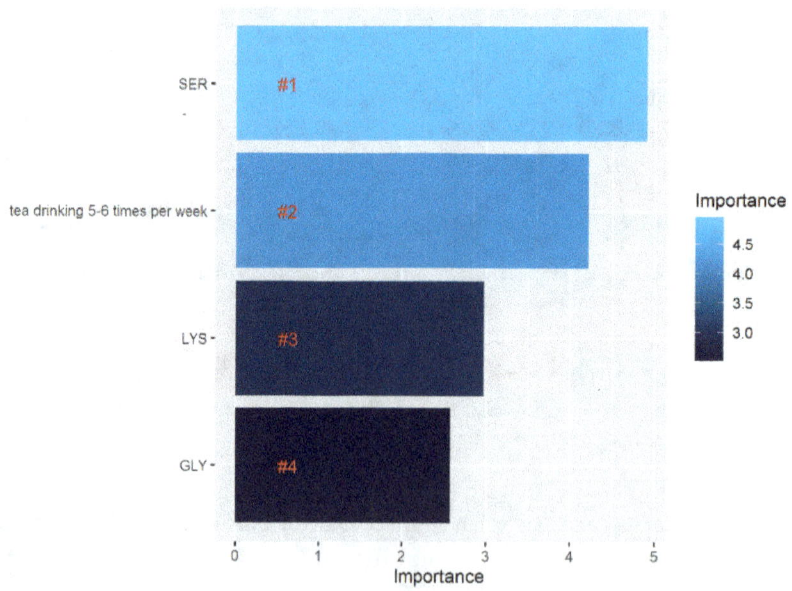

Figure 8. Variable importance assessing the relative importance of individual predictors in the random forest model. According to the legend on the right, the lighter the color, the higher the contribution of the variable to the classification between patients with and without impairment.

The accuracy, sensitivity, specificity, and AUC of the RF model is presented in Table 3.

Table 3. Performance of the random forest model, assessed by different metrics.

	Random Forest Model
Accuracy	0.72 (0.47–0.84)
Sensitivity	0.64 (0.38–0.83)
Specificity	0.78 (0.51–0.85)
AUC	0.74 (0.57–0.88)

Based on 16 amino acid concentrations, the greatest separation between both groups (healthy elderly subjects with no dementia diagnosed and patients with mild or moderate dementia) was served by arginine, serine, and isoleucine. Significantly increased concentrations of serine, isoleucine, and arginine were present in patients with dementia compared with the elderly subjects without dementia. In the RF model, serine appeared to be the most important, and in the logistic regression model, this variable appeared to be significant.

Based on the *p*-values, only the SER concentration and drinking tea 5–6 times per week appeared to be significant at $\alpha = 0.05$. An OR > 1 denotes a risk of mild-to-moderate dementia, while an OR < 1 represents a protective effect. A one-unit increase in the SER concentration led to a 1.51-fold increase in the odds of the presence of mild-to-moderate dementia. Tea drinking was negatively correlated with having mild-to-moderate dementia. There was a 74 percent reduction in the odds of having mild-to-moderate dementia for those with a tea drinking frequency of 5–6 times per week compared with patients with no CI or MCI (Table 4).

Table 4. Logistic regression estimates with the odds ratio (OR), 95% lower confidence intervals (LCIs), and 95% upper confidence intervals (UCIs) on the whole data set of 123 patients.

Variable	Estimate	OR [Exp(Estimate)]	*p*-Value
SER	1.51	4.53 (1.48–13.87)	0.008
GLY	0.38	1.46 (0.58–3.69)	0.417
LYS	0.17	1.19 (0.61–2.33)	0.6
Tea drinking 5–6 times/week	−1.33	0.26 (0.12–0.53)	0.0002

To further study the nature of amino acids, we checked correlations between the amino acids against each other. Since the distribution for each AA resembled a normal distribution and AA originate from similar pathways, we may expect a linear dependence between them. Thus, we used a Pearson correlation, which measures the linear dependence between variables.

In Figure 9, we present a correlation matrix demonstrating the degree of linear relationship between the AAs. Only positive relationships between amino acids were observed, which was expected, taking into account that AA origins might be driven by a similar mechanism. As observed in this figure, they carried essentially the same information.

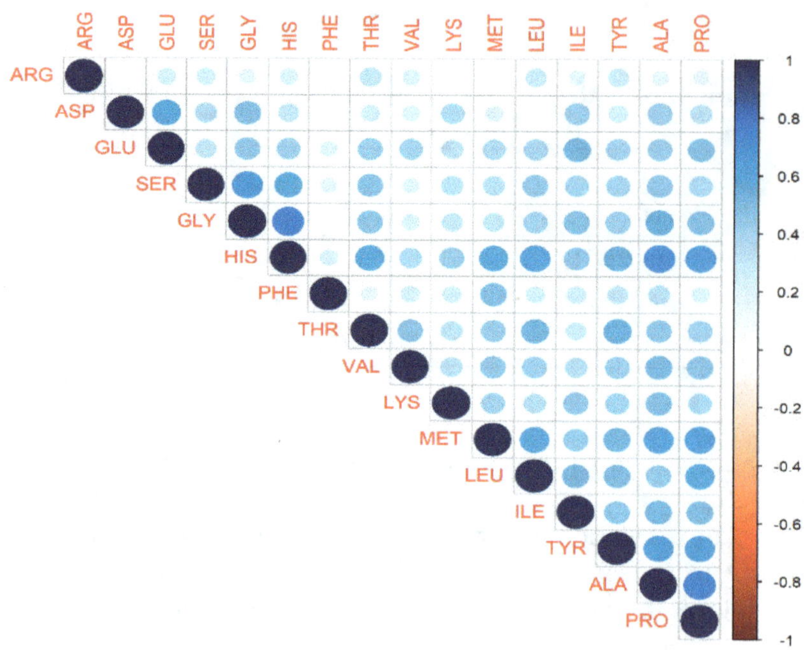

Figure 9. Correlation matrix demonstrating the degree of linear relationship between amino acids. The variables are ordered according to the value of the Pearson correlation coefficient. The lighter the color, the lesser the coefficient value between two variables. Only significant correlations are depicted; insignificant correlations are leaved blank. No negative correlation between amino acids was observed.

4. Discussion

Metabolomic approaches represent a promising, potent, and comprehensive tool for the identification of a wide range of biochemical changes that are associated with neurodegenerative diseases and their treatments. Recent scientific evidence associates metabolic dysfunctions with neurodegenerative development and the severity thereof. However, despite significant technological and research progress, there is as of yet no unequivocal evidence pointing to accurate biomarkers of the disease in human models. Several researchers support the assumption that AD is a systemic disorder characterized by mitochondrial dysfunction, glucose metabolism, and altered amino acid metabolism [6,22]. The results of this study indicate that the serum levels of three amino acids changed significantly in patients with the initial stages of dementia, in relation to elderly subjects without dementia.

In particular, we observed differences in concentrations for SER (significantly increased in patients with dementia compared with the control group), ARG (significantly increased in patients with dementia compared with the control group), and ILE (significantly increased in patients with dementia compared with the control group), which were supported by visual inspection. In the RF model, serine appeared to be the most important. Based on the *p*-values, a one-unit increase in SER concentration led to a 1.51-fold increase in the odds of the presence of dementia.

It is interesting to note that D-serine, formed from L-serine by serine racemase, is the physiologic main co-agonist at the N-methyl-D-aspartate receptors (NMDARs) subtype in the frontal brain areas. An association between the incorrect activation of the glutamate receptors of the NMDARs, synapse dysfunction, and neurotoxicity in AD was reported [23–32]. Researchers confirmed the serine implication in NMDAR-mediated neurotoxicity [23–33]. Previously, in vitro studies showed an increased release of D-serine from neuronal and glial cells and NMDAR activation under injury in AD model systems [23,34,35].

Madeira et al. measured the serine levels in post-mortem samples from subjects without dementia and AD patients, and they reported that D-serine levels were significantly higher in the CSF of AD patients than in the control group. They showed that increased levels of brain and CSF D-serine are associated with AD. Furthermore, they indicated the significant correlation between increased D-serine in CSF and poorer cognitive performance. They suggested that D-serine could be a novel AD biomarker [23]. The present findings seem to be consistent with other research, which found increased D-serine levels in the CSF of AD patients compared with the control group [36].

As mentioned in the literature review, increased serine levels in the CSF and brain tissue samples from patients with advanced neurodegenerative diseases were previously reported. However, in reviewing the literature, no data was found for serine measured in non-invasive material from patients with early stages of neurodegenerative diseases. In this study, we showed the increase level of serine in the initial stage of dementia (mild and moderate dementia) with a relatively easy method involving a non-invasive material sampling technique. We acknowledge that this is an introductory pilot study and, thus, a larger study on greater samples is warranted to extend the validity of our results. Isoleucine is one of the essential branched-chain amino acids (BCAAs). Larsson et al. noticed that the uptake of BCAAs into the brain occurs at the blood–brain barrier via a competitive transport carrier that they share with tryptophan. Tryptophan is the precursor of serotonin and other large, neutral amino acids. A long-term increase in the levels of branched-chain amino acids could lead to reduced levels of brain tryptophan, as well as the decreased synthesis of neuronal serotonin and serotonergic signaling. Finally, this may increase the risk of the development of neurodegenerative diseases such as AD [37,38]. In 2017, Larsson and a coworker demonstrated that a genetic predisposition to higher levels of isoleucine in plasma is positively associated with the occurrence of AD. They suggest that lifelong increased levels of isoleucine may raise the risk of AD [37]. The results of our study seem to be consistent with previous research and suggest that isoleucine increases in patients with dementia.

Finally, we observed the significant increase in concentration of arginine in patients with dementia (from mild to moderate) compared with the healthy control group. This finding is in agreement with Corso et al. and their findings, which showed the trend toward increased arginine concentration in dementia caused by AD [15]. Furthermore, our results are consistent with those of Olazaran, who found the trend of arginine growth along the continuum from the control group (healthy subjects) to mild cognitive impairment and to AD [39].

Fonteh et al. showed that an increase in the concentration of arginine in urine and plasma, accompanied by a decreased in the arginine concentration in CSF, is evidence of a change in nitrogen detoxification in AD [18]. Furthermore, a number of recent studies have found the implications of alterations in arginine metabolism in the pathogenesis of neurodegenerative disorders. In 2014, Liu et al. reported that arginine metabolism definitely changed in diverse regions of the brain in AD and emphasized that further research should be done to understand its role in the pathogenesis of the disease. It is important to note that arginine is a precursor for nitric oxide and polyamines. Both are essential modulators of neuronal physiology and are thought to be involved in the pathogenesis of neurodegenerative diseases such as dementia [40]. Nitric oxide is produced from L-arginine, and it has numerous physiological functions such as learning, memory, noradrenaline and dopamine release, and regulation of the cerebrovascular system. It also takes part in some pathologies, such as schizophrenia, stroke, cerebral ischemia, and Huntington's disease [41].

In 2015, Graham et al. published a paper in which they described the analysis of human plasma and how it indicated differentially affected polyamine and L-arginine metabolisms in mild cognitive impairment subjects converting to AD. Researchers found that the L-arginine metabolism and polyamine metabolism were interlinked, sharing common metabolite intermediates. They are connected via the urea cycle through the enzyme arginase, which converts L-arginine to urea and L-ornithine. Researchers indicated that enzyme arginase appeared to control the proliferation and apoptosis of neural cells. Their results demonstrated that, in MCI and in AD, there was a significant increase in L-arginine which was coupled with a decrease in L-ornithine. It has been suggested that this disturbance in the arginase pathway may potentially reflect alterations in neurogenesis [42–44]. These results and their interpretations, based on the literature, suggest that the metabolisms of some amino acids seem to be changed in patients with dementia. However, at this point, we highlight that the main limitation of this study relates to small and unbalanced sample sizes. Therefore, the obtained results should be confirmed with a larger sample size and should be interpreted with caution to fully confirm their validity. Furthermore, amino acid modifications could be a consequence and not a cause of AD, and they also should be considered as limitations. Factors affecting plasma amino acid concentrations should also be considered. Therefore, our findings need further validation, especially regarding potential alterations in energy metabolism in patients with dementia. It seems valuable for future studies to include different biological materials (tissue and fluid samples) from one patient for a more comprehensive analysis. Long-term studies to measure changes in amino acid concentrations versus dementia progression (from mild to advanced stages) would also allow for a more thorough analysis.

5. Conclusions

We conclude that amino acid profiling might be helpful in better understanding biochemical and metabolic changes related to the pathogenesis and progression of dementia. In the present study, we discovered significant changes in serine, isoleucine, and arginine concentrations in patients with dementia compared with elderly subjects without dementia. These changes may each play a different role in the disease, and this highlights the multifactorial, heterogenous, and complex nature of this disease.

While this information is very useful, it is not sufficient by itself for good understanding of the pathological changes associated with dementia. Considering the multifactorial, heterogenous, and complex nature of this disease, validation with a greater study sample in further research is required.

Author Contributions: Conceptualization, E.S., P.K. and M.K.; methodology, P.K. and E.S.; software and validation, P.K.; formal analysis, E.D.-W. and E.S.; investigation, E.S., P.K., K.M.-G., K.K.-K. and M.G.; resources, E.S, P.K. and M.K.; data curation, E.S.; writing—original draft preparation, E.S. and P.K.; writing—review M.K. and E.D.-W.; writing—editing, E.S.; visualization, E.D.-W.; supervision, E.S. and M.K.; project administration, E.S. and M.K.; funding acquisition, E.S. and M.K. This work is part of a PhD dissertation thesis by E.S. All authors have read and agreed to the published version of the manuscript.

References

1. National Collaborating Centre for Mental Health (UK). Dementia: A NICE-SCIE Guideline on Supporting People With Dementia and Their Carers in Health and Social Care. Leicester (UK): British Psychological Society; 2007. (NICE Clinical Guidelines, No. 42.) 4, DEMENTIA. Available online: https://www.ncbi.nlm.nih.gov/books/NBK55480/ (accessed on 27 November 2020).
2. Winblad, B.; Amouyel, P.; Andrieu, S. Defeating Alzheimer's disease and other dementias: A priority for European science and society. *Lancet Neurol.* **2016**, *15*, 455–532. [CrossRef]
3. Alzheimer's Association. 2020 Alzheimer's Disease Facts and Figures. *Alzheimers Dement* **2020**, *16*, 391. [CrossRef]
4. Griffin, J.W.D.; Bradshaw, P.C. Amino Acid Catabolism in Alzheimer's Disease Brain: Friend or Foe? *Hindawi Oxidative Med. Cell. Longev.* **2017**. [CrossRef]
5. Herrup, K. The case for rejecting the amyloid cascade hypothesis. *Nat. Neurosci.* **2015**, *18*, 794–799. [CrossRef] [PubMed]
6. Polis, B.; Samson, A.O. Role of the metabolism of branched-chain amino acids in the development of Alzheimer's disease and other metabolic disorders. *Neural. Regen. Res.* **2020**, *15*, 1460–1470. [CrossRef] [PubMed]
7. Alford, S.; Patel, D.; Perakakis, N.; Mantzoros, C.S. Obesity as a risk factor for Alzheimer's disease: Weighing the evidence. *Obes. Rev.* **2018**, *19*, 269–280. [CrossRef] [PubMed]
8. Craft, S.; Baker, L.D.; Montine, T.J.; Minoshima, S.; Watson, G.S.; Claxton, A.; Arbuckle, M.; Callaghan, M.; Tsai, E.; Plymate, S.R.; et al. Intranasal insulin therapy for Alzheimer disease and amnestic mild cognitive impairment: A pilot clinical trial. *Arch. Neurol.* **2012**, *69*, 29–38. [CrossRef]

9. Asadbegi, M.; Yaghmaei, P.; Salehi, I.; Ebrahim-Habibi, A.; Komaki, A. Neuroprotective effects of metformin against Aβ-mediated inhibition of long-term potentiation in rats fed a high-fat diet. *Brain Res. Bull.* **2016**, *121*, 178–185. [CrossRef]
10. Blennow, K. A Review of Fluid Biomarkers for Alzheimer's Disease: Moving from CSF to Blood. *Neurol. Ther.* **2017**, *6* (Suppl. 1), 15–24. [CrossRef]
11. Maciejczyk, M.; Zalewska, A.; Gerreth, K. Salivary Redox Biomarkers in Selected Neurodegenerative Diseases. *J. Clin. Med.* **2020**, *9*, 497. [CrossRef]
12. Klimiuk, A.; Maciejczyk, M.; Choromańska, M.; Fejfer, K.; Waszkiewicz, N.; Zalewska, A. Salivary Redox Biomarkers in Different Stages of Dementia Severity. *J. Clin. Med.* **2019**, *8*, 840. [CrossRef] [PubMed]
13. Assche, R.; Temmerman, L.; Dias, D.A.; Boughton, B.; Boonen, K.; Braeckman, B.P.; Schoofs, L.; Roessner, U. Metabolic profiling of a transgenic Caenorhabditis elegans Alzheimer model. *Metabolomics* **2015**, *11*, 477–486. [CrossRef] [PubMed]
14. Bateman, R.J.; Xiong, C.; Benzinger, T.L.; Fagan, A.M.; Goate, A.; Fox, N.C.; Marcus, D.S.; Cairns, N.J.; Xie, X.; Blazey, T.M.; et al. Oxidative stress and Parkinson's disease. *Front. Neuroanat.* **2015**, *9*, 91.
15. Corso, G.; Cristofano, A.; Sapere, N.; Marca, G.; Angiolillo, A.; Vitale, M.; Fratangelo, R.; Lombardi, T.; Porcile, C.; Intrieri, M.; et al. Serum Amino Acid Profiles in Normal Subjects and in Patients with or at Risk of Alzheimer Dementia. *Dement. Geriatr. Cogn. Disord. Extra* **2017**, *7*, 143–159. [CrossRef] [PubMed]
16. Gong, Y.; Liu, Y.; Zhou, L.; Di, X.; Li, W.; Li, Q.; Bi, K. A UHPLC-TOF/MS method based metabonomic study of total ginsenosides effects on Alzheimer disease mouse model. *J. Pharm. Biomed. Anal.* **2015**, *115*, 174–182. [CrossRef] [PubMed]
17. Inoue, K.; Tsutsui, H.; Akatsu, H.; Hashizume, Y.; Matsukawa, N.; Yamamoto, T.; Toyo'oka, T. Metabolic profiling of Alzheimer's disease brains. *Sci. Rep.* **2013**, *3*, 2364. [CrossRef] [PubMed]
18. Fonteh, A.N.; Harrington, R.J.; Tsai, A.; Liao, P.; Harrington, M.G. Free amino acid and dipeptide changes in the body fluids from Alzheimer's disease subjects. *Amino Acids* **2007**, *32*, 213–224. [CrossRef] [PubMed]
19. Adachi, Y.; Ono, N.; Imaizumi, A.; Muramatsu, T.; Andou, T.; Shimodaira, Y.; Nagao, K.; Kageyama, Y.; Mori, M.; Noguchi, Y.; et al. Plasma Amino Acid Profile in Severely Frail Elderly Patients in Japan. *Int. J. Gerontol.* **2018**. [CrossRef]
20. Figura, M.; Kuśmierska, K.; Bucior, E.; Szlufik, S.; Koziorowski, D.; Jamrozik, Z.; Janik, P. Serum Amino Acid Profile in patients with Parkinson's disease. *PLoS ONE* **2018**, *13*, e0191670. [CrossRef]
21. Lunardon, N.; Menardi, G.; Torelli, N. ROSE: A Package for Binary Imbalanced Learning. *R. J.* **2014**, *6*, 79–90. [CrossRef]
22. Gonzalez-Domınguez, R.; Garcıa-Barrera, T.; Vitorica, J.; Gomez-Ariza, J.L. Application of metabolomics based on direct mass spectrometry analysis for the elucidation of altered metabolic pathways in serum from the APP/PS1 transgenic model of Alzheimer's disease. *J. Pharm. Biomed. Anal.* **2015**, *107*, 378–385. [CrossRef] [PubMed]
23. Madeira, C.; Lourenco, M.V.; Vargas-Lopes, C.; Suemoto, C.K.; Brandão, C.O.; Reis, T.; Leite, R.E.; Laks, J.; Jacob-Filho, W.; Pasqualucci, C.A.; et al. d-serine levels in Alzheimer's disease: Implications for novel biomarker development. *Transl. Psychiatry* **2015**, *5*, e561. [CrossRef]
24. Paula-Lima, A.C.; Brito-Moreira, J.; Ferreira, S.T. Deregulation of excitatory neurotransmission underlying synapse failure in Alzheimer's disease. *J. Neurochem.* **2013**, *126*, 191–202. [CrossRef] [PubMed]
25. Li, S.; Jin, M.; Koeglsperger, T.; Shepardson, N.E.; Shankar, G.M.; Selkoe, D.J. Soluble Aβoligomers inhibit long-term potentiation through a mechanism involving excessive activation of extrasynaptic NR2B-containing NMDA receptors. *J. Neurosci.* **2011**, *31*, 6627–6638. [CrossRef] [PubMed]
26. Li, S.; Hong, S.; Shepardson, N.E.; Walsh, D.M.; Shankar, G.M.; Selkoe, D. Soluble oligomers of amyloid-β protein facilitate hippocampal long-term depression by disrupting neuronal glutamate uptake. *Neuron* **2009**, *62*, 788–801. [CrossRef]
27. Shankar, G.M.; Bloodgood, B.L.; Townsend, M.; Walsh, D.M.; Selkoe, D.J.; Sabatini, B.L. Natural oligomers of the Alzheimer amyloid-β protein induce reversible synapse loss by modulating an NMDA-type glutamate receptor-dependent signaling pathway. *J. Neurosci.* **2007**, *27*, 2866–2875. [CrossRef]
28. De Felice, F.G.; Velasco, P.T.; Lambert, M.P.; Viola, K.; Fernandez, S.J.; Ferreira, S.T.; Klein, W.L. Aβoligomers induce neuronal oxidative stress through an N-methyl-D-aspartate receptor-dependent mechanism that is blocked by the Alzheimer drug memantine. *J. Biol. Chem.* **2007**, *282*, 11590–11601. [CrossRef]

29. Talantova, M.; Sanz-Blasco, S.; Zhang, X.; Xia, P.; Akhtar, M.W.; Okamoto, S.I.; Dziewczapolski, G.; Nakamura, T.; Cao, G.; Pratt, A.E.; et al. Aβ induces astrocytic glutamate release, extrasynaptic NMDA receptor activation, and synaptic loss. *Proc. Natl. Acad. Sci. USA* **2013**, *110*, E2518–E2527. [CrossRef]
30. Wolosker, H.; Radzishevsky, I. The serine shuttle between glia and neurons: Implications for neurotransmission and neurodegeneration. *Biochem. Soc. Trans.* **2013**, *41*, 1546–1550. [CrossRef]
31. Wolosker, H.; Dumin, E.; Balan, L.; Foltyn, V.N. d-Amino acids in the brain: D-serine in neurotransmission and neurodegeneration. *FEBS J.* **2008**, *275*, 3514–3526. [CrossRef]
32. Radzishevsky, I.; Sason, H.; Wolosker, H. D-Serine: Physiology and pathology. *Curr. Opin. Clin. Nutr. Metab. Care* **2013**, *16*, 72–75. [CrossRef] [PubMed]
33. Mustafa, A.K.; Ahmad, A.S.; Zeynalov, E.; Gazi, S.K.; Sikka, G.; Ehmsen, J.T.; Barrow, R.K.; Coyle, J.T.; Snyder, S.H.; Doré, S. Serine racemase deletion protects against cerebral ischemia and excitotoxicity. *J. Neurosci.* **2010**, *30*, 1413–1416. [CrossRef] [PubMed]
34. Wu, S.Z.; Bodles, A.M.; Porter, M.M.; Griffin, W.S.; Basile, A.S.; Barger, S.W. Induction of serine racemase expression and D-serine release from microglia by amyloid-β peptide. *J. Neuroinflamm.* **2004**, *1*, 2. [CrossRef]
35. Brito-Moreira, J.; CPaula-Lima, A.; RBomfim, T.; FOliveira, F.; JSepulveda, F.; GDe Mello, F.; GAguayo, L.; Panizzutti, R.; TFerreira, S. Aβ oligomers induce glutamate release from hippocampal neurons. *Curr. Alzheimer Res.* **2011**, *8*, 552–562. [CrossRef]
36. Fisher, G.; Lorenzo, N.; Abe, H.; Fujita, E.; Frey, W.H.; Emory, C.; Di Fiore, M.M.; D'Aniello, A. Free D- and L-amino acids in ventricular cerebrospinal fluid from Alzheimer and normal subjects. *Amino Acids* **1998**, *15*, 263–269. [CrossRef]
37. Larsson, S.C.; Markus, H.S. Branched-chain amino acids and Alzheimer's disease: A Mendelian randomization analysis. *Sci. Rep.* **2017**, *7*, 13604. [CrossRef]
38. Choi, S.; Disilvio, B.; Fernstrom, M.H.; Fernstrom, J.D. Oral branched-chain amino acid supplements that reduce brain serotonin during exercise in rats also lower brain catecholamines. *Amino Acids* **2013**, *45*, 1133–1142. [CrossRef]
39. Olazarán, J.; Gil-de-Gómez, L.; Rodríguez-Martín, A.; Valentí-Soler, M.; Frades-Payo, B.; Marín-Muñoz, J.; Antúnez, C.; Frank-García, A.; Acedo-Jiménez, C.; Morlán-Gracia, L.; et al. A blood-based, 7-metabolite signature for the early diagnosis of Alzheimer's disease. *J. Alzheimers Dis.* **2015**, *45*, 1157–1173. [CrossRef] [PubMed]
40. Ravaglia, G.; Forti, P.; Maioli, F.; Bianchi, G.; Martelli, M.; Talerico, T.; Servadei, L.; Zoli, M.; Mariani, E. Plasma amino acid concentrations in patients with amnestic mild cognitive impairment or Alzheimer disease. *Am. J. Clin. Nutr.* **2004**, *80*, 483–488. [CrossRef] [PubMed]
41. Vural, H.; Sirin, B.; Yilmaz, N.; Eren, I.; Deliba, N. The Role of Arginine–Nitric Oxide Pathway in Patients with Alzheimer Disease. *Biol. Trace Elem. Res.* **2009**, *129*, 58–64. [CrossRef]
42. Graham, S.F.; Chevallier, O.P.; Elliott, C.T.; Hölscher, C.; Johnston, J.; McGuinness, B. Untargeted Metabolomic Analysis of Human Plasma Indicates Differentially Affected Polyamine and L-Arginine Metabolism in Mild Cognitive Impairment Subjects Converting to Alzheimer's Disease. *PLoS ONE* **2015**, *10*, e0119452. [CrossRef] [PubMed]
43. Calcia, M.A.; Madeira, C.; Alheira, F.V.; Silva, T.C.; Tannos, F.M.; Vargas-Lopes, C.; Goldenstein, N.; Brasil, M.A.; Ferreira, S.T.; Panizzutti, R. Plasma levels of D-serine in Brazilian individuals with schizophrenia. *Schizophr. Res.* **2012**, *142*, 83–87. [CrossRef] [PubMed]
44. Di Prisco, G.V.; Huang, W.; Buffington, S.A.; Hsu, C.C.; Bonnen, P.E.; Placzek, A.N.; Sidrauski, C.; Krnjević, K.; Kaufman, R.J.; Walter, P.; et al. Translational control of mGluR-dependent long-term depression and object-place learning by eIF2alpha. *Nat. Neurosci.* **2014**, *17*, 1073–1082. [CrossRef] [PubMed]

3

Age-Associated Changes in the Immune System and Blood–Brain Barrier Functions

Michelle A. Erickson [1,2,*] and **William A. Banks** [1,2,*]

1 VA Puget Sound Healthcare System, Geriatric Research Education and Clinical Center, Seattle, WA 98108, USA
2 Division of Gerontology and Geriatric Medicine, Department of Medicine, University of Washington, Seattle, WA 98104, USA
* Correspondence: mericks9@uw.edu (M.A.E.); wabanks1@uw.edu (W.A.B.)

Abstract: Age is associated with altered immune functions that may affect the brain. Brain barriers, including the blood–brain barrier (BBB) and blood–CSF barrier (BCSFB), are important interfaces for neuroimmune communication, and are affected by aging. In this review, we explore novel mechanisms by which the aging immune system alters central nervous system functions and neuroimmune responses, with a focus on brain barriers. Specific emphasis will be on recent works that have identified novel mechanisms by which BBB/BCSFB functions change with age, interactions of the BBB with age-associated immune factors, and contributions of the BBB to age-associated neurological disorders. Understanding how age alters BBB functions and responses to pathological insults could provide important insight on the role of the BBB in the progression of cognitive decline and neurodegenerative disease.

Keywords: blood–brain barrier; aging; inflammation

1. Introduction

Advances in modern medicine, nutrition, hygiene, and safety standards have doubled the life expectancy of humans worldwide over the last century and a half [1]. It has been estimated that in the next 50 years, the elderly will comprise approximately 20% of the world population [2]. Therefore, it is imperative that the scientific and medical communities investigate approaches that will minimize age-associated disease and maximize quality of life. Age-associated neurological and neurodegenerative diseases are especially debilitating to the afflicted and their families, having tremendous emotional and socioeconomic costs. Changes in the immune system have long been recognized to occur with aging, and it is now appreciated that neuroinflammation likely contributes to age-associated neurological diseases [3]. However, it is less well understood how specific changes in the immune system with aging may affect central nervous system (CNS) functions and contribute to neurological disease. We posit that brain barriers, especially the blood–brain barrier (BBB) and blood–CSF barrier (BCSFB), are important interfaces between CNS and peripheral tissues that are affected by age-associated changes in the immune system. The BBB/BCSFB may, in turn, affect homeostatic functions of the CNS, and/or exhibit more detrimental responses to pathological stimuli. In this review, we will provide a brief overview of changes known to occur in the peripheral immune system with aging, and then discuss recent works that have explored the relationships of BBB/BCSFB dysfunction, healthy aging, and the immune system. We will also briefly discuss how age might contribute to BBB/BCSFB dysfunction in different disease states.

2. Changes in the Immune System with Aging

Aging is associated with immune-related changes that come with clinical consequences. For example, as one ages, vulnerability to certain infections increases, and effectiveness of many vaccines decreases [4]. These clinical features of aging are attributed to an overall decline in protective immune responses, termed "immunosenescence" [1]. Aging is also associated with low-grade inflammation that occurs in the absence of overt infection, termed "inflammaging" [5]. Immunosenescence and inflammaging are interrelated processes [6], and may occur with age due to a number of factors that include latent infections, metabolic changes, and cell/tissue injury. Changes in the adaptive and innate immune systems, and related physiological processes that are detectable outside of the CNS are summarized below. Later sections will further discuss known relations of these changes to neuroimmune functions of the BBB and BCSFB.

2.1. Age-Associated Changes in the Adaptive Immune System

The main function of the adaptive immune system is to confer immunological memory to the organism, which facilitates the rapid recognition and neutralization of specific pathogens upon subsequent encounters. Changes in the cellular arm of the adaptive immune system with age have been described comprehensively by many groups [7–9]. One prominent feature of immunosenescence in the elderly is the change in T-cell composition. In particular, there is a decrease in the number of naïve T lymphocytes and an increase in memory and effector T cells with age, as well as a reduced diversity in T-cell receptors, and diminished functions of both naïve and memory T-cells [7,10]. The mechanistic underpinnings of these changes have been described elsewhere [7]. Changes in the B-cell compartment include reduced B-cell numbers, a reduced repertoire of B-cell receptors, reduced proliferative capacity, and decreases in immunoglobulin class-switch recombination [10,11]. The immunological consequences of reduced B-cell and T-cell functions include the reduced ability to generate immune memory to novel antigens, and thus, the reduced vaccine efficacy and increased vulnerability to certain infections in the elderly.

2.2. Age-Associated Changes in the Innate Immune System

The innate immune system is important for mounting initial protective responses against infections, and in sterile tissue injury and wound repair. The innate immune system also initiates cross-talk with the adaptive immune system through antigen presentation, co-stimulatory molecule expression, and cytokine production and so can contribute to adaptive immune responses [12]. The major changes in the innate immune system with aging include a heightened level of baseline inflammation, and an impaired ability to mount an efficient innate immune response against pathogenic stimuli. Specific changes in the function of innate immune cells have been comprehensively described elsewhere [13], and include impairments in phagocytosis, capacity to produce reactive oxygen and nitrogen species, T-cell priming, and signaling through pattern recognition receptors.

2.3. Age-Associated Changes in the Microbiome

A significant portion of the body's immune system resides in or near the gastrointestinal tract and can regulate the resident gut microbial populations. In young humans, the most numerous and diverse bacterial phylum is Firmicutes, with most in this phylum belonging to the Clostridia class. The second most abundant phylum is Bacteriodetes, which shows a high level of subject-to-subject variability in phylotypes detected [14]. In initial studies from the ELDERMET consortium that explored differences in gut microbial populations in young versus elderly subjects, it was found that elderly subjects had a lower proportion of Firmicutes, and atypical Bacteriodetes/Firmicutes ratios where Bacteriodetes predominated [15]. However, this study and others also demonstrated that elderly subjects show high variability in their microbiota profiles [15,16]. Notably, many of the Firmicutes are major producers of the short chain fatty acid, butyrate [17], which has histone deacetylase inhibitor activities and has been shown to protect against age-associated conditions such as sarcopenia and cognitive impairment in rodent models of neurodegenerative disease [18,19]. Increases in pathogenic bacteria that thrive in pro-inflammatory environments such as streptococci, staphylococci, enterococci, and enterobacteria have also been reported with aging [16], namely in centenarians [20].

Gut-associated lymphoid tissues (GALT) are the major immune interfaces of the gut that regulate the microbiome throughout lifespan. Age-associated changes in GALT include a reduction in antigen-specific IgA-immune responses which are, in part, mediated by aberrant cytokine responses of CD4+ T-cells [21]. It has also been shown that aging is associated with a reduced induction of immune tolerance to novel oral antigens [22]. Loss of the immunoregulatory environment within the gut with aging may have consequences, such as immune responses to novel antigens that would normally be tolerated, or a shift in gut microbial populations [16]. A pro-inflammatory environment within the gut could also result in microbial translocation and release of pathogenic microbes and/or their products (e.g., lipopolysaccharides) into the bloodstream, which could affect distal organs such as the CNS [23,24].

Dietary and environmental changes that are specifically associated with aging may also contribute to alterations in the microbiome. For example, dietary changes may occur upon new residence in assisted living institutions [16]. The elderly are also disproportionately affected by *Clostridium difficile* infection, and risk factors that may facilitate changes in the microbiome include increased use of antibiotics, and prior health care exposures where *C. difficile* may be contracted [25].

2.4. Age-Associated Changes in Peripheral Tissue Microenvironments and the Circulation

The transition of cells to a senescent phenotype is thought to be a protective mechanism against malignancies, and accumulation of senescent cells in multiple tissues occurs with aging [26]. Senescent cells are growth-arrested, but they remain metabolically active and undergo dramatic changes in protein expression and secretion, primarily in response to DNA damage [27]. The senescence-associated secretory phenotype (SASP) involves secretion of soluble cytokines, chemokines, and growth factors, proteases, extracellular matrix components, and reactive oxygen and nitrogen species which together modify the tissue microenvironment to promote local inflammation and tissue damage [26]. Therefore, cellular senescence may be one contributing factor to inflammaging. It has been proposed that cells of the CNS that have proliferative capacities such as endothelial cells and glia may also adopt a SASP, which could result in low-grade inflammation in the aging brain [28].

The BBB could also be affected by the accumulation of SASP cells in the periphery if exposed to pro-inflammatory secreted factors in the bloodstream. Many studies to date have demonstrated elevations in circulating inflammatory and acute phase proteins with aging [29–32]. We have also recently reviewed many aspects of neuroimmune interactions of the BBB and BCSFB with immune factors associated with SASP [33]. Recently, a novel aptamer-based proteomic approach was used to assess proteomic profiles in blood with healthy aging [34]. This study significantly detected an overall enrichment of SASP proteins in blood with aging, although some classical aging biomarkers such as interleukin-6 (IL-6), tumor necrosis factor-α (TNF-α), and insulin-like growth factor-1 (IGF-1) were not among the top-ranking age-associated proteins [34,35]. However, the proteins detected did reflect enriched signaling pathways such as cytokine/cytokine-receptor interactions, complement and coagulation cascades, and axon guidance. Notably, the protein that most strongly correlated with aging in this study was macrophage inhibitory cytokine-1 (MIC-1)/growth differentiation factor 15 (GDF15), which is a transforming growth factor-β (TGF-β) superfamily member that has anti-inflammatory activities in vitro [34,36]. Recent studies have also implicated GDF15 in obesity and the regulation of body weight, as well as frailty [37–39]. Overall, results from biomarker studies suggest that there may be differences in blood biomarkers that could signify healthy aging and predict SASP-associated disease.

3. Age-Associated Changes in Neuroimmune Functions

3.1. Altered Neuroimmune Phenotypes with Aging

Evidence supports that aging causes a pro-inflammatory environment in the CNS. Factors that have been proposed to contribute to increased baseline activation of inflammatory processes in the brain include reactive oxygen species, release of damage-associated molecular patterns (DAMPs) from injured or dying cells, increased abundance of cells with SASP phenotypes, and responses to peripheral inflammatory signals [40–44]. In humans, non-human primates, and rodents, aging is associated with increased numbers of reactive microglia and astrocytes [45]. The reactive phenotype of both astrocytes and microglia is typically determined by the expression levels of specific cell surface markers, as well as morphological changes of the cells. For example, there is an increased proportion of microglia in aged mice that stain positive for cell surface markers such as major histocompatibility complex II (MHCII), and cluster of differentiation (CD)11b, 86, and 68 [46]. Microglia in the healthy brain adopt a ramified morphology, characterized by long, branched extensions from the cell body that function in surveying the local environment [47]. With aging, microglia de-ramification is apparent: processes retract and thicken, and cell bodies enlarge [46,48]. Astrocytes also demonstrate morphological changes and increased expression of the inflammatory surface marker, glial fibrillary acidic protein (GFAP), with aging [46]. Aging also involves a shift in cytokine expression profiles, with increases in pro-inflammatory cytokines such as interleukin-1β (IL-1β) and IL-6, and decreases in anti-inflammatory cytokines such as interleukins 10 and 4 (IL-10 and IL-4) [46]. Overall, these pro-inflammatory phenotypes of glia at baseline are thought not only to reflect chronic, low-grade neuroinflammation, but also a "primed" phenotype whereby glia have more robust responses to immune stimuli [44].

3.2. Altered Neuroimmune Responses to Stimuli with Aging

It is appreciated that the aging brain may be more vulnerable to pathological changes in response to acute illness and infections. For example, urinary tract infections, which are not associated with cognitive symptoms in the young, can cause delirium and other neuropsychiatric conditions in the elderly [49]. Rodent models also suggest that aged mice have more severe neuroinflammatory responses and exacerbated behavioral outcomes following peripheral immune stimuli [50]. A prototypical stimulator of the innate immune system is lipopolysaccharide (LPS), which is a cell wall constituent of Gram-negative bacteria that activates inflammatory signaling cascades through the pattern recognition receptor Toll-like receptor 4 (TLR4) [51]. Young, healthy mice treated intraperitoneally with LPS exhibit a systemic cascade of cytokines and chemokines in the blood and brain [52], reactive gliosis, changes in body temperature and weight, and sickness behaviors. Intraperitoneal injection of LPS in aged mice causes increased pro-inflammatory cytokine responses and reactive microgliosis versus young mice [50,53,54]. Behavioral complications of peripheral infections and/or exposure to bacterial components is also more pronounced with age. For example, aged rodents are more vulnerable to cognitive impairment, sickness behavior, and depressive-like behavior following exposure to systemic inflammatory stimuli [50,54–56]. Neuroinflammatory stimuli, such as injection of the cytokines TNF-α and interferon-γ (IFN-γ) in the lateral ventricle, also result in increased reactive gliosis which occurs in the absence of apparent neurodegenerative changes [57].

4. The BBB as an Interface for Neuroimmune Communication

4.1. Anatomical, Cellular, and Subcellular Organization of Brain Barriers

4.1.1. The Vascular BBB

The primary anatomical unit of the vascular BBB is the brain endothelial cell (BEC). BECs have unique phenotypic properties that restrict the unregulated diffusion of molecules from blood into brain (barrier functions), and also those that regulate the passage of circulating nutrients, hormones, peptides, and proteins into and out of the brain (transport functions). In addition, the vascular BBB is an important signaling and secretory interface and uniquely regulates immune surveillance in the brain [33]. In Section 4.2, we will discuss how these functions of the BBB contribute to the immune-privileged status of the CNS and to unique aspects of neuroimmune communication.

Barrier functions of the vascular BBB are conferred by at least four distinct phenotypes of brain endothelial cells. These include expression of specialized tight junction proteins, reduced levels of pinocytosis, expression of efflux transporters, and expression of metabolic enzymes Tight junction protein complexes expressed by BECs localize to cell–cell junctions and prevent the diffusion of substances between cells (paracellular diffusion). Tight junctions are comprised of integral membrane proteins that include claudins (namely, claudin-5), occludin, and junctional adhesion molecules such as zonula occludens [58,59]. In addition to limiting paracellular diffusion, tight junctions can limit the lateral diffusion of membrane proteins and thus confer polarity to BECs. Tight junction proteins also interact with the cytoskeleton, adherens junctions, and the extracellular matrix, and are dynamically regulated by a range of stimuli at transcriptional and post-translational levels [58]. Relative reductions in fluid-phase pinocytosis also contribute to the BBB, and recent works have begun to elucidate molecular processes that are uniquely active in BECs and suppress formation of pinocytic vesicles. For example, the lipid transporter major facilitator superfamily domain containing 2A (Mfsd2a) confers a unique membrane lipid composition to brain endothelial cells that prevents assembly of caveolin-1 vesicles [60,61]. Finally, the BBB expresses specialized efflux transporters and metabolic enzymes that prevent the diffusion of circulating xenobiotics and other molecular substrates that would otherwise accumulate in the brain. Most efflux transporters at the BBB belong to the family of ATP-binding cassette transporters, and include P-glycoprotein (P-gp), multidrug resistance proteins (MRPs) and breast cancer resistance proteins (BCRPs) [62]. Examples of metabolic enzymes that contribute to BEC barrier functions include those that metabolize neurotransmitters (e.g., monoamine oxidases, cholinesterases, and aminopeptidases), and Phase I and II enzymes such as cytochrome P450s and transferases that are important for drug metabolism [63].

Like peripheral organs, the brain derives nutritive and trophic support from the circulation. However, energy and anabolic substrates such as glucose and amino acids that are derived from the circulation do not freely diffuse across BEC membranes, and so require transporters at the BBB to permit their passage from brain-to-blood in sufficient concentrations to support normal brain functions. Similarly, peptides and proteins such as insulin, leptin, ghrelin and some cytokines and chemokines can cross the intact BBB, and utilize specialized transport systems to do so. Transport systems at the BBB include solute carriers, which facilitate energy-independent transport down a concentration gradient, endocytic receptors, which bind ligands and transport them from one side of the membrane to the other in an energy-dependent process, and adsorptive endocytosis which involves interactions with the glycocalyx [33]. BBB transporters are important for conveying signals that relay aspects of metabolic status such as satiety and adipose mass, as well as inflammatory status which will be discussed in greater detail in Section 4.2. Also described in greater detail in Section 4.2 are the signaling and secretory interface functions of the BBB and their relevance to neuroimmune communication.

The specialized phenotype of BECs is greatly influenced by their local environment and closely associated supportive cells that are collectively termed the neurovascular unit (NVU). The most closely apposed cells to BECs are pericytes, which are found mostly around capillaries and post-capillary venules, and share a basement membrane with the brain endothelium. Pericytes are important for BBB induction and maintenance, as has been shown in mouse models with pericyte deficiencies [64]. Astrocyte end feet are also in very close proximity to the BBB, and ensheath the vessels. Astrocytes are also important for BBB induction and maintenance, as astrocyte conditioned medium is sufficient to promote BBB properties of BECs cultured in vitro [65]. Other components of the NVU include neurons, microglia, oligodendrocytes, and the extracellular matrix, which have been described for their contributions to BBB function under physiological and inflammatory states [33].

4.1.2. The Epithelial BCSFB

The BCSFB exists at the level of brain epithelial cells that comprise the choroid plexus (CP), which is located in each of the brain ventricles. Arachnoid epithelial cells also contribute to the BCSFB. Notably, endothelial cells comprising the vasculature in the CP do not have a BBB phenotype, and so permit leakage of serum components into the CP stroma [66]. The CP vasculature is also permissive to leukocyte trafficking, and so the stroma within the CP is a site where immune surveillance actively occurs. The CP epithelial cells of the BSCFB, similar to the BBB, express specialized tight junction proteins and efflux transporters that contribute to the barrier properties of the choroid plexus epithelium (CPE). The tight junction protein repertoire of the CPE is somewhat distinct from BECs in that they are comprised of distinct claudin proteins (1, 2, and 11) [59]. The CPE is the major site of cerebrospinal fluid (CSF) production, and CPE transporters are important for regulating CSF composition (reviewed in [67]). The arachnoid epithelium, while not a site for CSF production, does express the tight junction protein claudin 11, and efflux transporters such as P-gp and BCRP which may influence drug penetration in to the brain [33].

In contrast to the brain parenchyma, which has very low levels of blood-derived leukocytes under physiological conditions, the CSF and meninges do have resident populations of blood-derived leukocytes which must cross brain barriers to enter these compartments [68]. Indeed, the choroid plexus and arachnoid epithelial cells of the BCSFB are proposed to be major routes by which leukocytes gain entry to CSF under healthy conditions [68,69], and can also be a route of entry in injured states [70]. Aspects of leukocyte trafficking to the brain across brain barriers with aging will be discussed later in Section 5.1.4.

4.2. Neuroimmune Axes of the BBB

The BBB prevents the unregulated exchange of neuroimmune substances and cells between the CNS and blood. Hence, it is the BBB more than any other structure that secures the CNS as an immune-privileged tissue. However, the immune-privileged status of the CNS is relative as a number of mechanisms establish links between the peripheral components of the immune system and those of the CNS. These mechanisms are operational physiologically and, as discussed below, can be involved in aging and in aging-related diseases. Some of these mechanisms, such as vagal and other cranial nerve afferents, do not directly involve the BBB, whereas many others do. For convenience, mechanisms of BBB-neuroimmune interactions can be grouped into five categories or "axes" [33].

The first axis relates to the physiological regulation of the barrier properties that prevent leakage and is currently the least understood of the axes. As discussed above, much is known about how the barrier [71] is formed and even about how it can breakdown to once again become leaky [72–76]. However, there is some evidence that a degree of leakage may occur normally, if transiently. Hormones known to affect BBB tightness and that vary diurnally or with aging include insulin and dehydroepiandrosterone [77,78]. Such "physiological" leakage is probably at a very low level and its purpose is unknown.

A second axis is the alteration of other barrier functions, such as its transporter functions, by neuroimmune substances. There are many examples of these, such as TNF-α affecting the brain endothelial cell cytoskeleton [79], LPS increasing insulin transport [80], and granulocyte-macrophage colony-stimulating factor and IL-6 modulating BBB permeability to human immunodeficiency virus [81].

A third axis relates to the ability of the barriers to transport neuroimmune substances between the CNS and the blood. The best studied in this category are blood-to-brain transporters for cytokines, including IL-1α and β, IL-6, and TNF-α [82].

A fourth axis relates to immune cell trafficking as discussed above. This axis is clearly involved in both disease, as exemplified by multiple sclerosis, and in normal brain functioning [83]. The latter is illustrated by the belief that an impairment of immune cell surveillance in the brain can lead to progressive multifocal leukoencephalopathy [84].

The fifth axis relates to the ability of barrier cells themselves to secrete neuroimmune substances. For example, LPS acting at the luminal surface of brain endothelial cells induces release of prostaglandins into brain [85,86], resulting in fever. Barrier cells also secrete nitric oxide and cytokines [87]. Such release can be constitutive or induced. Secretion can be either from the same cell membrane surface (i.e., luminal–luminal or abluminal–abluminal) that receives the immune stimuli or, as in the case of LPS-prostaglandin-fever, from the opposite cell membrane surface [88].

These axes can interact in dynamic ways. As discussed below, they are known in some cases to be involved in aging and aging-related diseases.

5. Neuroimmune Mechanisms of Age-Associated Changes at the BBB

As was conveyed in Section 2, physiological aging is associated with changes in the immune system that may occur in response to the altered molecular environment of the aged organism. Although very few studies to date have explored direct relationships between BBB dysfunction and age-associated changes in peripheral components of the innate or adaptive immune systems (discussed in Section 5.1.5), emerging works have explored mechanistic changes at the BBB with aging that may contribute to altered neuroimmune functions. In this section, we will discuss changes at the BBB that are associated with aging in the absence of overt disease, and how physiological aging may affect BBB responses to immune stimuli. We will also consider activities of age-associated signaling pathways at the BBB and BCSFB, and how these might be affected using pharmacological approaches.

5.1. Changes in Brain Barrier Function with Aging

A challenge in the assessment of BBB dysfunction in healthy human aging is that many parameters can only be assessed in post-mortem tissues, and so it is difficult to distinguish changes at the BBB in humans that occur as a result of aging versus disease. Measurements of BBB dysfunction in living human subjects using imaging techniques such as PET, SPECT, and MRI are also becoming more robust with advances in instrumentation and analysis techniques, and have suggested that pathological changes at the BBB do occur progressively with aging, and predict clinical symptoms such as cognitive impairment. Findings in rodent models also corroborate general aging-associated phenotypes of the BBB and have elucidated possible mechanisms by which BBB functions are altered with age. These details are further described below.

5.1.1. Brain Barrier Disruption

One of the most-studied (and yet, poorly understood) aspects of BBB dysfunction is disruption [89], which is typically defined by the apparent leakage of normally BBB impenetrant molecules. Recent imaging results argue that BBB disruption does occur in healthy aging, and is worse in individuals with mild cognitive impairment, which is considered a prodrome of Alzheimer's disease (AD) [90,91]. One common approach to proxy BBB disruption in living humans is to measure the ratio of abundant, BBB-impermeant proteins such as albumin or immunoglobulin G (IgG) in CSF versus serum. However, these measures may be confounded by other known CNS deficits with aging, such as altered production and reabsorption of CSF, and inflammatory changes in the serum and CSF levels of these proteins, which have been discussed previously [57,92]. Further, there may be leakage of the BCSFB and altered protein synthesis at this site with age [93,94]. Recent studies have implemented advanced imaging technologies that can visualize leakage of intravenously injected tracers such as gadolinium via dynamic contrast MRI, and these have indicated that vascular BBB disruption does occur in the aging human brain, albeit at low levels [91].

In healthy aged mice (24 mo.), leakage of IgG into the parenchymal space of the cerebral cortex and hippocampus occurs when compared with young mice (3 mo.), suggesting that there is BBB disruption in this model. Increased IgG leakage in aged mice was associated with astrogliosis, endoplasmic reticulum (ER) stress, and increased endothelial cell levels of TNF-α; the latter measure significantly correlated with circulating levels of IL-6. In the same study, a significant reduction in occludin expression per brain endothelial cell was also observed in aged mice [95]. Other studies have corroborated findings of BBB disruption in aging mice [96]. Molecular mechanisms of BBB disruption in aging have been identified, and include reduced expression of sirtuin-1 [96], a de-acetylase enzyme which has been implicated in the regulation of lifespan, senescence, and inflammatory responses to environmental stress [97].

BBB disruption in the context of aging or disease could result in disease exacerbation through leakage of potentially harmful proteins into the brain [91]. However, it is not entirely clear that BBB disruption under any circumstance will always lead to brain damage. For example, certain therapeutic strategies for delivery of chemotherapeutics to the brain have relied on transiently disrupting the BBB, and are generally well-tolerated when brain cancers are the target [98]. Recent work has also indicated that repeated transient BBB disruption in humans with AD using focused ultrasound did not cause any serious clinical or radiological adverse events [99]. In contrast, healthy rodents with no prior brain abnormalities showed symptoms of reactive gliosis and neurodegeneration when transiently perfused with mannitol to cause widespread disruption of the BBB [100], and also had increased deposition of harmful serum proteins like fibrinogen in the CNS [101,102]. The apparent paradox in efforts to disrupt the BBB as a therapeutic strategy versus BBB disruption having known adverse consequences on the CNS and associations with many CNS diseases highlights the complexities of BEC barrier functions that are likely nuanced and context-specific. Why BBB disruption in and of itself is apparently innocuous under some conditions, but clearly detrimental in others remains to be understood in greater molecular detail.

5.1.2. Transporter Dysfunctions and Altered Signaling at Brain Barriers with Aging

Glucose transport: Glucose is the main energy source for the brain. The BBB regulates glucose uptake by the brain through expression of the glucose transporter GLUT1 on brain endothelial cells. GLUT1 is a uniporter that facilitates glucose diffusion from blood-to-brain. The amount of glucose uptake into brain is thus thought to depend on energy utilization by neurons which maintains a concentration gradient that drives glucose diffusion into the brain [103]. Under this assumption, neuronal dysfunction or neurodegeneration would result in reductions of glucose uptake by the brain due to reduced energy utilization and thus loss of the glucose concentration gradient. However, more recent works have suggested that reductions in brain glucose uptake could also reflect BBB dysfunction in glucose transport [103,104]. Brain glucose uptake can be measured in humans by imaging the uptake of ^{18}F-fludeoxyglucose into the brain with PET. Using this technique, it was shown that there is reduced glucose uptake into the brain in the frontal and temporal cortex with aging, even after correction for volume loss [105]. Aged rodents also show reduced brain glucose uptake, which is associated with cognitive impairment [106,107]. In mice, GLUT1 reductions at the BBB are apparent at 15 mo., and are even further reduced in an AD model of the same age [108].

Amyloid beta transport: Accumulation and deposition of the amyloid beta (Aβ) protein in the brain is a pathological hallmark of AD and contributes to neurodegeneration [109]. The BBB expresses transport systems for Aβ that mediate both transport into (influx) and transport out of (efflux) the CNS. Efflux transporters are thought to be important regulators of Aβ clearance from the brain, and these include the low-density lipoprotein receptor-related protein 1 (LRP-1) and P-gp [110–112]. The latter is also an important multidrug efflux transporter that can affect drug delivery to the brain. LRP-1 expression was shown to be decreased in brain microvessels with age, and in AD [110,113]. P-gp function is decreased in aged humans [114–116] as well as in aged mice [117]. Collectively, these changes at the BBB with age could contribute to Aβ accumulation in the brain with AD. It is also known that systemic inflammation in young mice can contribute to Aβ efflux deficits [118]; whether there is an inflammatory component to the Aβ efflux deficit in aging remains to be determined.

Insulin transport: Insulin is a trophic factor in the brain, and regulates critical functions such as feeding and learning and memory [119]. Brain insulin is not thought to be derived from CNS production, but rather from circulating insulin produced by the pancreas. Transport of insulin from blood-to-brain occurs through saturable transport mechanisms at the BBB [120–122]. In humans, it was recently shown that CSF/serum ratios of insulin decrease with aging [123], suggesting that BBB transport may be impaired. Reductions of insulin concentrations in brain tissues have also been reported with human aging [124]. In the senescence-accelerated mouse P8 (SAMP8) model of accelerated aging and AD-like cognitive decline, significant differences in the transport rate of insulin across the BBB were not observed in young versus aged mice. Increased insulin occupancy of vascular space was observed in aged SAMP8 mice in the parietal cortex, cerebellum, and thalamus, which indicates that there may be increased binding of insulin to brain endothelium with age in these regions [125]. It has not yet been determined whether commonly used mouse strains exhibit alterations in insulin transport across the BBB with age.

5.1.3. Interactions of Age-Associated Circulating Factors with Brain Barriers

Aging is associated with both increases in circulating factors that are harmful to the CNS, and decreases in circulating factors that are protective [29,126]. For example, circulating levels of growth differentiation factor 11 (GDF11, a member of the TGF-β superfamily), decline with age [127], and GDF11 treatments can stimulate vascular proliferation in vitro and in the subventricular zone of aged mice [128]. A circulating factor that increases in blood with aging is the chemokine CCL11, which has been shown through parabiosis studies to mediate cognitive impairment and to inhibit neurogenesis [29]. CCL11 in the circulation can access the CNS through a non-saturable or high capacity transport system at the BBB [129], indicating that increasing levels of circulating CCL11 in blood with age contribute to increased brain levels even when the BBB is intact. Another recent report has demonstrated that the enzyme acid sphingomyelinase (ASM) can contribute to BBB dysfunction [130]. This study showed that ASM concentrations increase in the circulation and in brain endothelial cells with aging. When compared with old mice that had reduced capillary density and evidence of BBB disruption, it was shown that mice heterozygous for sphingomyelin phosphodiesterase 1 (*Smpd1*) gene, which encodes ASM, were protected against these age-associated changes. It was further shown that ASM contributes to BBB disruption through induction of caveolae-cytoskeleton interactions that result in increased fluid-phase pinocytosis, but not through any apparent changes in paracellular/tight junction-regulated routes. ASM has enzymatic activity that facilitates the hydrolysis of sphingomyelin to ceramide and phosphorylcholine conversion [131], and thus altered membrane lipid composition could be contributing to the apparent changes in pinocytosis as well. Smpd1 heterozygosity also protected against age-associated deficits in learning and memory [130].

A summary of disruptive and non-disruptive changes at the vascular BBB with age and consequences to CNS function is depicted in Figure 1.

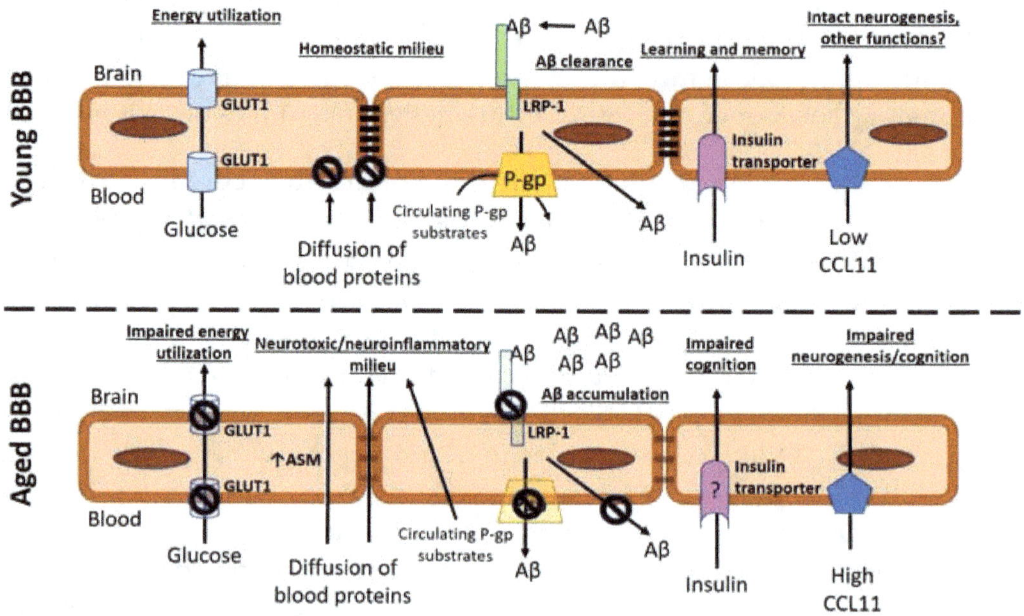

Figure 1. Changes in vascular blood–brain barrier (BBB) function that may lead to brain pathology with age. The upper panel depicts physiological functions of the BBB such as glucose transport, expression of intact tight junction complexes and suppression of vesicular processes that prevent the paracellular or transcellular leakage of blood proteins into the brain, intact functions of the efflux transporter P-gp, which contributes to barrier function by limiting diffusion of its substrates into the brain, and in concert with lipoprotein receptor-related protein 1 (LRP-1), facilitates amyloid beta (Aβ) clearance from the brain. Additionally, entry of insulin into the brain supports neuronal functions and contributes to learning and memory, and brain entry of circulating compounds with high-capacity transporters such as CCL11 is limited by low circulatory concentrations. The lower panel depicts aspects of BBB dysfunction that are either supported or suggested to occur with aging. Transparent appearance of transporters (GLUT1, LRP-1, and P-gp) indicates reduced protein expression levels at the BBB, and the interdictory circles over transporters indicate known functional impairments which may occur in the presence or absence of expression changes. The question mark on the insulin receptor suggests a possible mechanism by which aging influences brain insulin through altered function of the insulin transporter, which has not yet been definitively determined.

5.1.4. Age-Associated Changes in Inflammatory Signaling at the Choroid Plexus

The choroid plexus epithelium that comprises the BCSFB is an important immunological brain interface. The CSF is immunologically active, and contains cells of the adaptive immune system such as central memory T-cells which are thought to participate in CNS immune surveillance [132]. The BCSFB is an important site for leukocyte trafficking into CSF [132,133] and may regulate both protective and pathogenic types of immune cell recruitment to damaged tissues in the CNS and peripheral nervous system (PNS) [133]. Therefore, changes in BSCFB function with age may alter aspects of protective adaptive immunity in the CNS. We discuss this prospect in more detail in the following section.

Age-associated changes in gene expression profiles of the CPE have been found in both mice and humans, and some of the most robust changes in CPE gene expression were related to interferon (IFN)-associated pathways. With aging, there is an increased expression of type I IFN-response genes, and a decrease in type II IFN-response genes at the CP [134]. In the same study, it was found that circulating factors from aged mice reduced type II IFN gene expression, whereas factors in CSF increased type I IFN gene expression, suggesting that the aging brain and systemic compartments have distinct effects on CP gene expression. In aged mice that demonstrated deficits in spatial memory, it was shown that blocking signaling of the interferon α/β receptor, which binds type I IFN cytokines, could improve spatial memory. Aging also induces a shift in cytokine levels expressed at the CP, with increased expression of IL-4 and pro-inflammatory cytokines IL-1β and IL-6, and reduced expression of the type II interferon IFN-γ. It was also found that CPEs could express CCL11, which is induced by IL-4, when IFN-γ levels are low [134]. Therefore, the CP in addition to blood could be a source of CNS CCL11.

Another molecule thought to regulate the CPE with aging is the protein Klotho. Klotho is a transmembrane protein that facilitates signaling of fibroblast growth factor 23 (FGF23), and can also be secreted or cleaved from the membrane by a disintegrin and metalloproteinase domain-containing protein (ADAM) 10 or 17 and released as a soluble form to activate transient receptor potential cation channel subfamily V (TRPV5) signaling or inhibit IGF-1 and wnt signaling [134]. Mice lacking functional Klotho exhibit an accelerated aging phenotype which includes early thymic involution, osteopenia, skin atrophy, hearing loss, and neurodegeneration [135,136]. Klotho expression is not ubiquitous among tissues but is expressed at high levels in the CPE [136]. Expression of Klotho mRNA and protein is significantly reduced at the CPE with age [136]. Such reductions are also associated with increased expression of MHCII in CP stroma, increased levels of peripheral blood-derived macrophages in CP stroma and increased microglial activation, and NLRP3 inflammasome activation [137]. Therefore, Klotho may have important functions in suppressing activation of innate immunity in the CPE, and its reduction may be one mechanism by which neuroimmune functions change with age.

5.1.5. Immune Cell Trafficking

Immune cell trafficking in the brain under healthy conditions is largely compartmentalized to CSF and meningeal spaces, and is thought to be mediated in part through expression of P-selectins and intracellular adhesion molecule-1 (ICAM-1) expressed by the choroid plexus and arachnoid epithelium [68,138]. The post-capillary venules of the BBB are also interfaces for immune cell trafficking, particularly in disease states such as brain injury and multiple sclerosis. Detailed aspects of immune cell trafficking across brain barriers have been discussed by us in a recent review [33]. Relatively little is known about how immune cell populations in the CNS change with healthy aging, or how brain barriers may regulate such changes. However, it is plausible that relations do exist, since changes in peripheral leukocyte populations occur with aging (discussed in Section 2), and brain barriers are active sites of immune cell trafficking to the CNS in both healthy and injured/diseased states. Further, it should be considered whether peripheral changes in innate and adaptive immune cell composition with age could have important implications for CNS function. T-cells, which are the major blood-derived leukocyte population in the CNS (mostly residing in the CSF and meninges) have recently been shown to regulate aspects of learning and memory [138], but it is presently unclear whether age-related changes in T-cell subsets are associated with cognitive deficits.

Increases in T-cell and dendritic cell numbers have been observed in aged mice, starting at about 12 months [139]. One recent study in mice has explored relations among changes in leukocyte subsets in brain and blood [140]. The results of this study showed that numbers of T-cells, but not myeloid cells or other CD45+ cell types significantly increased in the brain with age. Further exploration of T-cell subsets demonstrated that in blood, the ratio of CD4+/CD8+ T-cells decreased with age, whereas age had no effect on the CD4+/CD8+ ratios in brain. In brain, the majority of T-cells detected were CD8+, and localized to perivascular spaces, brain parenchyma, and in the choroid plexus and meninges. Interestingly, the majority of T-cells in human CSF are CD4+ central memory T-cells [69], and so may reflect a different population than those found in brain parenchyma, although species differences may also explain the different abundances of CD4+ versus CD8+ T-cell subsets. The majority of the CD8+ T-cells in aged mouse brains had an effector memory phenotype, and the enrichment of these cells in the brain with age was not attributed to clonal expansion following exposure to brain antigens [140]. Age-associated increases in CD8+ T-cells positively correlated with microglia numbers, and phagocytosis, but negatively correlated with TNF-α positive microglia, suggesting that the CD8+ T-cells may be facilitating microglia polarization towards a phagocytic phenotype. However, it is also possible that the aged microglial phenotype could be driving T-cell recruitment. Finally, this study showed that CD8+ brain T-cells from aged mice produce greater levels of reactive oxygen species and pro-inflammatory cytokines following ischemic injury [140].

Overall, these data indicate that T-cell subsets in brain are distinct from those that predominate in blood, and that changes in T-cell subsets in aged blood are not necessarily reflected by the same population changes in the brain. Although it is presently not known which T-cell subsets in the circulation contribute to brain T-cell populations in parenchyma or CSF/meninges, findings from Ritzel et al. did indicate that T-cells from aged mice had elevated expression of adhesion molecules that are necessary for capture and diapedesis across brain barriers [140]. Future studies are needed to determine the contributions of brain barriers to age-associated increases in T-cell trafficking to the brain.

5.2. Effects of Aging on BBB Responses to Immune Stimuli

Dysfunction of the BBB can occur in concert with systemic and neuroinflammatory changes, however existing data suggest that the young, healthy BBB is relatively resistant to dysfunction caused by peripheral inflammatory insults, and relatively high doses of immune stimulators like LPS are required to elicit BBB disruption and dysfunction of transporters [118,141,142]. This is also supported in humans, where it was recently shown that in the absence of CSF abnormalities that would suggest disease, there were no correlations of systemic inflammatory markers with CSF/serum albumin ratios [143]. These findings further suggest that the healthy BBB of young adults is resistant to disruption induced by moderate systemic inflammation.

It is also understood that BBB dysfunction in response to neuroinflammatory stimuli may be regulated by the systemic inflammatory context. For example, intracerebroventricular (ICV) injection of IL-1β causes a robust influx of leukocytes into CNS parenchyma, but an intraperitoneal dose of LPS inhibits the ability of ICV IL-1β to recruit leukocytes to the brain [144]. The apparent resistance of the BBB to leukocyte trafficking in the presence of systemic inflammation in this context could be an adaptive advantage to protect the CNS from the systemic response to pathogen infections in the periphery.

As previously discussed, aging is associated with decreased BBB integrity and functional impairment of transporters. Aging may also exacerbate BBB responses to CNS injury and systemic inflammatory stimuli. In an LPS model that causes cerebral microhemorrhages (CMH), it was shown that mice aged 18 months had more numerous and severe CMH than young mice. This phenotype was associated with increased microgliosis and astrogliosis [145]. Aging also can cause dramatic changes in sleep, which is associated with increased production of pro-inflammatory cytokines such as TNF-α [146]. Cytokines such as TNF-α can cross the intact BBB, and so peripherally derived TNF-α may enter the brain to activate neuroinflammatory responses directly [147]. Sleep fragmentation in aged mice significantly increased the transport of TNF-α into the brain, but had no significant effect in young mice [146].

5.3. Interactions of the BBB with the Aging Microbiome

Interactions of the microbiome with the BBB have been reviewed recently [148]. Much of the current knowledge of these interactions is based on findings in germ-free mouse models, which exhibit increased BBB disruption that is apparently due to reduced tight junction protein expression and tight junction dysfunction [149]. It is therefore plausible that changes in the microbiome with age may affect BBB function. To date, no studies have directly tested this possibility, although emerging works suggest potential mechanisms. For example, short-chain fatty acids such as butyrate have been shown to protect against BBB disruption in germ-free mice [149]. Emerging evidence also supports that there is a reduced capacity of the microbiome to produce butyrate in the elderly [150], and so it may be that reduced butyrate levels contribute to age-associated BBB dysfunction. Recent studies have also begun to identify how age-associated changes in the microbiome might affect aspects of CNS function in which the BBB could be involved. For example, aged mice have altered cecal microbiota compositions, which is associated with increased gut permeability and higher levels of circulating pro-inflammatory cytokines in the periphery versus young mice. The same aged mouse cohort also demonstrated increased anxiety-like behaviors and impaired object–place recognition memory and social recognition [151]. Although altered BBB functions were not examined in this study, future works could further elucidate relationships of BBB dysfunction and aging with microbiome alterations. However, we also acknowledge that other plausible neuroimmune mechanisms, such as altered gut-to-brain signals as mediated by the vagus nerve or the BSCFB, could also be contributing to CNS changes caused by gut microbiome dyshomeostasis [152,153].

5.4. Effects of Aging on Non-Endothelial Cells of the Neurovascular Unit

Endothelial cells of the BBB develop and maintain their specialized phenotype through interactions with other associated cell types in the CNS that include pericytes, astrocytes, neurons, and also other glial cell types such as microglia and oligodendrocytes [33]. Pericytes and astrocytes are the most extensively studied for their roles in promoting and maintaining BBB functions and may contribute to BBB dysfunction with aging. Detailed aspects of these changes are discussed below.

Pericyte loss/dysfunction: Numerous functions have been ascribed to brain pericytes, including contractility, pluripotent stem cell-like properties, phagocytosis, and induction and maintenance of the BBB [154,155]. Platelet-derived growth factor receptor beta (PDGFRβ) heterozygous mice, which show an age-dependent loss of brain pericytes, also have increased evidence of BBB disruption with aging which coincides with pericyte loss and precedes associated neuroinflammation and learning and memory impairment in this model [156]. In studies of wild-type mice and humans, pericyte loss has been reported with age, but not consistently [156–159]. However, it is more clear that pericyte damage can occur with age, perhaps through phagocytosis of increasing amounts of cell debris [159], which also occurs under inflammatory conditions [160]. Recent studies have reported an increase of soluble PDGFRβ in CSF, a proposed marker of pericyte damage, with aging, BBB disruption, and cognitive impairment in humans [91,161,162].

Astrocyte changes: Astrocyte endfeet ensheath brain capillaries, and contribute to BBB maturation and maintenance [65]. Phenotypic changes have been observed in astrocytes with aging, such as reduced vascular coverage, increased GFAP expression, enlarged size, and reduced aquaporin-4 (AQP4) expression [157,158,163]. Such changes indicate increased reactive astrogliosis, which is also a process that occurs in response to pro-inflammatory stimuli. Given the important role of AQP4 in facilitating paravascular clearance of brain solutes [164], AQP4 reductions on astrocytes with aging could contribute to the neurotoxic accumulation of solutes in the brain.

6. The BBB in Age-Associated Neurological Diseases

Aging increases the risk of developing disease, and many neurological conditions in which the BBB has been implicated are also associated with aging. This section discusses some of these diseases in context of age-associated BBB dysfunction that may predispose or exacerbate the molecular mechanisms of disease.

6.1. Alzheimer's Disease

AD is the most common neurodegenerative disorder, and the greatest risk factor for AD is aging. There have been many recent reviews on the relations of BBB, inflammation, and AD that are beyond the scope of this review [57,165]. This section will focus on some recent conceptual advancements in the AD field that may relate inflammatory changes with aging and the BBB.

Evolving concepts in AD: Under a new research framework proposed by the National Institute on Aging and Alzheimer's Association, it was proposed that AD should be redefined by biological markers of disease, which include neurodegeneration and markers of deposition of two pathological proteins in the brain: amyloid beta and tau [166]. Whereas previous definitions of AD required a clinical diagnosis of dementia, it is now appreciated that pathological changes in AD precede onset of clinical symptoms by years, or even decades [167]. Although Aβ and tau are used to define AD as a unique neurodegenerative disease, it is now being considered that disease modifiers other than Aβ and tau may act in concert to regulate disease progression and manifestation of clinical symptoms. In previous sections, we have discussed aspects of BBB dysfunction that may be causal in AD, and here refer the reader to a recent detailed commentary on the importance of considering the neurovasculature as a possible driver of and therapeutic target for AD [104]. We also consider some additional timely findings that implicate interactions of the BBB, inflammation, and aging in AD.

ApoE isoform-dependent immunomodulatory activities: In humans, there are three major alleles of the apolipoprotein E (*APOE*) gene, which are *APOE2*, *APOE3*, and *APOE4*. *APOE4* is the strongest genetic risk factor for late-onset forms of Alzheimer's disease, which may be due to a number of distinct functions of ApoE4 protein versus the more prevalent ApoE3 protein. ApoE4 may be contributing to AD in part via limiting Aβ clearance from the brain [168], and also through tau-dependent effects [169]. ApoE4 also has diverse functions in regulating the immune system that may be independent or synergistic with Aβ and tau-driven brain pathology [170]. For example, transgenic ApoE4 mice have BBB disruption through the loss of interaction of ApoE4 with LRP-1 in pericytes, which is preserved in mice expressing ApoE3 or ApoE2. As a result, matrix metalloproteinase 9 (MMP9) activation occurring in brain endothelial cells contributes to BBB disruption in the model [74]. This molecular route of BBB disruption in APOE4 carriers has also been reported in human AD [171].

Low-grade CNS infections and AD: Since the discovery of AD by Alois Alzheimer, there have been speculations and a few studies supporting that CNS infections could be causal in AD [172,173]. Although this concept has been largely overshadowed by the amyloid cascade hypotheses and is still controversial, emerging studies have supported that CNS bacterial and viral infections may contribute to or exacerbate AD. Early works have shown that herpes simplex virus-1 (HSV-1) DNA is present in brains of humans with and without AD [174,175], but it was also questioned whether HSV-1 infection was directly involved in AD [176]. Subsequently, it was shown that HSV-1 infection of cultured neurons and glia and mouse brain can increase the production of Aβ [177], and induce cytoskeletal abnormalities in neurons that include tau hyperphosphorylation [178]. Recent works have indicated that Aβ has antimicrobial properties against bacteria and viruses [179,180], and have substantiated the associations of herpes virus infections and AD or dementia [181–185]. These findings suggest that Aβ and/or tau may be protective responses to CNS infections that would be more likely to occur with age-associated immunosenescence and a dysfunctional BBB. It remains to be determined whether antimicrobial strategies such as antibiotics, antivirals, or vaccines could protect the infected against AD progression.

Preclinical animal models of AD: Mouse models of AD have been used extensively to define mechanisms of disease pathology and therapeutic efficacy. Most of these models are based on genetic mutations which cause Aβ plaque deposition, and so are really models of Aβ-driven brain injury [186]. However, other factors such as extraphysiological expression of transgenes and individual or combinations of mutations that are not observed in sporadic AD could further confound these models. Additionally, the AD-like sequalae (plaques, neuroinflammation, cognitive deficits, and neuronal/synaptic loss) in most transgenic mouse models of AD occur when the mice are considered to be young (3–6 mo.) or middle-aged (10–14 mo.), and so exclude the aging component of AD. Accelerated aging models, such as SAMP8 mice which have modest increases in brain Aβ, deficits in Aβ clearance, and impaired learning and memory by 12 months of age [187,188] are less widely used, but have utility in studying the synergy of aging and AD. Along these lines, BBB disruption variably occurs in mouse models of Aβ-driven brain pathology and is not apparent in SAMP8 mice [125,189–192], and recent works have also indicated that tauopathies may also drive BBB disruption in rodents [193,194]. BBB efflux systems have also been identified for truncated forms of tau [195]. Inclusion of an aging component in preclinical AD models may reveal important therapeutic considerations of treatment, or novel aspects of disease progression that may improve the chances of success in drug development.

6.2. Depression

Depression affects individuals of all ages, but poses unique considerations in the aging population. Although depression is less prevalent in older versus younger adults, it is notable that over half of depression diagnoses in the aged are in those who have not previously been afflicted [196]. Depression in the aged is also associated with cognitive dysfunction, dementia risk, and vascular dysfunction [196]. Notably, cardiovascular disease (CVD) and depression are inter-related in that major depressive disorder (MDD) prevalence is more prevalent in individuals with CVD, and MDD increases CVD morbidity and mortality [197]. Systemic inflammation may also be a factor that drives MDD, with studies showing associations of MDD and cytokines and acute phase proteins in blood [198,199]. The BBB has recently been implicated as a possible mediator of depressive behaviors in mice. Mice that were vulnerable to depressive-like behaviors following chronic social defeat stress were shown to have reductions in the tight junction protein claudin-5 and BBB leakiness in the nucleus accumbens (NAc), as well as increased leukocyte trafficking and IL-6 accumulation in this region. Knock-down of claudin-5 in the NAc recapitulated depressive-like behaviors [200]. Notably, aged mice have increased inflammatory responses to social defeat stress [201], suggesting that synergy of BBB dysfunction, glial cell priming, and increased peripheral cytokine responses could all contribute to depressive responses to stress in the aged.

Another possible link between aging, the BBB, and depression is the microbiome. In humans with major depressive disorder, and in rodents subjected to a variety of stressors that can cause depressive-like behavior, composition of the gut microbiome is altered [202–204]. Humans with active MDD were shown to have an increase in Bacteroidetes and a reduction in Firmicutes, similar to age-associated microbiome changes that were discussed in Section 2.3. Recent work has also shown that the transplantation of microbiota from MDD patients into germ-free mice caused depressive-like behaviors, and altered metabolites of carbohydrates and amino acids [205]. Interestingly, the current data suggest that there is bidirectional regulation of the brain and gut microbiome in MDD. Future work is needed to determine how brain barriers may be contributing to gut-brain communication in MDD and other diseases.

6.3. Metabolic Syndrome

Metabolic syndrome is defined by a cluster of risk factors that increases risk of developing CVD, type II diabetes, stroke, and other co-morbid diseases [206,207]. These risk factors include insulin resistance, abdominal obesity, high serum triglycerides, high blood pressure, and hyperglycemia [208]. In the United States, metabolic syndrome is most prevalent in individuals aged 60 and older [209]. Age-associated factors such as low testosterone in males, and low levels of vitamin D may contribute to components of metabolic syndrome in the elderly, such as insulin resistance [209]. Testosterone depletion was recently linked to BBB dysfunction. Orchiectomized mice were shown to have increased BBB disruption, which was in part attributed to reduced expression of the tight junction proteins claudin-5 and zonula occludens-1. Castrated mice from this study also had evidence of reactive astrogliosis [210]. BBB deficits in castrated mice could be rescued by testosterone supplementation, but it was unclear whether the BBB effects occurred through direct actions of testosterone on the BBB, or indirect consequences of testosterone depletion. Notably, in mice, metabolic effects of orchidectomy are very minor or absent on a standard chow diet, but androgen deprivation can exacerbate adipose hypertrophy, glucose intolerance, insulin insensitivity, and systemic inflammation when fed a high-fat diet [211], suggesting that interactions between hormone changes with aging could synergize with diet and obesity to affect BBB disruption.

Obesity is associated with increased systemic inflammation with aging and can exacerbate autoimmune diseases such as rheumatoid arthritis [212]. Obesity can also contribute to BBB dysfunction. Mice that are made to become obese through high-fat diet feeding have evidence of BBB disruption in the hippocampus, which is also associated with learning and memory deficits. BBB disruption in mice fed a high-fat also have reduced levels of tight junction proteins at the BBB and BCSFB [213]. Obesity is also associated with reduced transport of proteins across the BBB that act on the CNS to regulate feeding, such as leptin, insulin, and ghrelin. Whereas insulin and leptin signal satiety to the brain and stimulate anorexia, ghrelin is an orexigenic signal. However, levels of circulating leptin increase with obesity, whereas ghrelin levels decrease with obesity and aging [214]. In the case of ghrelin, age and obesity were also shown to have synergistic suppressive effects on transport across the BBB [215]. Transport of lipids such as palmitate and free fatty acids across the BBB is increased with obesity [213]. Triglycerides, which are elevated in obesity, are known inhibitors of leptin transport, and so may contribute to a feed-forward cycle of leptin deficiency in the brain that leads to hyperphagia and further increases in triglycerides [216]. Obesity induced by a genetic mutation in the leptin receptor has also been associated with increased neuroinflammation, which included monocyte trafficking across the BBB [217].

Type II diabetes mellitus (T2DM), a consequence of metabolic syndrome, is also associated with aging and BBB dysfunction. Studies in rodents and monkeys have shown that increased BBB disruption occurs in T2DM, and is associated with reduced levels of tight junction proteins [218–220]. T2DM is associated with an increased risk of AD [221], and recent work has demonstrated a mechanistic link that implicates BBB dysfunction in this process. In a mouse model of type II diabetes with hyperinsulinemia, it was shown that BBB transport of Aβ into the brain was increased, and transport of Aβ out of the brain was decreased when compared with non-diabetic controls. Antidiabetic drugs reduced Aβ influx and increased Aβ efflux in diabetic mice, and these changes appeared to be mediated through decreases of the Aβ influx transporter, receptor for advanced glycation endproducts (RAGE), and increases in the Aβ efflux transporter, LRP-1 [222]. The BBB dysfunction that occurs as a result of obesity alone, or in combination with T2DM may be further exacerbated by aging, or vice-versa [213,223,224].

7. Conclusions

Inflammatory changes with aging are important drivers of CNS dysfunction, and we have described mechanisms by which BBB dysfunction in healthy aging could predispose to neurological disease. Clearly, more work is necessary to further explore how aging and associated inflammatory changes could affect brain barrier functions in health, infection, and injury. Developing a better understanding of the interactions of aging with known pathogenic mechanisms of disease is important in the development of novel therapies for neurological disorders.

Author Contributions: Writing—Original Draft Preparation, M.A.E. and W.A.B.; Writing—Review & Editing, M.A.E. and W.A.B.; Funding Acquisition, M.A.E. and W.A.B.

References

1. Aw, D.; Silva, A.B.; Palmer, D.B. Immunosenescence: Emerging challenges for an ageing population. *Immunology* **2007**, *120*, 435–446. [CrossRef]
2. Ellison, D.; White, D.; Farrar, F.C. Aging population. *Nurs. Clin. North. Am.* **2015**, *50*, 185–213. [CrossRef]
3. Ransohoff, R.M. How neuroinflammation contributes to neurodegeneration. *Science* **2016**, *353*, 777–783. [CrossRef]
4. Weinberger, B.; Herndler-Brandstetter, D.; Schwanninger, A.; Weiskopf, D.; Grubeck-Loebenstein, B. Biology of immune responses to vaccines in elderly persons. *Clin. Infect. Dis.* **2008**, *46*, 1078–1084. [CrossRef] [PubMed]
5. Franceschi, C.; Bonafe, M.; Valensin, S.; Olivieri, F.; De Luca, M.; Ottaviani, E.; De Benedictis, G. Inflamm-aging. An evolutionary perspective on immunosenescence. *Ann. N. Y. Acad. Sci.* **2000**, *908*, 244–254. [CrossRef]

6. Fulop, T.; Larbi, A.; Dupuis, G.; Le Page, A.; Frost, E.H.; Cohen, A.A.; Witkowski, J.M.; Franceschi, C. Immunosenescence and Inflamm-Aging As Two Sides of the Same Coin: Friends or Foes? *Front. Immunol.* **2017**, *8*, 1960. [CrossRef]
7. Arnold, C.R.; Wolf, J.; Brunner, S.; Herndler-Brandstetter, D.; Grubeck-Loebenstein, B. Gain and loss of T cell subsets in old age–age-related reshaping of the T cell repertoire. *J. Clin. Immunol.* **2011**, *31*, 137–146. [CrossRef]
8. Nikolich-Zugich, J.; Li, G.; Uhrlaub, J.L.; Renkema, K.R.; Smithey, M.J. Age-related changes in CD8 T cell homeostasis and immunity to infection. *Semin. Immunol.* **2012**, *24*, 356–364. [CrossRef] [PubMed]
9. Frasca, D.; Diaz, A.; Romero, M.; Landin, A.M.; Blomberg, B.B. Age effects on B cells and humoral immunity in humans. *Ageing Res. Rev.* **2011**, *10*, 330–335. [CrossRef] [PubMed]
10. Poland, G.A.; Ovsyannikova, I.G.; Kennedy, R.B.; Lambert, N.D.; Kirkland, J.L. A systems biology approach to the effect of aging, immunosenescence and vaccine response. *Curr. Opin. Immunol.* **2014**, *29*, 62–68. [CrossRef] [PubMed]
11. Frasca, D.; Landin, A.M.; Lechner, S.C.; Ryan, J.G.; Schwartz, R.; Riley, R.L.; Blomberg, B.B. Aging down-regulates the transcription factor E2A, activation-induced cytidine deaminase, and Ig class switch in human B cells. *J. Immunol.* **2008**, *180*, 5283–5290. [CrossRef]
12. Jain, A.; Pasare, C. Innate Control of Adaptive Immunity: Beyond the Three-Signal Paradigm. *J. Immunol.* **2017**, *198*, 3791–3800. [CrossRef]
13. Shaw, A.C.; Goldstein, D.R.; Montgomery, R.R. Age-dependent dysregulation of innate immunity. *Nat. Rev. Immunol.* **2013**, *13*, 875–887. [CrossRef]
14. Eckburg, P.B.; Bik, E.M.; Bernstein, C.N.; Purdom, E.; Dethlefsen, L.; Sargent, M.; Gill, S.R.; Nelson, K.E.; Relman, D.A. Diversity of the human intestinal microbial flora. *Science* **2005**, *308*, 1635–1638. [CrossRef] [PubMed]
15. Claesson, M.J.; Cusack, S.; O'Sullivan, O.; Greene-Diniz, R.; de Weerd, H.; Flannery, E.; Marchesi, J.R.; Falush, D.; Dinan, T.; Fitzgerald, G.; et al. Composition, variability, and temporal stability of the intestinal microbiota of the elderly. *Proc. Natl. Acad. Sci. USA* **2011**, *108* (Suppl. 1), 4586–4591. [CrossRef] [PubMed]
16. Biagi, E.; Candela, M.; Turroni, S.; Garagnani, P.; Franceschi, C.; Brigidi, P. Ageing and gut microbes: Perspectives for health maintenance and longevity. *Pharmacol. Res.* **2013**, *69*, 11–20. [CrossRef] [PubMed]
17. Pryde, S.E.; Duncan, S.H.; Hold, G.L.; Stewart, C.S.; Flint, H.J. The microbiology of butyrate formation in the human colon. *FEMS Microbiol. Lett.* **2002**, *217*, 133–139. [CrossRef] [PubMed]
18. Walsh, M.E.; Bhattacharya, A.; Sataranatarajan, K.; Qaisar, R.; Sloane, L.; Rahman, M.M.; Kinter, M.; Van Remmen, H. The histone deacetylase inhibitor butyrate improves metabolism and reduces muscle atrophy during aging. *Aging Cell* **2015**, *14*, 957–970. [CrossRef] [PubMed]
19. Bourassa, M.W.; Alim, I.; Bultman, S.J.; Ratan, R.R. Butyrate, neuroepigenetics and the gut microbiome: Can a high fiber diet improve brain health? *Neurosci. Lett.* **2016**, *625*, 56–63. [CrossRef] [PubMed]
20. Biagi, E.; Nylund, L.; Candela, M.; Ostan, R.; Bucci, L.; Pini, E.; Nikkila, J.; Monti, D.; Satokari, R.; Franceschi, C.; et al. Through ageing, and beyond: Gut microbiota and inflammatory status in seniors and centenarians. *PLoS ONE* **2010**, *5*, e10667. [CrossRef]
21. Kawanishi, H.; Senda, S.; Ajitsu, S. Aging-associated intrinsic defects in IgA production by murine Peyer's patch B cells stimulated by autoreactive Peyer's patch T cell hybridoma-derived B cell stimulatory factors (BSF). *Mech. Ageing Dev.* **1989**, *49*, 61–78. [CrossRef]
22. Fujihashi, K.; McGhee, J.R. Mucosal immunity and tolerance in the elderly. *Mech. Ageing Dev.* **2004**, *125*, 889–898. [CrossRef] [PubMed]
23. D'Ettorre, G.; Douek, D.; Paiardini, M.; Ceccarelli, G.; Vullo, V. Microbial translocation and infectious diseases: What is the link? *Int. J. Microbiol.* **2012**, *2012*, 356981. [CrossRef] [PubMed]
24. Brenchley, J.M.; Price, D.A.; Schacker, T.W.; Asher, T.E.; Silvestri, G.; Rao, S.; Kazzaz, Z.; Bornstein, E.; Lambotte, O.; Altmann, D.; et al. Microbial translocation is a cause of systemic immune activation in chronic HIV infection. *Nat. Med.* **2006**, *12*, 1365–1371. [CrossRef] [PubMed]
25. Asempa, T.E.; Nicolau, D.P. Clostridium difficile infection in the elderly: An update on management. *Clin. Interv. Aging* **2017**, *12*, 1799–1809. [CrossRef] [PubMed]
26. Coppe, J.P.; Desprez, P.Y.; Krtolica, A.; Campisi, J. The senescence-associated secretory phenotype: The dark side of tumor suppression. *Annu. Rev. Pathol.* **2010**, *5*, 99–118. [CrossRef]

27. Tchkonia, T.; Zhu, Y.; van Deursen, J.; Campisi, J.; Kirkland, J.L. Cellular senescence and the senescent secretory phenotype: Therapeutic opportunities. *J. Clin. Investig.* **2013**, *123*, 966–972. [CrossRef]
28. Chinta, S.J.; Woods, G.; Rane, A.; Demaria, M.; Campisi, J.; Andersen, J.K. Cellular senescence and the aging brain. *Exp. Gerontol.* **2015**, *68*, 3–7. [CrossRef]
29. Villeda, S.A.; Luo, J.; Mosher, K.I.; Zou, B.; Britschgi, M.; Bieri, G.; Stan, T.M.; Fainberg, N.; Ding, Z.; Eggel, A.; et al. The ageing systemic milieu negatively regulates neurogenesis and cognitive function. *Nature* **2011**, *477*, 90–94. [CrossRef]
30. Byerley, L.O.; Leamy, L.; Tam, S.W.; Chou, C.W.; Ravussin, E.; Louisiana Healthy Aging Study. Development of a serum profile for healthy aging. *Age (Dordr)* **2010**, *32*, 497–507. [CrossRef] [PubMed]
31. Maggio, M.; Guralnik, J.M.; Longo, D.L.; Ferrucci, L. Interleukin-6 in aging and chronic disease: A magnificent pathway. *J. Gerontol. A Biol. Sci. Med. Sci.* **2006**, *61*, 575–584. [CrossRef]
32. Bruunsgaard, H.; Andersen-Ranberg, K.; Jeune, B.; Pedersen, A.N.; Skinhoj, P.; Pedersen, B.K. A high plasma concentration of TNF-alpha is associated with dementia in centenarians. *J. Gerontol. A Biol. Sci. Med. Sci.* **1999**, *54*, M357–M364. [CrossRef]
33. Erickson, M.A.; Banks, W.A. Neuroimmune Axes of the Blood-Brain Barriers and Blood-Brain Interfaces: Bases for Physiological Regulation, Disease States, and Pharmacological Interventions. *Pharmacol. Rev.* **2018**, *70*, 278–314. [CrossRef] [PubMed]
34. Tanaka, T.; Biancotto, A.; Moaddel, R.; Moore, A.Z.; Gonzalez-Freire, M.; Aon, M.A.; Candia, J.; Zhang, P.; Cheung, F.; Fantoni, G.; et al. Plasma proteomic signature of age in healthy humans. *Aging Cell* **2018**, *17*, e12799. [CrossRef] [PubMed]
35. Krabbe, K.S.; Pedersen, M.; Bruunsgaard, H. Inflammatory mediators in the elderly. *Exp. Gerontol.* **2004**, *39*, 687–699. [CrossRef] [PubMed]
36. Bootcov, M.R.; Bauskin, A.R.; Valenzuela, S.M.; Moore, A.G.; Bansal, M.; He, X.Y.; Zhang, H.P.; Donnellan, M.; Mahler, S.; Pryor, K.; et al. MIC-1, a novel macrophage inhibitory cytokine, is a divergent member of the TGF-beta superfamily. *Proc. Natl. Acad. Sci. USA* **1997**, *94*, 11514–11519. [CrossRef]
37. Villanueva, M.T. Obesity: GDF15 tells the brain to lose weight. *Nat. Rev. Drug Discov.* **2017**, *16*, 827. [CrossRef]
38. Xiong, Y.; Walker, K.; Min, X.; Hale, C.; Tran, T.; Komorowski, R.; Yang, J.; Davda, J.; Nuanmanee, N.; Kemp, D.; et al. Long-acting MIC-1/GDF15 molecules to treat obesity: Evidence from mice to monkeys. *Sci. Transl. Med.* **2017**, *9*. [CrossRef]
39. Cardoso, A.L.; Fernandes, A.; Aguilar-Pimentel, J.A.; de Angelis, M.H.; Guedes, J.R.; Brito, M.A.; Ortolano, S.; Pani, G.; Athanasopoulou, S.; Gonos, E.S.; et al. Towards frailty biomarkers: Candidates from genes and pathways regulated in aging and age-related diseases. *Ageing Res. Rev.* **2018**, *47*, 214–277. [CrossRef] [PubMed]
40. Floyd, R.A.; Hensley, K. Oxidative stress in brain aging. Implications for therapeutics of neurodegenerative diseases. *Neurobiol. Aging* **2002**, *23*, 795–807. [CrossRef]
41. Bhat, R.; Crowe, E.P.; Bitto, A.; Moh, M.; Katsetos, C.D.; Garcia, F.U.; Johnson, F.B.; Trojanowski, J.Q.; Sell, C.; Torres, C. Astrocyte senescence as a component of Alzheimer's disease. *PLoS ONE* **2012**, *7*, e45069. [CrossRef] [PubMed]
42. Fulop, G.A.; Kiss, T.; Tarantini, S.; Balasubramanian, P.; Yabluchanskiy, A.; Farkas, E.; Bari, F.; Ungvari, Z.; Csiszar, A. Nrf2 deficiency in aged mice exacerbates cellular senescence promoting cerebrovascular inflammation. *Geroscience* **2018**, *40*, 513–521. [CrossRef]
43. Wilhelm, I.; Nyul-Toth, A.; Kozma, M.; Farkas, A.E.; Krizbai, I.A. Role of pattern recognition receptors of the neurovascular unit in inflamm-aging. *Am. J. Physiol. Heart Circ. Physiol* **2017**, *313*, H1000–H1012. [CrossRef] [PubMed]
44. Perry, V.H.; Teeling, J. Microglia and macrophages of the central nervous system: The contribution of microglia priming and systemic inflammation to chronic neurodegeneration. *Semin. Immunopathol.* **2013**, *35*, 601–612. [CrossRef]
45. Godbout, J.P.; Johnson, R.W. Age and neuroinflammation: A lifetime of psychoneuroimmune consequences. *Immunol. Allergy Clin. N. Am.* **2009**, *29*, 321–337. [CrossRef]
46. Norden, D.M.; Godbout, J.P. Review: Microglia of the aged brain: Primed to be activated and resistant to regulation. *Neuropathol. Appl. Neurobiol.* **2013**, *39*, 19–34. [CrossRef] [PubMed]

47. Nimmerjahn, A.; Kirchhoff, F.; Helmchen, F. Resting microglial cells are highly dynamic surveillants of brain parenchyma in vivo. *Science* **2005**, *308*, 1314–1318. [CrossRef] [PubMed]
48. Karperien, A.; Ahammer, H.; Jelinek, H.F. Quantitating the subtleties of microglial morphology with fractal analysis. *Front. Cell Neurosci.* **2013**, *7*, 3. [CrossRef]
49. Chae, J.H.; Miller, B.J. Beyond Urinary Tract Infections (UTIs) and Delirium: A Systematic Review of UTIs and Neuropsychiatric Disorders. *J. Psychiatr. Pract.* **2015**, *21*, 402–411. [CrossRef]
50. Godbout, J.P.; Chen, J.; Abraham, J.; Richwine, A.F.; Berg, B.M.; Kelley, K.W.; Johnson, R.W. Exaggerated neuroinflammation and sickness behavior in aged mice following activation of the peripheral innate immune system. *FASEB J.* **2005**, *19*, 1329–1331. [CrossRef]
51. Lu, Y.C.; Yeh, W.C.; Ohashi, P.S. LPS/TLR4 signal transduction pathway. *Cytokine* **2008**, *42*, 145–151. [CrossRef]
52. Erickson, M.A.; Banks, W.A. Cytokine and chemokine responses in serum and brain after single and repeated injections of lipopolysaccharide: Multiplex quantification with path analysis. *Brain Behav. Immun.* **2011**, *25*, 1637–1648. [CrossRef] [PubMed]
53. Henry, C.J.; Huang, Y.; Wynne, A.M.; Godbout, J.P. Peripheral lipopolysaccharide (LPS) challenge promotes microglial hyperactivity in aged mice that is associated with exaggerated induction of both pro-inflammatory IL-1beta and anti-inflammatory IL-10 cytokines. *Brain Behav. Immun.* **2009**, *23*, 309–317. [CrossRef] [PubMed]
54. Chen, J.; Buchanan, J.B.; Sparkman, N.L.; Godbout, J.P.; Freund, G.G.; Johnson, R.W. Neuroinflammation and disruption in working memory in aged mice after acute stimulation of the peripheral innate immune system. *Brain Behav. Immun.* **2008**, *22*, 301–311. [CrossRef] [PubMed]
55. Barrientos, R.M.; Higgins, E.A.; Biedenkapp, J.C.; Sprunger, D.B.; Wright-Hardesty, K.J.; Watkins, L.R.; Rudy, J.W.; Maier, S.F. Peripheral infection and aging interact to impair hippocampal memory consolidation. *Neurobiol. Aging* **2006**, *27*, 723–732. [CrossRef] [PubMed]
56. Godbout, J.P.; Moreau, M.; Lestage, J.; Chen, J.; Sparkman, N.L.; O'Connor, J.; Castanon, N.; Kelley, K.W.; Dantzer, R.; Johnson, R.W. Aging exacerbates depressive-like behavior in mice in response to activation of the peripheral innate immune system. *Neuropsychopharmacology* **2008**, *33*, 2341–2351. [CrossRef]
57. Erickson, M.A.; Banks, W.A. Blood-brain barrier dysfunction as a cause and consequence of Alzheimer's disease. *J. Cereb. Blood Flow Metab.* **2013**, *33*, 1500–1513. [CrossRef]
58. Luissint, A.C.; Artus, C.; Glacial, F.; Ganeshamoorthy, K.; Couraud, P.O. Tight junctions at the blood brain barrier: Physiological architecture and disease-associated dysregulation. *Fluids Barriers CNS* **2012**, *9*, 23. [CrossRef]
59. Tietz, S.; Engelhardt, B. Brain barriers: Crosstalk between complex tight junctions and adherens junctions. *J. Cell Biol.* **2015**, *209*, 493–506. [CrossRef] [PubMed]
60. Andreone, B.J.; Chow, B.W.; Tata, A.; Lacoste, B.; Ben-Zvi, A.; Bullock, K.; Deik, A.A.; Ginty, D.D.; Clish, C.B.; Gu, C. Blood-Brain Barrier Permeability Is Regulated by Lipid Transport-Dependent Suppression of Caveolae-Mediated Transcytosis. *Neuron* **2017**, *94*, 581–594.e5. [CrossRef]
61. Ben-Zvi, A.; Lacoste, B.; Kur, E.; Andreone, B.J.; Mayshar, Y.; Yan, H.; Gu, C. Mfsd2a is critical for the formation and function of the blood-brain barrier. *Nature* **2014**, *509*, 507–511. [CrossRef]
62. Begley, D.J. ABC transporters and the blood-brain barrier. *Curr. Pharm. Des.* **2004**, *10*, 1295–1312. [CrossRef] [PubMed]
63. Agundez, J.A.; Jimenez-Jimenez, F.J.; Alonso-Navarro, H.; Garcia-Martin, E. Drug and xenobiotic biotransformation in the blood-brain barrier: A neglected issue. *Front. Cell Neurosci.* **2014**, *8*, 335. [CrossRef] [PubMed]
64. Sweeney, M.D.; Ayyadurai, S.; Zlokovic, B.V. Pericytes of the neurovascular unit: Key functions and signaling pathways. *Nat. Neurosci.* **2016**, *19*, 771–783. [CrossRef] [PubMed]
65. Abbott, N.J.; Ronnback, L.; Hansson, E. Astrocyte-endothelial interactions at the blood-brain barrier. *Nat. Rev. Neurosci.* **2006**, *7*, 41–53. [CrossRef] [PubMed]
66. Johanson, C.E.; Stopa, E.G.; McMillan, P.N. The blood-cerebrospinal fluid barrier: Structure and functional significance. *Methods Mol. Biol.* **2011**, *686*, 101–131. [CrossRef]
67. Damkier, H.H.; Brown, P.D.; Praetorius, J. Cerebrospinal fluid secretion by the choroid plexus. *Physiol. Rev.* **2013**, *93*, 1847–1892. [CrossRef] [PubMed]
68. Engelhardt, B.; Ransohoff, R.M. The ins and outs of T-lymphocyte trafficking to the CNS: Anatomical sites and molecular mechanisms. *Trends Immunol.* **2005**, *26*, 485–495. [CrossRef] [PubMed]

69. Kivisakk, P.; Mahad, D.J.; Callahan, M.K.; Trebst, C.; Tucky, B.; Wei, T.; Wu, L.; Baekkevold, E.S.; Lassmann, H.; Staugaitis, S.M.; et al. Human cerebrospinal fluid central memory CD4+ T cells: Evidence for trafficking through choroid plexus and meninges via P-selectin. *Proc. Natl. Acad. Sci. USA* **2003**, *100*, 8389–8394. [CrossRef] [PubMed]
70. Llovera, G.; Benakis, C.; Enzmann, G.; Cai, R.; Arzberger, T.; Ghasemigharagoz, A.; Mao, X.; Malik, R.; Lazarevic, I.; Liebscher, S.; et al. The choroid plexus is a key cerebral invasion route for T cells after stroke. *Acta Neuropathol.* **2017**, *134*, 851–868. [CrossRef]
71. Daneman, R.; Zhou, L.; Agalliu, D.; Cahoy, J.D.; Kaushal, A.; Barres, B.A. The mouse blood-brain barrier transcriptome: A new resource for understanding the development and function of brain endothelial cells. *PLoS ONE* **2010**, *5*, e13741. [CrossRef]
72. Stamatovic, S.M.; Shakui, P.; Keep, R.F.; Moore, B.B.; Kunkel, S.L.; Van Rooijen, N.; Andjelkovic, A.V. Monocyte chemoattractant protein-1 regulation of blood-brain barrier permeability. *J. Cereb. Blood Flow Metab.* **2005**, *25*, 593–606. [CrossRef]
73. Higashida, T.; Kreipke, C.W.; Rafols, J.A.; Peng, C.; Schafer, S.; Schafer, P.; Ding, J.Y.; Dornbos, D.; LI, X.; Guthikonda, M.; et al. The role of hypoxia-inducible factor-1alpha, aquaporin-4, and matrix metalloproteinase-9 in blood-brain barrier disruption and brain edema after traumatic brain injury. *J. Neurosurg.* **2011**, *114*, 92–101. [CrossRef]
74. Bell, R.D.; Winkler, E.A.; Singh, I.; Sagare, A.P.; Deane, R.; Wu, Z.; Holtzman, D.M.; Betsholtz, C.; Armulik, A.; Sallstrom, J.; et al. Apolipoprotein E controls cerebrovascular integrity via cyclophilin A. *Nature* **2012**, *485*, 512–516. [CrossRef] [PubMed]
75. Persidsky, Y.; Dykstra, F.S.; Reichenbach, N.L.; Rom, S.; Rameriz, S.H. Activation of cannabinoid type two receptors (CB2) diminish inflammatory responses in macrophages and brain endothelium. *J. Neuroimmune Pharmacol.* **2015**, *10*, 302–308. [CrossRef]
76. Zhang, J.; Sadowska, G.B.; Chen, X.; Park, S.Y.; Kim, J.E.; Bodge, C.A.; Cummings, E.E.; Lim, Y.P.; Makeyev, O.; Besio, W.G.; et al. Anti-IL-6 neutralizing antibody modulates blood-brain barrier function in the ovine fetus. *FASEB J.* **2015**, *29*, 1739–1753. [CrossRef] [PubMed]
77. Papadopoulos, D.; Scheiner-Bobis, G. Dehydroepiandrosterone sulfate augments blood-brain barrier and tight junction protein expression in brain endothelial cells. *Biochim. Biophys. Acta Mol. Cell Res.* **2017**, *8*, 1382–1392. [CrossRef] [PubMed]
78. Ito, S.; Yanai, M.; Yamaguchi, S.; Couraud, P.O.; Ohtsuki, S. Regulation of tight-junction integrity by insulin in an in vitro model of human blood-brain barrier. *J. Pharm. Sci.* **2017**, *106*, 2599–2605. [CrossRef] [PubMed]
79. Megyeri, P.; Abraham, C.S.; Temesvari, P.; Kovacs, J.; Vas, T.; Speer, C.P. Recombinant human tumor necrosis factor alpha constricts pial arterioles and increases blood-brain barrier permeability in newborn piglets. *Neurosci. Lett.* **1992**, *148*, 137–140. [CrossRef]
80. Xaio, H.; Banks, W.A.; Niehoff, M.L.; Morley, J.E. Effect of LPS on the permeability of the blood-brain barrier to insulin. *Brain Res.* **2001**, *896*, 36–42. [CrossRef]
81. Dohgu, S.; Fleegal-DeMotta, M.A.; Banks, W.A. Lipopolysaccharide-enhanced transcellular transport of HIV-1 across the blood-brain barrier is mediated by luminal microvessel IL-6 and GM-CSF. *J. Neuroinflamm.* **2011**, *8*, 167. [CrossRef] [PubMed]
82. Banks, W.A.; Kastin, A.J.; Broadwell, R.D. Passage of cytokines across the blood-brain barrier. *Neuroimmunomodulation* **1995**, *2*, 241–248. [CrossRef]
83. Greenwood, J.; Heasman, S.J.; Alvarez, J.I.; Pratt, A.; Lyck, R.; Engelhardt, B. Review: Leukocyte-endothelial cell crosstalk at the blood-brain barrier: A prerequisite for successful immune cell entry to the brain. *Neuropathol. Appl. Neurobiol.* **2011**, *37*, 24–39. [CrossRef]
84. Warnke, C.; Menge, T.; Hartung, H.-P.; Racke, M.K.; Cravens, P.D.; Bennett, J.L.; Frohman, E.M.; Greenberg, B.M.; Zamvil, S.S.; Gold, R.; et al. Natalizumab and progressive mutifocal leukoencephalopathy. *JAMA Neurol.* **2010**, *67*, 923–930.
85. Engstrom, L.; Ruud, J.; Eskilsson, A.; Larsson, A.; Mackerlova, L.; Kugelberg, U.; Qian, H.; Vasilache, A.M.; Larsson, P.; Engblom, D.; et al. Lipopolysaccharide-induced fever depends on prostaglandin E2 production specifically in brain endothelial cells. *Endocrinology* **2012**, *153*, 4849–4861. [CrossRef]
86. Nilsson, A.; Wilhelms, D.B.; Mirrasekhian, E.; Jaarola, M.; Blomqvist, A.; Engblom, D. Inflammation-induced anorexia and fever are elicited by distinct prostaglandin dependent mechanisms, whereas conditioned taste aversion is prostaglandin independent. *Brain Behav. Immun.* **2017**, *61*, 236–243. [CrossRef]

87. Banks, W.A.; Kovac, A.; Morofuji, Y. Neurovascular unit crosstalk: Pericytes and astrocytes modify cytokine secretion patterns of brain endothelial cells. *J. Cereb. Blood Flow Metab.* **2017**, *38*, 1104–1118. [CrossRef] [PubMed]
88. Verma, S.; Nakaoke, R.; Dohgu, S.; Banks, W.A. Release of cytokines by brain endothelial cells: A polarized response to lipopolysaccharide. *Brain Behav. Immun.* **2006**, *20*, 449–455. [CrossRef]
89. Varatharaj, A.; Galea, I. The blood-brain barrier in systemic inflammation. *Brain Behav. Immun.* **2017**, *60*, 1–12. [CrossRef] [PubMed]
90. Farrall, A.J.; Wardlaw, J.M. Blood-brain barrier: Ageing and microvascular disease–systematic review and meta-analysis. *Neurobiol. Aging* **2009**, *30*, 337–352. [CrossRef]
91. Montagne, A.; Barnes, S.R.; Sweeney, M.D.; Halliday, M.R.; Sagare, A.P.; Zhao, Z.; Toga, A.W.; Jacobs, R.E.; Liu, C.Y.; Amezcua, L.; et al. Blood-brain barrier breakdown in the aging human hippocampus. *Neuron* **2015**, *85*, 296–302. [CrossRef] [PubMed]
92. Chen, R.L. Is it appropriate to use albumin CSF/plasma ratio to assess blood brain barrier permeability? *Neurobiol. Aging* **2011**, *32*, 1338–1339. [CrossRef] [PubMed]
93. Chen, R.L.; Kassem, N.A.; Redzic, Z.B.; Chen, C.P.; Segal, M.B.; Preston, J.E. Age-related changes in choroid plexus and blood-cerebrospinal fluid barrier function in the sheep. *Exp. Gerontol.* **2009**, *44*, 289–296. [CrossRef]
94. Chen, R.L.; Athauda, S.B.; Kassem, N.A.; Zhang, Y.; Segal, M.B.; Preston, J.E. Decrease of transthyretin synthesis at the blood-cerebrospinal fluid barrier of old sheep. *J. Gerontol. A Biol. Sci. Med. Sci.* **2005**, *60*, 852–858. [CrossRef]
95. Elahy, M.; Jackaman, C.; Mamo, J.C.; Lam, V.; Dhaliwal, S.S.; Giles, C.; Nelson, D.; Takechi, R. Blood-brain barrier dysfunction developed during normal aging is associated with inflammation and loss of tight junctions but not with leukocyte recruitment. *Immun. Ageing* **2015**, *12*, 2. [CrossRef]
96. Stamatovic, S.M.; Martinez-Revollar, G.; Hu, A.; Choi, J.; Keep, R.F.; Andjelkovic, A.V. Decline in Sirtuin-1 expression and activity plays a critical role in blood-brain barrier permeability in aging. *Neurobiol. Dis.* **2018**. [CrossRef] [PubMed]
97. Rahman, S.; Islam, R. Mammalian Sirt1: Insights on its biological functions. *Cell Commun. Signal.* **2011**, *9*, 11. [CrossRef] [PubMed]
98. Doolittle, N.D.; Muldoon, L.L.; Culp, A.Y.; Neuwelt, E.A. Delivery of chemotherapeutics across the blood-brain barrier: Challenges and advances. *Adv. Pharmacol.* **2014**, *71*, 203–243. [CrossRef] [PubMed]
99. Lipsman, N.; Meng, Y.; Bethune, A.J.; Huang, Y.; Lam, B.; Masellis, M.; Herrmann, N.; Heyn, C.; Aubert, I.; Boutet, A.; et al. Blood-brain barrier opening in Alzheimer's disease using MR-guided focused ultrasound. *Nat. Commun.* **2018**, *9*, 2336. [CrossRef] [PubMed]
100. Salahuddin, T.S.; Johansson, B.B.; Kalimo, H.; Olsson, Y. Structural changes in the rat brain after carotid infusions of hyperosmolar solutions: A light microscopic and immunohistochemical study. *Neuropathol. Appl. Neurobiol.* **1988**, *14*, 467–482. [CrossRef]
101. Salahuddin, T.S.; Kalimo, H.; Johansson, B.B.; Olsson, Y. Observations on exsudation of fibronectin, fibrinogen and albumin in the brain after carotid infusion of hyperosmolar solutions. An immunohistochemical study in the rat indicating longlasting changes in the brain microenvironment and multifocal nerve cell injuries. *Acta Neuropathol.* **1988**, *76*, 1–10.
102. Merlini, M.; Rafalski, V.A.; Rios Coronado, P.E.; Gill, T.M.; Ellisman, M.; Muthukumar, G.; Subramanian, K.S.; Ryu, J.K.; Syme, C.A.; Davalos, D.; et al. Fibrinogen Induces Microglia-Mediated Spine Elimination and Cognitive Impairment in an Alzheimer's Disease Model. *Neuron* **2019**. [CrossRef] [PubMed]
103. Patching, S.G. Glucose Transporters at the Blood-Brain Barrier: Function, Regulation and Gateways for Drug Delivery. *Mol. Neurobiol.* **2017**, *54*, 1046–1077. [CrossRef]
104. Sweeney, M.D.; Montagne, A.; Sagare, A.P.; Nation, D.A.; Schneider, L.S.; Chui, H.C.; Harrington, M.G.; Pa, J.; Law, M.; Wang, D.J.J.; et al. Vascular dysfunction-The disregarded partner of Alzheimer's disease. *Alzheimers Dement.* **2019**, *15*, 158–167. [CrossRef] [PubMed]
105. Bonte, S.; Vandemaele, P.; Verleden, S.; Audenaert, K.; Deblaere, K.; Goethals, I.; Van Holen, R. Healthy brain ageing assessed with 18F-FDG PET and age-dependent recovery factors after partial volume effect correction. *Eur. J. Nucl. Med. Mol. Imaging* **2017**, *44*, 838–849. [CrossRef]

106. Jiang, T.; Yin, F.; Yao, J.; Brinton, R.D.; Cadenas, E. Lipoic acid restores age-associated impairment of brain energy metabolism through the modulation of Akt/JNK signaling and PGC1alpha transcriptional pathway. *Aging Cell* **2013**, *12*, 1021–1031. [CrossRef] [PubMed]
107. Gage, F.H.; Kelly, P.A.; Bjorklund, A. Regional changes in brain glucose metabolism reflect cognitive impairments in aged rats. *J. Neurosci.* **1984**, *4*, 2856–2865. [CrossRef] [PubMed]
108. Ding, F.; Yao, J.; Rettberg, J.R.; Chen, S.; Brinton, R.D. Early decline in glucose transport and metabolism precedes shift to ketogenic system in female aging and Alzheimer's mouse brain: Implication for bioenergetic intervention. *PLoS ONE* **2013**, *8*, e79977. [CrossRef]
109. Selkoe, D.J.; Hardy, J. The amyloid hypothesis of Alzheimer's disease at 25 years. *EMBO Mol. Med.* **2016**, *8*, 595–608. [CrossRef]
110. Shibata, M.; Yamada, S.; Kumar, S.R.; Calero, M.; Bading, J.; Frangione, B.; Holtzman, D.M.; Miller, C.A.; Strickland, D.K.; Ghiso, J.; et al. Clearance of Alzheimer's amyloid-ss(1-40) peptide from brain by LDL receptor-related protein-1 at the blood-brain barrier. *J. Clin. Investig.* **2000**, *106*, 1489–1499. [CrossRef] [PubMed]
111. Storck, S.E.; Hartz, A.M.S.; Bernard, J.; Wolf, A.; Kachlmeier, A.; Mahringer, A.; Weggen, S.; Pahnke, J.; Pietrzik, C.U. The concerted amyloid-beta clearance of LRP1 and ABCB1/P-gp across the blood-brain barrier is linked by PICALM. *Brain Behav. Immun.* **2018**, *73*, 21–33. [CrossRef] [PubMed]
112. Hartz, A.M.; Miller, D.S.; Bauer, B. Restoring blood-brain barrier P-glycoprotein reduces brain amyloid-beta in a mouse model of Alzheimer's disease. *Mol. Pharmacol.* **2010**, *77*, 715–723. [CrossRef] [PubMed]
113. Ramanathan, A.; Nelson, A.R.; Sagare, A.P.; Zlokovic, B.V. Impaired vascular-mediated clearance of brain amyloid beta in Alzheimer's disease: The role, regulation and restoration of LRP1. *Front. Aging Neurosci.* **2015**, *7*, 136. [CrossRef]
114. Toornvliet, R.; van Berckel, B.N.; Luurtsema, G.; Lubberink, M.; Geldof, A.A.; Bosch, T.M.; Oerlemans, R.; Lammertsma, A.A.; Franssen, E.J. Effect of age on functional P-glycoprotein in the blood-brain barrier measured by use of (R)-[(11)C]verapamil and positron emission tomography. *Clin. Pharmacol. Ther.* **2006**, *79*, 540–548. [CrossRef]
115. van Assema, D.M.; Lubberink, M.; Boellaard, R.; Schuit, R.C.; Windhorst, A.D.; Scheltens, P.; Lammertsma, A.A.; van Berckel, B.N. P-glycoprotein function at the blood-brain barrier: Effects of age and gender. *Mol. Imaging Biol.* **2012**, *14*, 771–776. [CrossRef] [PubMed]
116. Chiu, C.; Miller, M.C.; Monahan, R.; Osgood, D.P.; Stopa, E.G.; Silverberg, G.D. P-glycoprotein expression and amyloid accumulation in human aging and Alzheimer's disease: Preliminary observations. *Neurobiol. Aging* **2015**, *36*, 2475–2482. [CrossRef]
117. Hoffman, J.D.; Parikh, I.; Green, S.J.; Chlipala, G.; Mohney, R.P.; Keaton, M.; Bauer, B.; Hartz, A.M.S.; Lin, A.L. Age Drives Distortion of Brain Metabolic, Vascular and Cognitive Functions, and the Gut Microbiome. *Front. Aging Neurosci.* **2017**, *9*, 298. [CrossRef]
118. Jaeger, L.B.; Dohgu, S.; Sultana, R.; Lynch, J.L.; Owen, J.B.; Erickson, M.A.; Shah, G.N.; Price, T.O.; Fleegal-Demotta, M.A.; Butterfield, D.A.; et al. Lipopolysaccharide alters the blood-brain barrier transport of amyloid beta protein: A mechanism for inflammation in the progression of Alzheimer's disease. *Brain Behav. Immun.* **2009**, *23*, 507–517. [CrossRef] [PubMed]
119. Banks, W.A.; Owen, J.B.; Erickson, M.A. Insulin in the brain: There and back again. *Pharmacol. Ther.* **2012**, *136*, 82–93. [CrossRef] [PubMed]
120. Duffy, K.R.; Pardridge, W.M. Blood-brain barrier transcytosis of insulin in developing rabbits. *Brain Res.* **1987**, *420*, 32–38. [CrossRef]
121. Banks, W.A.; Jaspan, J.B.; Huang, W.; Kastin, A.J. Transport of insulin across the blood-brain barrier: Saturability at euglycemic doses of insulin. *Peptides* **1997**, *18*, 1423–1429. [CrossRef]
122. Baura, G.D.; Foster, D.M.; Porte, D., Jr.; Kahn, S.E.; Bergman, R.N.; Cobelli, C.; Schwartz, M.W. Saturable transport of insulin from plasma into the central nervous system of dogs in vivo. A mechanism for regulated insulin delivery to the brain. *J. Clin. Investig.* **1993**, *92*, 1824–1830. [CrossRef] [PubMed]
123. Sartorius, T.; Peter, A.; Heni, M.; Maetzler, W.; Fritsche, A.; Haring, H.U.; Hennige, A.M. The brain response to peripheral insulin declines with age: A contribution of the blood-brain barrier? *PLoS ONE* **2015**, *10*, e0126804. [CrossRef] [PubMed]

124. Frolich, L.; Blum-Degen, D.; Bernstein, H.G.; Engelsberger, S.; Humrich, J.; Laufer, S.; Muschner, D.; Thalheimer, A.; Turk, A.; Hoyer, S.; et al. Brain insulin and insulin receptors in aging and sporadic Alzheimer's disease. *J. Neural. Transm (Vienna)* **1998**, *105*, 423–438. [CrossRef] [PubMed]
125. Banks, W.A.; Farr, S.A.; Morley, J.E. Permeability of the blood-brain barrier to albumin and insulin in the young and aged SAMP8 mouse. *J. Gerontol. A Biol. Sci. Med. Sci.* **2000**, *55*, B601–B606. [CrossRef] [PubMed]
126. Yates, D. Brain ageing: Blood-derived rejuvenation. *Nat. Rev. Neurosci.* **2014**, *15*, 352–353. [CrossRef] [PubMed]
127. Poggioli, T.; Vujic, A.; Yang, P.; Macias-Trevino, C.; Uygur, A.; Loffredo, F.S.; Pancoast, J.R.; Cho, M.; Goldstein, J.; Tandias, R.M.; et al. Circulating Growth Differentiation Factor 11/8 Levels Decline With Age. *Circ. Res.* **2016**, *118*, 29–37. [CrossRef]
128. Katsimpardi, L.; Litterman, N.K.; Schein, P.A.; Miller, C.M.; Loffredo, F.S.; Wojtkiewicz, G.R.; Chen, J.W.; Lee, R.T.; Wagers, A.J.; Rubin, L.L. Vascular and neurogenic rejuvenation of the aging mouse brain by young systemic factors. *Science* **2014**, *344*, 630–634. [CrossRef]
129. Erickson, M.A.; Morofuji, Y.; Owen, J.B.; Banks, W.A. Rapid transport of CCL11 across the blood-brain barrier: Regional variation and importance of blood cells. *J. Pharmacol. Exp. Ther.* **2014**, *349*, 497–507. [CrossRef]
130. Park, M.H.; Lee, J.Y.; Park, K.H.; Jung, I.K.; Kim, K.T.; Lee, Y.S.; Ryu, H.H.; Jeong, Y.; Kang, M.; Schwaninger, M.; et al. Vascular and Neurogenic Rejuvenation in Aging Mice by Modulation of ASM. *Neuron* **2018**, *100*, 167–182. [CrossRef] [PubMed]
131. Li, C.; Wang, A.; Wu, Y.; Gulbins, E.; Grassme, H.; Zhao, Z. Acid Sphingomyelinase-Ceramide System in Bacterial Infections. *Cell Physiol. Biochem.* **2019**, *52*, 280–301. [CrossRef]
132. Ransohoff, R.M.; Engelhardt, B. The anatomical and cellular basis of immune surveillance in the central nervous system. *Nat. Rev. Immunol.* **2012**, *12*, 623–635. [CrossRef] [PubMed]
133. Baruch, K.; Schwartz, M. CNS-specific T cells shape brain function via the choroid plexus. *Brain Behav. Immun.* **2013**, *34*, 11–16. [CrossRef] [PubMed]
134. Baruch, K.; Deczkowska, A.; David, E.; Castellano, J.M.; Miller, O.; Kertser, A.; Berkutzki, T.; Barnett-Itzhaki, Z.; Bezalel, D.; Wyss-Coray, T.; et al. Aging. Aging-induced type I interferon response at the choroid plexus negatively affects brain function. *Science* **2014**, *346*, 89–93. [CrossRef] [PubMed]
135. Kuro-o, M. Klotho and aging. *Biochim. Biophys. Acta* **2009**, *1790*, 1049–1058. [CrossRef] [PubMed]
136. Kuro-o, M.; Matsumura, Y.; Aizawa, H.; Kawaguchi, H.; Suga, T.; Utsugi, T.; Ohyama, Y.; Kurabayashi, M.; Kaname, T.; Kume, E.; et al. Mutation of the mouse klotho gene leads to a syndrome resembling ageing. *Nature* **1997**, *390*, 45–51. [CrossRef] [PubMed]
137. Zhu, L.; Stein, L.R.; Kim, D.; Ho, K.; Yu, G.Q.; Zhan, L.; Larsson, T.E.; Mucke, L. Klotho controls the brain-immune system interface in the choroid plexus. *Proc. Natl. Acad. Sci. USA* **2018**, *115*, E11388–E11396. [CrossRef] [PubMed]
138. Schwartz, M.; Baruch, K. Breaking peripheral immune tolerance to CNS antigens in neurodegenerative diseases: Boosting autoimmunity to fight-off chronic neuroinflammation. *J. Autoimmun.* **2014**, *54*, 8–14. [CrossRef]
139. Stichel, C.C.; Luebbert, H. Inflammatory processes in the aging mouse brain: Participation of dendritic cells and T-cells. *Neurobiol. Aging* **2007**, *28*, 1507–1521. [CrossRef]
140. Ritzel, R.M.; Crapser, J.; Patel, A.R.; Verma, R.; Grenier, J.M.; Chauhan, A.; Jellison, E.R.; McCullough, L.D. Age-Associated Resident Memory CD8 T Cells in the Central Nervous System Are Primed to Potentiate Inflammation after Ischemic Brain Injury. *J. Immunol.* **2016**, *196*, 3318–3330. [CrossRef]
141. Erickson, M.A.; Liang, W.S.; Fernandez, E.G.; Bullock, K.M.; Thysell, J.A.; Banks, W.A. Genetics and sex influence peripheral and central innate immune responses and blood-brain barrier integrity. *PLoS ONE* **2018**, *13*, e0205769. [CrossRef] [PubMed]
142. Banks, W.A.; Gray, A.M.; Erickson, M.A.; Salameh, T.S.; Damodarasamy, M.; Sheibani, N.; Meabon, J.S.; Wing, E.E.; Morofuji, Y.; Cook, D.G.; et al. Lipopolysaccharide-induced blood-brain barrier disruption: Roles of cyclooxygenase, oxidative stress, neuroinflammation, and elements of the neurovascular unit. *J. Neuroinflamm.* **2015**, *12*, 223. [CrossRef] [PubMed]
143. Elwood, E.; Lim, Z.; Naveed, H.; Galea, I. The effect of systemic inflammation on human brain barrier function. *Brain Behav. Immun.* **2017**, *62*, 35–40. [CrossRef] [PubMed]
144. Ching, S.; Zhang, H.; Lai, W.; Quan, N. Peripheral injection of lipopolysaccharide prevents brain recruitment of leukocytes induced by central injection of interleukin-1. *Neuroscience* **2006**, *137*, 717–726. [CrossRef]

145. Sumbria, R.K.; Grigoryan, M.M.; Vasilevko, V.; Paganini-Hill, A.; Kilday, K.; Kim, R.; Cribbs, D.H.; Fisher, M.J. Aging exacerbates development of cerebral microbleeds in a mouse model. *J. Neuroinflamm.* **2018**, *15*, 69. [CrossRef]
146. Opp, M.R.; George, A.; Ringgold, K.M.; Hansen, K.M.; Bullock, K.M.; Banks, W.A. Sleep fragmentation and sepsis differentially impact blood-brain barrier integrity and transport of tumor necrosis factor-alpha in aging. *Brain Behav. Immun.* **2015**, *50*, 259–265. [CrossRef]
147. Gutierrez, E.G.; Banks, W.A.; Kastin, A.J. Murine tumor necrosis factor alpha is transported from blood to brain in the mouse. *J. Neuroimmunol* **1993**, *47*, 169–176. [CrossRef]
148. Logsdon, A.F.; Erickson, M.A.; Rhea, E.M.; Salameh, T.S.; Banks, W.A. Gut reactions: How the blood-brain barrier connects the microbiome and the brain. *Exp. Biol. Med. (Maywood)* **2018**, *243*, 159–165. [CrossRef] [PubMed]
149. Braniste, V.; Al-Asmakh, M.; Kowal, C.; Anuar, F.; Abbaspour, A.; Toth, M.; Korecka, A.; Bakocevic, N.; Ng, L.G.; Kundu, P.; et al. The gut microbiota influences blood-brain barrier permeability in mice. *Sci. Transl. Med.* **2014**, *6*, 263ra158. [CrossRef]
150. Hippe, B.; Zwielehner, J.; Liszt, K.; Lassl, C.; Unger, F.; Haslberger, A.G. Quantification of butyryl CoA:acetate CoA-transferase genes reveals different butyrate production capacity in individuals according to diet and age. *FEMS Microbiol. Lett.* **2011**, *316*, 130–135. [CrossRef] [PubMed]
151. Scott, K.A.; Ida, M.; Peterson, V.L.; Prenderville, J.A.; Moloney, G.M.; Izumo, T.; Murphy, K.; Murphy, A.; Ross, R.P.; Stanton, C.; et al. Revisiting Metchnikoff: Age-related alterations in microbiota-gut-brain axis in the mouse. *Brain Behav. Immun.* **2017**, *65*, 20–32. [CrossRef] [PubMed]
152. Gorle, N.; Blaecher, C.; Bauwens, E.; Vandendriessche, C.; Balusu, S.; Vandewalle, J.; Van Cauwenberghe, C.; Van Wonterghem, E.; Van Imschoot, G.; Liu, C.; et al. The choroid plexus epithelium as a novel player in the stomach-brain axis during Helicobacter infection. *Brain Behav. Immun.* **2018**, *69*, 35–47. [CrossRef] [PubMed]
153. Dinan, T.G.; Cryan, J.F. The Microbiome-Gut-Brain Axis in Health and Disease. *Gastroenterol. Clin. N. Am.* **2017**, *46*, 77–89. [CrossRef] [PubMed]
154. Dore-Duffy, P. Pericytes: Pluripotent cells of the blood brain barrier. *Curr. Pharm. Des.* **2008**, *14*, 1581–1593. [CrossRef]
155. Winkler, E.A.; Sagare, A.P.; Zlokovic, B.V. The pericyte: A forgotten cell type with important implications for Alzheimer's disease? *Brain Pathol.* **2014**, *24*, 371–386. [CrossRef] [PubMed]
156. Bell, R.D.; Winkler, E.A.; Sagare, A.P.; Singh, I.; LaRue, B.; Deane, R.; Zlokovic, B.V. Pericytes control key neurovascular functions and neuronal phenotype in the adult brain and during brain aging. *Neuron* **2010**, *68*, 409–427. [CrossRef]
157. Duncombe, J.; Lennen, R.J.; Jansen, M.A.; Marshall, I.; Wardlaw, J.M.; Horsburgh, K. Ageing causes prominent neurovascular dysfunction associated with loss of astrocytic contacts and gliosis. *Neuropathol. Appl. Neurobiol.* **2017**, *43*, 477–491. [CrossRef]
158. Goodall, E.F.; Wang, C.; Simpson, J.E.; Baker, D.J.; Drew, D.R.; Heath, P.R.; Saffrey, M.J.; Romero, I.A.; Wharton, S.B. Age-associated changes in the blood-brain barrier: Comparative studies in human and mouse. *Neuropathol. Appl. Neurobiol.* **2018**, *44*, 328–340. [CrossRef]
159. Erdo, F.; Denes, L.; de Lange, E. Age-associated physiological and pathological changes at the blood-brain barrier: A review. *J. Cereb. Blood Flow Metab.* **2017**, *37*, 4–24. [CrossRef]
160. Pieper, C.; Marek, J.J.; Unterberg, M.; Schwerdtle, T.; Galla, H.J. Brain capillary pericytes contribute to the immune defense in response to cytokines or LPS in vitro. *Brain Res.* **2014**, *1550*, 1–8. [CrossRef] [PubMed]
161. Sagare, A.P.; Sweeney, M.D.; Makshanoff, J.; Zlokovic, B.V. Shedding of soluble platelet-derived growth factor receptor-beta from human brain pericytes. *Neurosci. Lett.* **2015**, *607*, 97–101. [CrossRef] [PubMed]
162. Nation, D.A.; Sweeney, M.D.; Montagne, A.; Sagare, A.P.; D'Orazio, L.M.; Pachicano, M.; Sepehrband, F.; Nelson, A.R.; Buennagel, D.P.; Harrington, M.G.; et al. Blood-brain barrier breakdown is an early biomarker of human cognitive dysfunction. *Nat. Med.* **2019**, *25*, 270–276. [CrossRef]
163. Middeldorp, J.; Hol, E.M. GFAP in health and disease. *Prog. Neurobiol.* **2011**, *93*, 421–443. [CrossRef] [PubMed]
164. Iliff, J.J.; Wang, M.; Liao, Y.; Plogg, B.A.; Peng, W.; Gundersen, G.A.; Benveniste, H.; Vates, G.E.; Deane, R.; Goldman, S.A.; et al. A paravascular pathway facilitates CSF flow through the brain parenchyma and the clearance of interstitial solutes, including amyloid beta. *Sci. Transl. Med.* **2012**, *4*, 147ra111. [CrossRef]

165. Zenaro, E.; Piacentino, G.; Constantin, G. The blood-brain barrier in Alzheimer's disease. *Neurobiol. Dis.* **2017**, *107*, 41–56. [CrossRef] [PubMed]
166. Jack, C.R., Jr.; Bennett, D.A.; Blennow, K.; Carrillo, M.C.; Dunn, B.; Haeberlein, S.B.; Holtzman, D.M.; Jagust, W.; Jessen, F.; Karlawish, J.; et al. NIA-AA Research Framework: Toward a biological definition of Alzheimer's disease. *Alzheimers Dement.* **2018**, *14*, 535–562. [CrossRef] [PubMed]
167. Jack, C.R., Jr.; Knopman, D.S.; Jagust, W.J.; Petersen, R.C.; Weiner, M.W.; Aisen, P.S.; Shaw, L.M.; Vemuri, P.; Wiste, H.J.; Weigand, S.D.; et al. Tracking pathophysiological processes in Alzheimer's disease: An updated hypothetical model of dynamic biomarkers. *Lancet Neurol.* **2013**, *12*, 207–216. [CrossRef]
168. Castellano, J.M.; Kim, J.; Stewart, F.R.; Jiang, H.; DeMattos, R.B.; Patterson, B.W.; Fagan, A.M.; Morris, J.C.; Mawuenyega, K.G.; Cruchaga, C.; et al. Human apoE isoforms differentially regulate brain amyloid-beta peptide clearance. *Sci. Transl. Med.* **2011**, *3*, 89ra57. [CrossRef] [PubMed]
169. Shi, Y.; Yamada, K.; Liddelow, S.A.; Smith, S.T.; Zhao, L.; Luo, W.; Tsai, R.M.; Spina, S.; Grinberg, L.T.; Rojas, J.C.; et al. ApoE4 markedly exacerbates tau-mediated neurodegeneration in a mouse model of tauopathy. *Nature* **2017**, *549*, 523–527. [CrossRef] [PubMed]
170. Tai, L.M.; Ghura, S.; Koster, K.P.; Liakaite, V.; Maienschein-Cline, M.; Kanabar, P.; Collins, N.; Ben-Aissa, M.; Lei, A.Z.; Bahroos, N.; et al. APOE-modulated Abeta-induced neuroinflammation in Alzheimer's disease: Current landscape, novel data, and future perspective. *J. Neurochem.* **2015**, *133*, 465–488. [CrossRef]
171. Halliday, M.R.; Rege, S.V.; Ma, Q.; Zhao, Z.; Miller, C.A.; Winkler, E.A.; Zlokovic, B.V. Accelerated pericyte degeneration and blood-brain barrier breakdown in apolipoprotein E4 carriers with Alzheimer's disease. *J. Cereb. Blood Flow Metab.* **2016**, *36*, 216–227. [CrossRef]
172. Fulop, T.; Witkowski, J.M.; Bourgade, K.; Khalil, A.; Zerif, E.; Larbi, A.; Hirokawa, K.; Pawelec, G.; Bocti, C.; Lacombe, G.; et al. Can an Infection Hypothesis Explain the Beta Amyloid Hypothesis of Alzheimer's Disease? *Front. Aging Neurosci.* **2018**, *10*, 224. [CrossRef]
173. Itzhaki, R.F.; Lathe, R.; Balin, B.J.; Ball, M.J.; Bearer, E.L.; Braak, H.; Bullido, M.J.; Carter, C.; Clerici, M.; Cosby, S.L.; et al. Microbes and Alzheimer's Disease. *J. Alzheimers Dis.* **2016**, *51*, 979–984. [CrossRef] [PubMed]
174. Deatly, A.M.; Haase, A.T.; Fewster, P.H.; Lewis, E.; Ball, M.J. Human herpes virus infections and Alzheimer's disease. *Neuropathol. Appl. Neurobiol.* **1990**, *16*, 213–223. [CrossRef]
175. Ball, M.J.; Lewis, E.; Haase, A.T. Detection of herpes virus genome in Alzheimer's disease by in situ hybridization: A preliminary study. *J. Neural. Transm. Suppl.* **1987**, *24*, 219–225.
176. Walker, D.G.; O'Kusky, J.R.; McGeer, P.L. In situ hybridization analysis for herpes simplex virus nucleic acids in Alzheimer disease. *Alzheimer Dis. Assoc. Disord.* **1989**, *3*, 123–131. [CrossRef] [PubMed]
177. Wozniak, M.A.; Itzhaki, R.F.; Shipley, S.J.; Dobson, C.B. Herpes simplex virus infection causes cellular beta-amyloid accumulation and secretase upregulation. *Neurosci. Lett.* **2007**, *429*, 95–100. [CrossRef]
178. Zambrano, A.; Solis, L.; Salvadores, N.; Cortes, M.; Lerchundi, R.; Otth, C. Neuronal cytoskeletal dynamic modification and neurodegeneration induced by infection with herpes simplex virus type 1. *J. Alzheimers Dis.* **2008**, *14*, 259–269. [CrossRef]
179. Eimer, W.A.; Vijaya Kumar, D.K.; Navalpur Shanmugam, N.K.; Rodriguez, A.S.; Mitchell, T.; Washicosky, K.J.; Gyorgy, B.; Breakefield, X.O.; Tanzi, R.E.; Moir, R.D. Alzheimer's Disease-Associated beta-Amyloid Is Rapidly Seeded by Herpesviridae to Protect against Brain Infection. *Neuron* **2018**, *99*, 56–63. [CrossRef] [PubMed]
180. Kumar, D.K.; Choi, S.H.; Washicosky, K.J.; Eimer, W.A.; Tucker, S.; Ghofrani, J.; Lefkowitz, A.; McColl, G.; Goldstein, L.E.; Tanzi, R.E.; et al. Amyloid-beta peptide protects against microbial infection in mouse and worm models of Alzheimer's disease. *Sci. Transl. Med.* **2016**, *8*, 340ra372. [CrossRef]
181. Readhead, B.; Haure-Mirande, J.V.; Funk, C.C.; Richards, M.A.; Shannon, P.; Haroutunian, V.; Sano, M.; Liang, W.S.; Beckmann, N.D.; Price, N.D.; et al. Multiscale Analysis of Independent Alzheimer's Cohorts Finds Disruption of Molecular, Genetic, and Clinical Networks by Human Herpesvirus. *Neuron* **2018**, *99*, 64–82. [CrossRef] [PubMed]
182. Wozniak, M.A.; Mee, A.P.; Itzhaki, R.F. Herpes simplex virus type 1 DNA is located within Alzheimer's disease amyloid plaques. *J. Pathol.* **2009**, *217*, 131–138. [CrossRef]
183. Tsai, M.C.; Cheng, W.L.; Sheu, J.J.; Huang, C.C.; Shia, B.C.; Kao, L.T.; Lin, H.C. Increased risk of dementia following herpes zoster ophthalmicus. *PLoS ONE* **2017**, *12*, e0188490. [CrossRef]

184. Chen, V.C.; Wu, S.I.; Huang, K.Y.; Yang, Y.H.; Kuo, T.Y.; Liang, H.Y.; Huang, K.L.; Gossop, M. Herpes Zoster and Dementia: A Nationwide Population-Based Cohort Study. *J. Clin. Psychiatry* **2018**, *79*. [CrossRef] [PubMed]
185. Tzeng, N.S.; Chung, C.H.; Lin, F.H.; Chiang, C.P.; Yeh, C.B.; Huang, S.Y.; Lu, R.B.; Chang, H.A.; Kao, Y.C.; Yeh, H.W.; et al. Anti-herpetic Medications and Reduced Risk of Dementia in Patients with Herpes Simplex Virus Infections-a Nationwide, Population-Based Cohort Study in Taiwan. *Neurotherapeutics* **2018**, *15*, 417–429. [CrossRef] [PubMed]
186. Elder, G.A.; Gama Sosa, M.A.; De Gasperi, R. Transgenic mouse models of Alzheimer's disease. *Mt. Sinai. J. Med.* **2010**, *77*, 69–81. [CrossRef] [PubMed]
187. Banks, W.A.; Robinson, S.M.; Verma, S.; Morley, J.E. Efflux of human and mouse amyloid beta proteins 1-40 and 1-42 from brain: Impairment in a mouse model of Alzheimer's disease. *Neuroscience* **2003**, *121*, 487–492. [CrossRef]
188. Kumar, V.B.; Farr, S.A.; Flood, J.F.; Kamlesh, V.; Franko, M.; Banks, W.A.; Morley, J.E. Site-directed antisense oligonucleotide decreases the expression of amyloid precursor protein and reverses deficits in learning and memory in aged SAMP8 mice. *Peptides* **2000**, *21*, 1769–1775. [CrossRef]
189. Bien-Ly, N.; Boswell, C.A.; Jeet, S.; Beach, T.G.; Hoyte, K.; Luk, W.; Shihadeh, V.; Ulufatu, S.; Foreman, O.; Lu, Y.; et al. Lack of Widespread BBB Disruption in Alzheimer's Disease Models: Focus on Therapeutic Antibodies. *Neuron* **2015**, *88*, 289–297. [CrossRef]
190. Gustafsson, S.; Gustavsson, T.; Roshanbin, S.; Hultqvist, G.; Hammarlund-Udenaes, M.; Sehlin, D.; Syvanen, S. Blood-brain barrier integrity in a mouse model of Alzheimer's disease with or without acute 3D6 immunotherapy. *Neuropharmacology* **2018**, *143*, 1–9. [CrossRef] [PubMed]
191. Dickstein, D.L.; Biron, K.E.; Ujiie, M.; Pfeifer, C.G.; Jeffries, A.R.; Jefferies, W.A. Abeta peptide immunization restores blood-brain barrier integrity in Alzheimer disease. *FASEB J.* **2006**, *20*, 426–433. [CrossRef]
192. Montagne, A.; Zhao, Z.; Zlokovic, B.V. Alzheimer's disease: A matter of blood-brain barrier dysfunction? *J. Exp. Med.* **2017**, *214*, 3151–3169. [CrossRef] [PubMed]
193. Kovac, A.; Zilkova, M.; Deli, M.A.; Zilka, N.; Novak, M. Human truncated tau is using a different mechanism from amyloid-beta to damage the blood-brain barrier. *J. Alzheimers Dis.* **2009**, *18*, 897–906. [CrossRef] [PubMed]
194. Blair, L.J.; Frauen, H.D.; Zhang, B.; Nordhues, B.A.; Bijan, S.; Lin, Y.C.; Zamudio, F.; Hernandez, L.D.; Sabbagh, J.J.; Selenica, M.L.; et al. Tau depletion prevents progressive blood-brain barrier damage in a mouse model of tauopathy. *Acta Neuropathol. Commun.* **2015**, *3*, 8. [CrossRef] [PubMed]
195. Banks, W.A.; Kovac, A.; Majerova, P.; Bullock, K.M.; Shi, M.; Zhang, J. Tau Proteins Cross the Blood-Brain Barrier. *J. Alzheimers Dis.* **2017**, *55*, 411–419. [CrossRef] [PubMed]
196. Fiske, A.; Wetherell, J.L.; Gatz, M. Depression in older adults. *Annu. Rev. Clin. Psychol.* **2009**, *5*, 363–389. [CrossRef]
197. Seligman, F.; Nemeroff, C.B. The interface of depression and cardiovascular disease: Therapeutic implications. *Ann. N. Y. Acad. Sci.* **2015**, *1345*, 25–35. [CrossRef]
198. Chamberlain, S.R.; Cavanagh, J.; de Boer, P.; Mondelli, V.; Jones, D.N.C.; Drevets, W.C.; Cowen, P.J.; Harrison, N.A.; Pointon, L.; Pariante, C.M.; et al. Treatment-resistant depression and peripheral C-reactive protein. *Br. J. Psychiatry* **2019**, *214*, 11–19. [CrossRef]
199. Hodes, G.E.; Kana, V.; Menard, C.; Merad, M.; Russo, S.J. Neuroimmune mechanisms of depression. *Nat. Neurosci.* **2015**, *18*, 1386–1393. [CrossRef]
200. Menard, C.; Pfau, M.L.; Hodes, G.E.; Kana, V.; Wang, V.X.; Bouchard, S.; Takahashi, A.; Flanigan, M.E.; Aleyasin, H.; LeClair, K.B.; et al. Social stress induces neurovascular pathology promoting depression. *Nat. Neurosci.* **2017**, *20*, 1752–1760. [CrossRef] [PubMed]
201. Kinsey, S.G.; Bailey, M.T.; Sheridan, J.F.; Padgett, D.A. The inflammatory response to social defeat is increased in older mice. *Physiol. Behav.* **2008**, *93*, 628–636. [CrossRef]
202. Jiang, H.; Ling, Z.; Zhang, Y.; Mao, H.; Ma, Z.; Yin, Y.; Wang, W.; Tang, W.; Tan, Z.; Shi, J.; et al. Altered fecal microbiota composition in patients with major depressive disorder. *Brain Behav. Immun.* **2015**, *48*, 186–194. [CrossRef] [PubMed]
203. O'Mahony, S.M.; Marchesi, J.R.; Scully, P.; Codling, C.; Ceolho, A.M.; Quigley, E.M.; Cryan, J.F.; Dinan, T.G. Early life stress alters behavior, immunity, and microbiota in rats: Implications for irritable bowel syndrome and psychiatric illnesses. *Biol. Psychiatry* **2009**, *65*, 263–267. [CrossRef]

204. Bailey, M.T.; Dowd, S.E.; Galley, J.D.; Hufnagle, A.R.; Allen, R.G.; Lyte, M. Exposure to a social stressor alters the structure of the intestinal microbiota: Implications for stressor-induced immunomodulation. *Brain Behav. Immun.* **2011**, *25*, 397–407. [CrossRef]
205. Zheng, P.; Zeng, B.; Zhou, C.; Liu, M.; Fang, Z.; Xu, X.; Zeng, L.; Chen, J.; Fan, S.; Du, X.; et al. Gut microbiome remodeling induces depressive-like behaviors through a pathway mediated by the host's metabolism. *Mol. Psychiatry* **2016**, *21*, 786–796. [CrossRef] [PubMed]
206. Mauro, C.; De Rosa, V.; Marelli-Berg, F.; Solito, E. Metabolic syndrome and the immunological affair with the blood-brain barrier. *Front. Immunol.* **2014**, *5*, 677. [CrossRef]
207. Dominguez, L.J.; Barbagallo, M. The biology of the metabolic syndrome and aging. *Curr. Opin. Clin. Nutr. Metab. Care* **2016**, *19*, 5–11. [CrossRef] [PubMed]
208. Kaur, J. A comprehensive review on metabolic syndrome. *Cardiol Res Pract* **2014**, *2014*, 943162. [CrossRef] [PubMed]
209. Morley, J.E.; Sinclair, A. The metabolic syndrome in older persons: A loosely defined constellation of symptoms or a distinct entity? *Age Ageing* **2009**, *38*, 494–497. [CrossRef] [PubMed]
210. Atallah, A.; Mhaouty-Kodja, S.; Grange-Messent, V. Chronic depletion of gonadal testosterone leads to blood-brain barrier dysfunction and inflammation in male mice. *J. Cereb. Blood Flow Metab.* **2017**, *37*, 3161–3175. [CrossRef]
211. Dubois, V.; Laurent, M.R.; Jardi, F.; Antonio, L.; Lemaire, K.; Goyvaerts, L.; Deldicque, L.; Carmeliet, G.; Decallonne, B.; Vanderschueren, D.; et al. Androgen Deficiency Exacerbates High-Fat Diet-Induced Metabolic Alterations in Male Mice. *Endocrinology* **2016**, *157*, 648–665. [CrossRef]
212. Frasca, D.; Blomberg, B.B.; Paganelli, R. Aging, Obesity, and Inflammatory Age-Related Diseases. *Front. Immunol.* **2017**, *8*, 1745. [CrossRef]
213. Rhea, E.M.; Salameh, T.S.; Logsdon, A.F.; Hanson, A.J.; Erickson, M.A.; Banks, W.A. Blood-Brain Barriers in Obesity. *AAPS J.* **2017**, *19*, 921–930. [CrossRef]
214. Klok, M.D.; Jakobsdottir, S.; Drent, M.L. The role of leptin and ghrelin in the regulation of food intake and body weight in humans: A review. *Obes. Rev.* **2007**, *8*, 21–34. [CrossRef] [PubMed]
215. Banks, W.A.; Burney, B.O.; Robinson, S.M. Effects of triglycerides, obesity, and starvation on ghrelin transport across the blood-brain barrier. *Peptides* **2008**, *29*, 2061–2065. [CrossRef]
216. Banks, W.A.; Farr, S.A.; Morley, J.E. The effects of high fat diets on the blood-brain barrier transport of leptin: Failure or adaptation? *Physiol. Behav.* **2006**, *88*, 244–248. [CrossRef]
217. Stranahan, A.M.; Hao, S.; Dey, A.; Yu, X.; Baban, B. Blood-brain barrier breakdown promotes macrophage infiltration and cognitive impairment in leptin receptor-deficient mice. *J. Cereb. Blood Flow Metab.* **2016**, *36*, 2108–2121. [CrossRef]
218. Fujihara, R.; Chiba, Y.; Nakagawa, T.; Nishi, N.; Murakami, R.; Matsumoto, K.; Kawauchi, M.; Yamamoto, T.; Ueno, M. Albumin microvascular leakage in brains with diabetes mellitus. *Microsc. Res. Tech.* **2016**, *79*, 833–837. [CrossRef]
219. Xu, Z.; Zeng, W.; Sun, J.; Chen, W.; Zhang, R.; Yang, Z.; Yao, Z.; Wang, L.; Song, L.; Chen, Y.; et al. The quantification of blood-brain barrier disruption using dynamic contrast-enhanced magnetic resonance imaging in aging rhesus monkeys with spontaneous type 2 diabetes mellitus. *Neuroimage* **2017**, *158*, 480–487. [CrossRef] [PubMed]
220. Salameh, T.S.; Mortell, W.G.; Logsdon, A.F.; Butterfield, D.A.; Banks, W.A. Disruption of the hippocampal and hypothalamic blood-brain barrier in a diet-induced obese model of type II diabetes: Prevention and treatment by the mitochondrial carbonic anhydrase inhibitor, topiramate. *Fluids Barriers CNS* **2019**, *16*, 1. [CrossRef] [PubMed]
221. Arnold, S.E.; Arvanitakis, Z.; Macauley-Rambach, S.L.; Koenig, A.M.; Wang, H.Y.; Ahima, R.S.; Craft, S.; Gandy, S.; Buettner, C.; Stoeckel, L.E.; et al. Brain insulin resistance in type 2 diabetes and Alzheimer disease: Concepts and conundrums. *Nat. Rev. Neurol.* **2018**, *14*, 168–181. [CrossRef] [PubMed]
222. Chen, F.; Dong, R.R.; Zhong, K.L.; Ghosh, A.; Tang, S.S.; Long, Y.; Hu, M.; Miao, M.X.; Liao, J.M.; Sun, H.B.; et al. Antidiabetic drugs restore abnormal transport of amyloid-beta across the blood-brain barrier and memory impairment in db/db mice. *Neuropharmacology* **2016**, *101*, 123–136. [CrossRef] [PubMed]
223. Tucsek, Z.; Toth, P.; Sosnowska, D.; Gautam, T.; Mitschelen, M.; Koller, A.; Szalai, G.; Sonntag, W.E.; Ungvari, Z.; Csiszar, A. Obesity in aging exacerbates blood-brain barrier disruption, neuroinflammation,

and oxidative stress in the mouse hippocampus: Effects on expression of genes involved in beta-amyloid generation and Alzheimer's disease. *J. Gerontol. A Biol. Sci. Med. Sci.* **2014**, *69*, 1212–1226. [CrossRef] [PubMed]

224. Goldwaser, E.L.; Acharya, N.K.; Sarkar, A.; Godsey, G.; Nagele, R.G. Breakdown of the Cerebrovasculature and Blood-Brain Barrier: A Mechanistic Link Between Diabetes Mellitus and Alzheimer's Disease. *J. Alzheimers Dis.* **2016**, *54*, 445–456. [CrossRef] [PubMed]

4

Activating the Anaphase Promoting Complex to Enhance Genomic Stability and Prolong Lifespan

Troy A. A. Harkness

Department of Anatomy and Cell Biology, University of Saskatchewan, Saskatoon, SK S7N 5E5, Canada; troy.harkness@usask.ca

Abstract: In aging cells, genomic instability is now recognized as a hallmark event. Throughout life, cells encounter multiple endogenous and exogenous DNA damaging events that are mostly repaired, but inevitably DNA mutations, chromosome rearrangements, and epigenetic deregulation begins to mount. Now that people are living longer, more and more late life time is spent suffering from age-related disease, in which genomic instability plays a critical role. However, several major questions remain heavily debated, such as the following: When does aging start? How long can we live? In order to minimize the impact of genomic instability on longevity, it is important to understand when aging starts, and to ensure repair mechanisms remain optimal from the very start to the very end. In this review, the interplay between the stress and nutrient response networks, and the regulation of homeostasis and genomic stability, is discussed. Mechanisms that link these two networks are predicted to be key lifespan determinants. The Anaphase Promoting Complex (APC), a large evolutionarily conserved ubiquitin ligase, can potentially serve this need. Recent work demonstrates that the APC maintains genomic stability, mounts a stress response, and increases longevity in yeast. Furthermore, inhibition of APC activity by glucose and nutrient response factors indicates a tight link between the APC and the stress/nutrient response networks.

Keywords: Anaphase Promoting Complex; lifespan; cancer; yeast; human cell culture

---

1. Introduction

When does the aging process begin? How long can we live? Why do we age? These questions are highly debated with no distinct, definitive answers. Does aging begin when our skin starts to wrinkle, or when our hair commences to turn grey? Or perhaps aging begins after the completion of growth [1]. Aging has also been defined as a shift in an organism's aging reality. The aging reality has been described as a mutually enslaved system of DNA and its environment in which signaling failures within this DNA environment occur over time [2]. Much of the debate reflects the fact that we have not perceived children as aging; however, acquired somatic mutations are recognized in infants and children, leading to the development of childhood cancers [3–5]. More compelling support for childhood aging comes from premature aging syndromes, such as progeria, in which children age in a very similar manner to normal aging individuals but at an 8-fold accelerated rate [6]. Even Hayflick considered when aging begins, weighing the possibilities that aging starts before or at conception or, alternatively, when maximum strength and stamina is achieved [7]. Hayflick eventually concluded that aging is a stochastic program that begins after reproductive maturity in animals, resulting in the loss of molecular fidelity. This loss of fidelity ultimately surpasses repair capacity, leaving individuals prone to age-related diseases [8,9]. The idea that aging is a random stochastic program is supported by many researchers in the field [10,11]. The stochastic idea of aging gained traction when the free radical theory of aging was proposed. This theory states that aging occurs due to the natural wear and tear of cellular machinery and biological substances due to exposure to free radicals generated within the cell [12]. Biological systems are constantly fighting a battle with its environment, both internally and externally, to ward off damage. The simple generation of mitochondrial-dependent energy and DNA replication expose cells to damage that must be repaired. Evidence for a stochastic program of aging also comes from inorganic compounds that age over time; for example, rusting of metal and peeling of paint (discussed in [13]), implying that something beyond genetics controls aging. From this work comes the idea that entropy drives aging, while genes drive longevity.

This review will summarize the current ideas describing our thoughts on the aging process. Molecular mechanisms will then be described that facilitate cellular aging. The notion that genomic instability is the driving force leading to aging and age-related disease will be discussed. Finally, the novel concept that activation of a cell cycle regulator, the Anaphase Promoting Complex, which is required for maintenance of cell health, inhibition of cancer progression, and enhanced longevity, will be explored.

2. Genetic Control of Longevity

Longevity depends on how long our cells remain functional, which is countered by the many insults faced by cells. Pathways that maintain cellular homeostasis are genetically controlled; thus, it clearly follows that a genetic program would be in place to control longevity. A recent review links proteostasis (a housekeeping phenomenon that controls the integrity of protein structure and function) with lifespan determination, and suggests the failure of the proteostatic network occurs early in life and marks the beginning of aging [14]. A global network encompassing maintenance of genomic stability, as well as enhancing proteostasis, would involve, for example, genes and proteins that repair DNA, scavenge free radicals, and the proteins that run these programs. Thus, the genetic and stochastic models appear to oppose one another. On the one hand, the stochastic model dictates that over time, our cells randomly accumulate damage, such as the accumulation of DNA mutations and genomic instability, and eventually succumb to the damage. On the other hand, the genetic program is in place to provide cells with options to survive the intrinsic and extrinsic environmental assaults that chronically bombard the cell and the biological system as a whole. Evolutionary biologists have argued that selection of lifespan-extending genes is unlikely, since the effects of these genes would only be seen long after reproduction has ceased, with the force of natural selection that declines with age leaving no valid reason to remain alive [2,15]. However, when these genes are viewed as controlling cell repair in the face of a damaging environment in order to survive, then it becomes clear that enhanced longevity may only be an indirect benefit accompanying the ability to survive unfavorable life events. Thus, evolution may not be selecting for longevity genes at all, but simply looking for genes that increase survival under trying times, with increased longevity simply a lucky side effect. This idea forms the foundation of the theory describing the response to nutrients versus stress as a driving force defining one's lifespan, as suggested earlier [16]. The concept of Hormesis, in which a potentially life-threatening stress, when given in a low dose, increases health or extends lifespan, is an example of a stress response providing a favorable and beneficial reaction [17,18].

One genetic theory of aging that is appealing to evolutionary biologists is the idea of pleiotropic antagonism. Antagonistic pleiotropy suggests that genes that are beneficial in the early years become harmful in later life [19–21]. A similar idea is described in the Disposable Soma theory [15]. It was proposed that because of high environmental mortality, resources are primarily spent on growth and reproduction, rather than on the soma, which would leave the soma exposed to environmental and intrinsic stresses. Nonetheless, the idea has been used to describe a Darwinian-evolutionary concept of aging in which the deleterious effects of previously beneficial genes in later life leads to the development of age-related disease [22]. Examples of antagonistic pleiotropy and how it could contribute to a Darwinian-evolutionary concept include the calcification of bones, which enables strength in early life, but eventually leads to deleterious calcification of arteries in late life. The erosion of telomeres, often considered a clear mechanism of aging, is also considered as support of a Darwinian-evolutionary model. While expression of telomerase extends telomere length in stem cell populations, it also contributes to tumor formation [23]. Thus, in early life, longer telomeres maintain the health and vitality of the cell. However, in later life, the inactivation of telomerase is proposed to ward off cancer, but at the cost of continued telomere erosion, and likely cellular senescence [24]. Darwinian selection of stress sensing and Darwinian selection of antagonistic pleiotropy genes are both used as examples of alternative mechanisms of lifespan determination, as both provide benefits in early life. However, the selection of stress sensing genes, but not antagonistic pleiotropy genes, provides an indirect longevity benefit in later life.

3. Genetic Control of Aging

The genetic model of lifespan determination is not at odds with the stochastic model, and involves a genetic program that determines the length of time that our cells and bodies can function. In the end, the more capable the cell is at damage repair, occurring through stochastic intrinsic and extrinsic events, the better the odds of surviving harsh environments and living to pass on genes to descendants. Longevity of the organism starts with the health of the cells. If cell health cannot be maintained, then health of the tissues and the animal itself will suffer. Cell type, in particular, is determined by programmed genetic and epigenetic networks. In the human body, for example, each cell harbors the same sequence of DNA, yet different cells carry out very different functions. Alterations to any of these networks can signal the end to that cell. Maintenance of the cellular equilibrium supporting tissue renewal is critical to the longevity of the organism. Over time, equilibrium and cell renewal begins to fail, leading to reduced replacement of cells lost due to attrition or senescence. Thus, the failing of the genetic system, contributing to the loss of cell equilibrium and renewal through accumulating mutations, is considered a hallmark of aging. Hallmarks of aging consist of the following attributes: genomic instability, telomere attrition, epigenetic alterations, and loss of proteostasis, leading to deregulated nutrient sensing, altered mitochondrial function, and cellular senescence [25,26].

Specific genes, many of which were first described and characterized in the simple lower eukaryotic yeast system (i.e., *SIR2* (yeast *SIRT* gene), *SNF1* (yeast *AMPK*), *FKH1/2* (yeast *FOXO*), *SCH9* (yeast *AKT/S6K*), *TOR1*, and *RAS2*, have been shown to be evolutionarily conserved genes that respond to stress or nutrients, influencing longevity [27–32]. Thus, genes (such as *SIR2*) clearly play a significant role in promoting lifespan from single cells to humans, but do genes also drive the loss of homeostasis and the aging process? While the stress response genes drive cell health and longevity in the presence of low-level stress, an example of Hormesis [17,18], the nutrient response genes do the opposite, and act as pro-aging genes. Thus, genes provide the impetus for both longevity and aging. Unlike the stochastic model, which relies on random factors to drive the aging process, the genetic program promoting aging relies on the activation of a web of nutrient response genes that inhibit the stress response network in the presence of usable resources [33]. Lifespan extension through caloric restriction is a classic example of Hormesis, and can be mimicked in yeast by mutating genes, such as *SCH9*, *TOR1*, or *RAS2*, which encode nutrient response proteins [29]. Ultimately, the longevity of an organism depends on the effectiveness of the counterbalanced stress and nutrient sensing pathways.

4. A Ceiling on a Maximum Lifespan?

Support for a predetermined program delineating our lifespan has been around for decades and is derived from the knowledge that human mean lifespan has increased dramatically over the past century, but the maximum lifespan has not [34]. The longest verified living human, Jeanne Calment, died at age 122 in 1997 [35], which is consistent with the idea that the maximum attainable human lifespan is not increasing and is likely capped at 125 years [36,37]. Indeed, few humans have ever lived past 115 years [38]. A maximum of 125 years is nonetheless controversial, as some feel there is no limit to our lifespan [8,39–43]. Further evidence supporting the idea that a predetermined genetic program dictates our maximum lifespan is provided by observations that maximum achievable lifespans are observed across evolutionary boundaries, as each specific organism seems to have a built in maximum possible lifespan [44]. The ever-increasing mean lifespan observed over the past century has also been used as evidence that human maximum lifespan will also continue unimpeded. Of course, this rise in expected lifespan is largely attributable to new developments in medical care, improved diet, less exposure to toxins, and regular exercise, which may only increase healthspan, and not lifespan. Regardless of how people feel about the dramatic rise in global expected lifespans, time is needed to fully realize the effect of improved human well-being, and thought should be put into policy development to deal with the likelihood that people will be living longer, healthier lives. Thus, if maximum lifespans have reached a ceiling, with mean life expectancy continuing to rise, lifespan curves may soon be considered lifespan cliffs, with increased human productivity a likely benefit.

5. So When Does Aging Begin?

It now seems quite clear that cellular aging is largely dependent on the degree to which genomic instability has affected DNA-dependent processes. Many studies, from yeast to humans, have repeatedly shown that during aging, senescent cells that exit the cell cycle or cease to function harbor large accumulations of DNA mutation, rearrangements, and epigenetic alterations. There are numerous sources of DNA damage, both endogenous and exogenous, that the cell must deal with. It is thought that a somatic cell may receive as many as 100,000 lesions daily [45,46]. It is not a coincidence that most age-dependent diseases, such as cancer, type II diabetes, and cardiopulmonary and neurodegenerative diseases are associated with increasingly elevated levels of genomic instability that occur over time [47–51]. When a cell is born, it is presumably at its functional apex, performing at its highest level. In yeast, the mother cell sequesters damage so that the daughter does not receive it, having a much better chance to begin life in a pristine state [52,53]. However, eventually the damage is too much for the yeast mother cell to fully sequester, with the daughter born with accumulating damage. If similar mechanisms that occur in yeast are occurring in higher eukaryotic systems, then it is easier to understand how a newly born cell would be at its best to repair damage and maintain proteostasis. With this in mind, the answer for when aging begins might be when the cells that form the zygote are first born; thus, aging of an individual may begin much earlier than conception, such as at the very moment when the mother develops oocytes in utero [54].

6. Connecting Stress Sensing with Nutrient Sensing

Genomic instability appears to be the gateway to aging and age-related disease. Genomic stability is threatened as soon as a cell is born due to the intrinsic damage caused by energy generation and the errors inflicted by DNA replication. The damage repair processes are presumably functioning at their best in these new cells, so genomic instability likely does not become an obstacle until much later in life. As discussed above, multiple antagonistic molecular networks are vying for available resources to respond to either stress and/or nutrients. It should be clear that the opposition of these pathways should not be all or none, as aspects of nutrient availability may be present even in an unfavorable environment. Thus, the question becomes how are nutrient and stress sensing networks regulated? What mediates the end of stress signaling when the stress is gone, or the stalling of the nutrient sensing pathways when the food source is used up?

7. The Anaphase Promoting Complex, Using Chromatin Assembly during Mitosis to Maintain Genome Stability

To answer these questions, it is important to identify components that connect stress and nutrient-sensing pathways. The Anaphase Promoting Complex (APC) has come to light as a potential link between the stress and nutrient sensing networks. The APC is an evolutionarily conserved large ubiquitin-protein ligase (E3) that targets proteins that inhibit mitotic entrance and exit, as well as proteins that inhibit G1 maintenance, for ubiquitin and proteasome-dependent degradation [55]. The APC is controlled by 2 co-activators, CDC20 and CDH1, which control mitotic progression, and G1 maintenance (Figures 1 and 2). CDC20 binds with the APC to initiate mitosis, and is then targeted for degradation by the APC^{CDH1} complex at the M/G1 transition [56,57]. CDH1 is then targeted for degradation at the G1/S transition by a second large E3 complex called the SCF (Skp-Cullin-F-box complex) [58]. The APC is largely known for its role in cell cycle progression, but we and others have identified it as a central player in stress sensing and lifespan determination using the simple brewing yeast eukaryotic model system (Figure 3) [31,59–65]. Mitosis is a time during the cell cycle when DNA damage can become permanent and lead to further chromosome erosion and genomic instability [66]. The APC is also required for replication-independent chromatin assembly and histone modifications [60,67–70]. Considering that replication-independent chromatin assembly is required for DNA repair [71,72], we speculate that the APC may be involved in repair of DNA damage incurred during chromosome segregation (Figure 3). The chromatin assembly factors Asf1, and the CAF-1 complex, have been shown in yeast and human cells to be involved in assembly of histones onto repaired DNA duplexes [73–76]. The link between repair of DNA during mitosis and the APC may be the CAF-1 and Asf1 chaperones, as the APC genetically interacts with both Asf1 and CAF-1 mutants in yeast (mutant combinations have worse phenotypes), and increased expression of any one of the CAF-1 subunits, or Asf1, rescues APC defects [67]. Consistent with a role in maintaining genomic stability, APC defects result in elevated sensitivity to UV radiation, increased loss of centromere based plasmids, and increased rDNA instability [60,64].

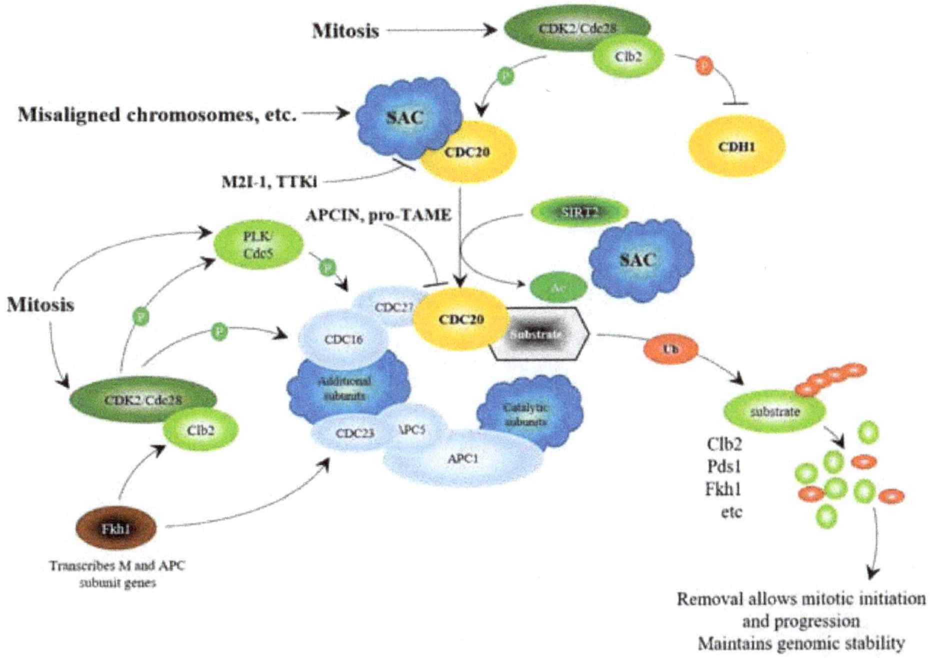

Figure 1. Regulation of the APC at the G2/M transition. The schematic considers results from mammalian and yeast studies. Yeast proteins are written as Cdc20, whereas mammalian proteins are written as CDC20. Genomic stability and segregation of replicated and repaired chromosomes is established via the Spindle Assembly Checkpoint (SAC) that sequesters Cdc20/CDC20 away from the APC, thus inhibiting APC function as cells enter mitosis [77,78]. When the SAC is satisfied, the cyclin Clb2 (Cyclin B), synthesized during G2 by Fkh1 [79], interacts with cyclin-dependent kinase Cdc28 (CDK2) to phosphorylate a series of proteins needed for mitotic progression: Cdc5 (PLK), Cdc16, Cdc23, and Cdc27 [80,81]. Once PLK is active, it further activates the APC by phosphorylating Apc9 (or APC1 in mammalian cells), Cdc16 and Cdc27 [80,81]. Cdc28-Clb2 also phosphorylates the co-activators Cdc20 for activation [80], and Cdh1 for inhibition [82]. A further activating stimulus is provided by SIRT2, which deacetylates CDC20 [83]. APC^{Cdc20} then targets proteins for degradation, such as Pds1 (PTTG1/Securin), to allow chromosome segregation, and Clb2 and Fkh1 to complete a negative feedback loop that prepares the cell for mitotic exit and G1 maintenance [65,84,85]. Degradation of Clb2

stops inhibition of Cdh1, allowing replacement of the APC^{Cdc20} complex with APC^{Cdh1}. APC chemical inhibitors, APCIN and pro-TAME, disrupt the CDC20-APC interaction [86,87], whereas the small molecule APC activators (M2I-1, TTKi) disrupt the CDC20-SAC interaction [88–90]. Protein degradation is shown by Ub, shaded with a red oval, attached to the target protein to build poly-Ub chains, followed by break down of the protein, shown in smaller circles. Inhibitory phosphorylation is shown with a red shaded "P", and activating phosphorylation is shown with a green shaded "P".

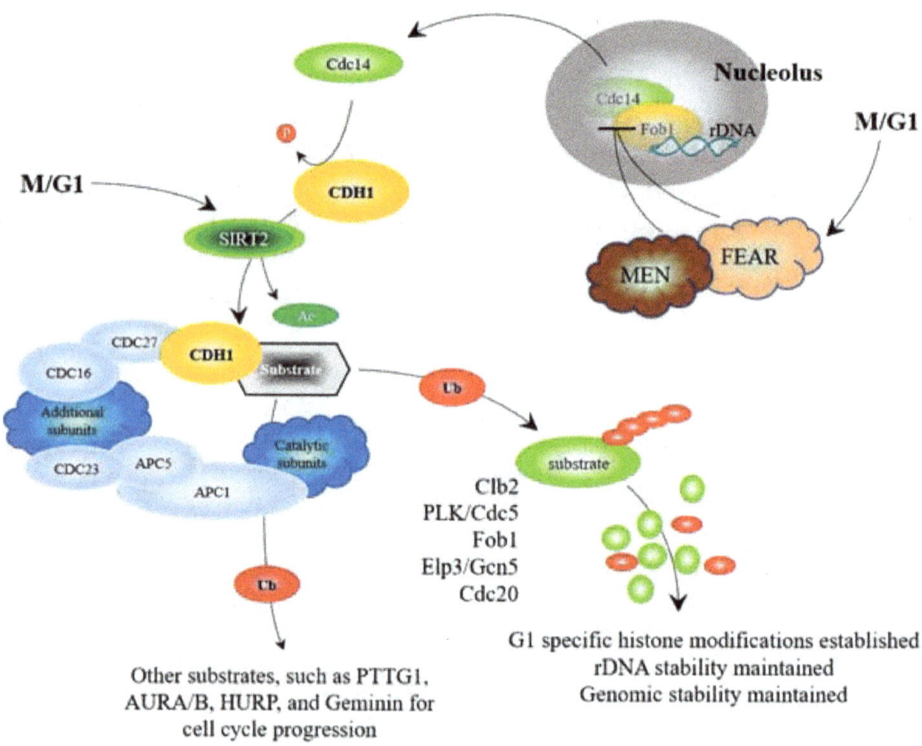

Figure 2. Regulation of the APC at the M/G1 transition. As mitosis comes to an end, the phosphatase Cdc14 is activated and released from sequestration within the nucleolus by Fob1, through a biphasic interaction involving the FEAR and MEN pathways [91,92]. Cdc14 dephosphorylates Cdh1, thus facilitating the interaction between Cdh1 and the APC [93]. Further activation is accomplished by deacetylation of CDH1 by SIRT2 [83]. APC^{Cdh1} function then leads to wholesale changes required for mitotic exit and transition into G1. Residual Pds1 and Clb2 are targeted for degradation by APC^{Cdh1}, as are Cdc20, Cdc5, and other targets, which puts an end to the pattern of proteins required for mitotic progression [56,57,94–100]. Degradation of Fob1, a negative regulator of FEAR, is required for G1 progression, as Fob1 [64] is required for rDNA condensation during mitosis. Gcn5 (and likely Elp3) is also required for G1 progression [69], as it presumably acetylates histones during mitosis to establish an epigenetic pattern required for G1 progression. Once this pattern is established during mitosis, Gcn5 (and likely Elp3) must be degraded. Ubiquitinated and degraded proteins are depicted as described above.

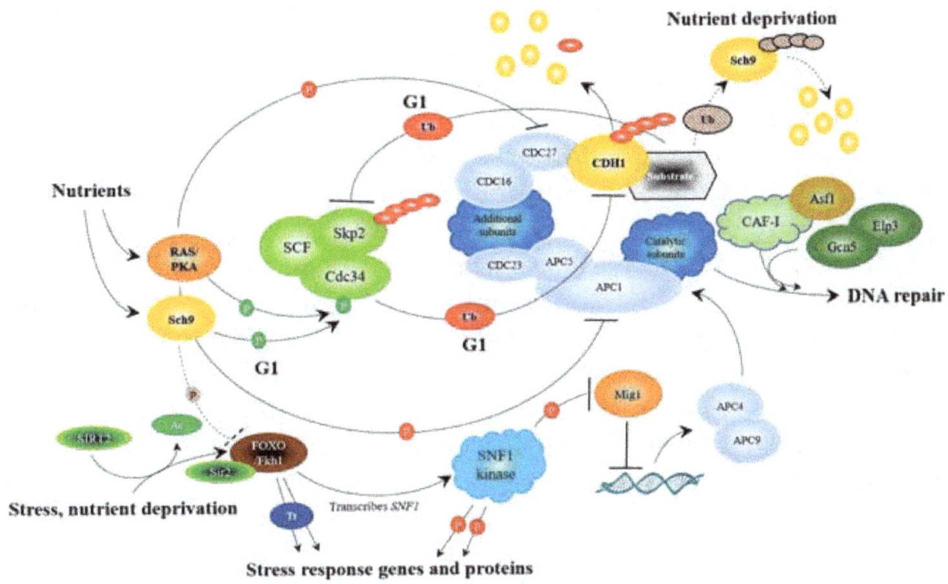

Figure 3. APC activity is decreased under nutrient conditions, and increased when nutrients are limiting. Inhibition of APC activity by glucose is mediated by the Ras/PKA pathway [81,101–103]. Recent work suggests that this is accomplished by driving the activity of the SCF ubiquitin ligase by the phosphorylation and activation of the SCF E2 component Cdc34 by the nutrient response kinases PKA and Sch9 (AKT/S6K) [104]. This could mediate APC inhibition, as it has been shown that the SCF targets the degradation of CDH1 during mitosis [58,105]. Our unpublished data also reveals that Sch9 likely inhibits Fkh1 function, and the subsequent induction of the stress pathways. Upon encountering stress, SIRT2 deacetylates and activates FOXO proteins [106], and in yeast, Sir2 physically associates with Fkh1 to facilitate inhibition of *CLB2* transcription in late M/G1 [107]. Fkh1 transcribes stress response genes (depicted by a a blue shaded "Tr"), including *SNF1*, which encodes the catalytic component of the SNF1 kinase, the yeast AMPK [79,108]. FOXO and AMPK interact across evolutionary boundaries to deal with stress [108–110]. The SNF1 kinase then enters the nucleus and inhibits the glucose responsive repressor Mig1, which represses the expression of the APC subunits *APC4* and *APC9* under nutrient conditions [61]. DNA repair is likely mediated, at least in part, by the APC, which controls the deposition and modification of histones during mitosis, which plays a pivotal role in DNA repair [67,69,71–74]. Inhibition of SCF-Cdc34 following APC activation is accomplished in two ways: first, the APC targets the SCF F-box protein Skp2 for degradation in G1 [111,112], and second, our unpublished data shows that the APC targets Sch9 for degradation once nutrients are depleted. Preliminary unpublished data is shown using dashed lines.

8. Maintaining Genomic Stability via APC-Mediated Histone Modifications

Histone post-translational modifications are involved in cell cycle progression, particularly mitosis [113], and in DNA repair. In yeast, DNA repair requires Asf1, CAF-1, and acetylation of H3 Lys56 (H3K56^{Ac}), mediated by the Asf1/Rtt109 complex [71,74]. Cells with impaired APC function have reduced H3K9^{Ac}, H3K79^{Me}, and H3K56^{Ac} [69]. H3K79^{Me} accumulates during mitosis [114], while H3K56^{Ac} and H3K9^{Ac} are reduced during mitosis but increase as cells enter G1 [115,116]. H3K9^{Ac} is important for transcriptional activation [117,118], H3K56^{Ac} is involved in histone deposition and DNA repair [74,119], while H3K79^{Me} is required for a variety of activities including transcriptional elongation, DNA repair, and cell cycle checkpoints [120,121]. Thus, the loss of these modifications due to impaired APC has a dramatic impact on chromatin and chromosome structure, transcription, and DNA repair. Furthermore, the histone acetyltransferase (HAT) that mediates H3K9^{Ac}, Gcn5, interacts genetically and functionally with the APC [69,70]. Increased expression of *GCN5* rescued APC defects and deletion of *GCN5* in APC mutants exacerbated growth defects. Furthermore, Gcn5 is targeted by the APC for degradation at the M/G1 transition [69]. Acetylation of histones during mitosis may be important to reset the epigenome as cells re-enter G1, leading to the appropriate activation of specific genes. The correlation of Gcn5 degradation at G1, just after the accumulation of $H3K9^{Ac}$ as cells exit mitosis, with APC mitotic function, is at the crux of establishing an active transcriptome for continued cell cycle progression. Furthermore, if targeted degradation of Gcn5 by the APC is conserved from yeast to humans, then this may be critical for tumor suppression and maintenance of genomic stability, as increased $H3K9^{Ac}$ is associated with DNA damage, genomic instability, and progression of multiple myeloma [122]. Consistent with this, APC defects lead to elevated genomic instability in yeast [60,64,65] and in human cells [123,124]. Thus, although the APC is required for mitotic progression, it is also required to guard against damage that can occur during chromosome segregation, and to ensure that histones are acetylated to enable proper transcription as cells enter G1. These activities are all critical to ensure that cells remain healthy, leading to enhanced lifespan. On the other hand, the inability to maintain cellular homeostasis is linked with genomic instability associated with cancer development and progression

9. Targeting APC Inhibition for Anticancer Therapy

Because of the role the APC plays in cell cycle progression, initial work focused on the inhibition of the APC as a means to block tumor growth [125–127]. The evolutionarily conserved Spindle Assembly Checkpoint (SAC) complex, consisting of the proteins MAD1, MAD2, BUB1, BUBR1, BUB3 and MPS1, binds and sequesters the APC co-activator CDC20 prior to mitosis [77,78], inhibiting APC activation until all chromosomes are ready for segregation (Figure 1). It was suggested that activation of the SAC, and inhibition of the APC, would protect the cell from inappropriate chromosome segregation and mitotic catastrophe in the presence of damaged chromosomes, which is often observed in cancer cells. Furthermore, *CDC20* mRNA expression is observed to be elevated in cancer cells, which is associated with a poor prognosis; *CDC20* knockdown is required for mitotic arrest and inhibition of cell growth [94,128,129]. Specific (APCIN and pro-TAME [86,87]) and non-specific (Velcade [126]) APC inhibitors have been developed recently and inhibit tumor growth in vitro [86,130]. Both APCIN and pro-TAME act by inhibiting the interaction of CDC20 with the APC (Figure 1). Thus, inhibition of the APC was believed to be a viable anti-tumor strategy.

10. Targeting APC Activation for Anticancer Therapy

Recent work in mammalian cancer cells provides evidence that APC activation, rather than inhibition, may be a potent anticancer therapy that antagonizes genomic instability. As discussed above, CDC20 is an APC coactivator, and high APC^{CDC20} may be inappropriately driving cells through mitosis to promote genomic instability and cancer progression, inferring that APC inhibition will be beneficial. Regulation of CDC20 is highly coordinated (Figure 1). As discussed above, CDC20 is sequestered and inhibited by the SAC until all chromosomes are aligned along the metaphase plate and ready for segregation [77,78]. Cdc20 in yeast is activated by Cdc28-Clb2-dependent phosphorylation [80]. Cdc28-Clb2 also phosphorylates the APC subunits Cdc16, Cdc23, and Cdc27 [81], the yeast Polo-like kinase, Cdc5 [131], and Cdh1 to maintain its inactivity [82]. Once Cdc5 is activated, it then potentially targets Cdc16, Cdc27, and Apc9 for phosphorylation to further activate the APC [80,81]. Cdc5 is later targeted by APC^{Cdh1} to exit mitosis [132]. CDC20 is also deacetylated by SIRT2, adding another level of activation [83]. Additional activation signals in yeast come from the Forkhead transcription factors Fkh1 and Fkh2. The *FKH1* and *FKH2* genes are transcribed during G2 by Hcm1 [133], and are required for the transcription of the "CLB2 cluster" of genes, which contains genes required for APC activity, such as *CLB2, CDC5, CDC20,* and *APC1* [79].

The APC is essential, and this is conserved from yeast to humans, as yeast deletion mutants are lethal and mouse models lacking APC subunits, or CDC20, die in embryogenesis [84,134–136]. The APC is also essential for the prevention of aneuploidy, which contributes to tumorigenesis [84].

Thus, the systemic in vivo use of APC inhibitors may be highly toxic, limiting this approach to cancer therapy. However, an alternative interpretation is possible to explain why CDC20 accumulates in cancer cells. CDC20 itself is targeted by APC^{CDH1} for degradation once mitosis is complete [56,57]. Therefore, elevated *CDC20* expression could reflect APC^{CDH1} impairment in cancer cells, inferring that APC activation will be beneficial to cell health. Our in vitro and in vivo work (Davies, Arnason and Harkness, unpublished), and findings from others, have noted that many APC^{CDH1} mitotic substrate genes and proteins are elevated in cancer cells, including CDC20 [94], PLK1 [95], AURA/B [96,97], HURP (*DLGAP* gene [98]), Securin (*PTTG1* gene [99]), and Geminin [100], hinting that impaired APC activity as a whole is involved, rather than isolated CDC20 elevation. Moreover, using the Cancer Genome Atlas database [137], we observed that the expression of the APC substrate genes *PTTG1* and *DLGAP5* in cancer patients is differentially regulated between normal tissues and tumor tissues, across 24 different types of cancer (Figure 4).

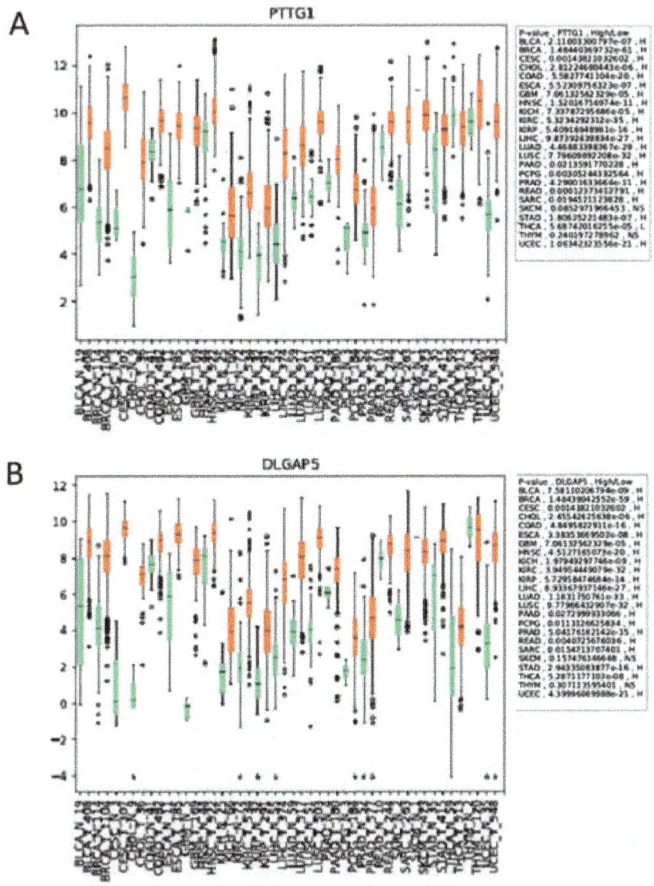

Figure 4. The APC substrate mRNAs PTTG1 and DLGAP5 are overexpressed in multiple cancer types. Expression scores for (**A**) PTTG1 and (**B**) DLGAP5 within 24 different types of cancer and normal tissue from TCGA [134]. The numbers in x-axis labels denote the number of patient samples in each cancer type. Statistical significance of the difference in expression between the normal and tumor samples is depicted for each cancer type. N.S. not significant. The abbreviation of each cancer in the axis label is represented as described in the TCGA portal [137].

While CDC20 has been linked to cancer progression, the second APC co-activator, CDH1, has been linked to tumor suppression, with earlier work demonstrating that cells lacking CDH1 have a shortened G1 phase, accumulate DNA damage, and undergo apoptosis [85]. CDH1 is also regulated through a complex web of interactions (Figure 2). As discussed above, the yeast Cdh1 is maintained in an inactive form by Cdc28-Clb2 phosphorylation until the end of mitosis, when Clb2 is targeted for degradation and the phosphatase Cdc14 is released from the nucleolus to undo the work of Cdc28-Clb2 [82,91,93]. The mammalian CDH1 is further activated by deacetylation by SIRT2 [83]. Recent work has demonstrated that cells with low levels of CDH1 accumulated in G1 with elevated mitotic APC substrates, causing genome instability [123,124]. Furthermore, entire loss of CDH1 increased DNA damage accumulation, driving progression of murine and human B-cell acute leukemia [138]. It was also revealed that many cancer cell lines lack the ability to activate APC^{Cdh1} when under replication stress [139,140], and that CDH1-depleted cells undergo senescence in G2, suggesting that APC^{Cdh1} may normally act as a barrier to genome instability [123]. Support for this idea comes from studies using SIRT2, an antitumor and lifespan-extending protein, which activates the APC by deacetylating CDC20 and CDH1; SIRT2-deficient mice exhibited higher levels of cancer and elevated levels of APC substrates [83]. Thus, impaired APC function appears linked with genomic instability and cancer development, providing strong therapeutic potential through targeted activation in cancer cells.

APC dysfunction and cancer development could occur in several ways. Loss of either CDC20 or CDH1 is deleterious; CDC20 deletion is lethal, while loss of CDH1 leads to genomic instability [123,124]. In addition, mutations have been observed in several APC subunit genes (APC3, APC6/CDC16, and APC8/CDC23) in cancer cells [141]. Inappropriate expression of the CDC23ΔTPR mutant disrupted cell cycle progression and led to elevated levels of APC substrates. Loss of the APC7 subunit has also been implicated in various tumors [142,143]. Furthermore, silencing of a variety of APC subunits causes cells to survive treatment with compounds that inhibit the SAC, providing a mechanism for the development of drug resistance [88,89]. Thus, evidence is accumulating to support the idea that APC activity is required for cell health, while loss of normal APC function leads to genomic instability and cancer.

11. APC Activation Reduces Substrate Levels and Inhibits Cancer Cell Growth

Recently, focus has shifted towards the creation of compounds that activate the APC. To do so, SAC inhibition has been targeted. Prolonged SAC, or impaired APC activity, can lead to inappropriate mitotic progression in a process called mitotic slippage [144,145]. This potentially provides time for cells to respond to increased toxic levels of genomic instability common in cancer cells. Furthermore, because of the aneuploid nature of cancer cells, cancer cells are heavily reliant on the SAC for proper segregation of chromosomes; inhibition of the SAC in cancer cells produces intolerable levels of genomic instability, killing these cells [146,147]. One compound, called Mad2-inhibitor-1, or M2I-1, blocks the MAD2/CDC20 interaction (Figure 1) and weakens the SAC, leading to early activation of the APC [90]. We have subsequently used M2I-1 in vitro and in vivo, and have found that, in vitro, M2I-1 synergizes with Doxorubicin to reduce the growth of drug resistant MCF7 breast cancer cells, while growth of patient-derived triple negative breast cancer cells in mice was stalled by M2I-1 (Davies, Arnason, and Harkness, unpublished). Both in vitro and in vivo, APC substrate mRNA and protein levels were reduced, showing that M2I-1 does indeed activate the APC. Additional SAC inhibitors have been developed that inhibit the kinase MPS1/TTK (TTKi's), a SAC component [88,89]. Kaplan-Meier plots revealed that overexpression of MPS1/TTK is correlated with poor overall and relapse-free survival in breast cancer patients [148]. Interestingly, as mentioned above, silencing of APC subunits generates resistance to the MPS1/TTK inhibitors (TTKi's) reversine and CFI-402257 [88,89]. This suggests that the lethal mitotic segregation errors induced by TTK inhibition can be overcome by prolonging the onset of anaphase.

12. APC Activity, via the Fkh/SNF Kinase/Sir2 Pathway, is Required for Prolonged Longevity

We have reported that the yeast APC prolongs longevity (increased expression of only *APC10* increased replicative lifespan [61]), responds to stress, and interacts with multiple conserved stress response pathways highlighted by the Forkhead (FOXO) and Snf1 (AMPK) pathways [31,32,61,63–65,108] (Figure 3). It is already clear that the FOXO and AMPK pathways intersect under stress in mammalian cells and drive the activity of several other stress response networks [109,110]. In yeast, *snf1Δ* mutants were also shown to interact genetically with the *apc5*^{CA} mutant; deletion of *SNF1* worsened the *apc5*^{CA} defect, whereas overexpression rescued it [61]. Furthermore, Mig1, a glucose responsive transcriptional repressor inhibited by Snf1 phosphorylation, repressed the expression of the APC subunits *APC4* and *APC9* [61]. Subsequent work showed that Fkh1 transcribed *SNF1*, and that increased longevity observed in the Snf1^{UBA} mutant depended on Fkh1 or Fkh2 [32]. This stress response network is further bolstered by the anti-aging protein deacetylase SIRT2, which deacetylates FOXO3a to increase its DNA binding ability in mammalian cells [106]. SIRT2 also binds to the APC^{CDC20} and APC^{CDH1} complexes and deacetylates both CDC20 and CDH1 to turn on the APC [83]. The SIRT2-FOXO interaction is also conserved in yeast, as the yeast Forkhead proteins, Fkh1 and Fkh2, physically associate with Sir2 during late M and G1 to repress the expression of the Fkh target gene Clb2 [107]. In addition, under stress conditions, Sir2 assists in APC function by inhibiting *CLB2* transcription; overexpression of *CLB2* under stress conditions is toxic [107]. However, it was not shown whether Sir2 deacetylates the Fkh proteins in this study. In yeast, the Fkh1 and Fkh2 transcription factors, like in mammalian cells, are involved in cell cycle progression, stress response, and longevity [63]. *FKH1* and *FKH2* are expressed during G2 to drive the expression of mitotic specific genes [79,149]. The *FKH* genes are activated by a third Forkhead protein called Hcm1, which is expressed at the G1/S boundary [133]. Interestingly, Hcm1 nuclear translocation is facilitated by the SNF1 kinase [150], defining a positive feedforward loop involving Snf1, Hcm1, and the Fkh proteins. Furthermore, the ubiquitin conjugating enzyme, Ubc1, interacts with the APC [151] and is required for SNF1 kinase function [108]. It was revealed that in yeast *ubc1Δ* mutants, Hcm1 remains cytosolic, *FKH1* and *FKH2* transcription is reduced, and SNF1 kinase activity is decreased [108]. Fkh1 action is then reduced at the onset of mitosis, as the bulk of Fkh1 is targeted for degradation by the APC^{Cdc20} complex [65] (Figure 1). Interestingly, Fkh1 and the APC subunit Apc5 physically interacted throughout the cell cycle [65]. Deletion of both *FKH1* and *FKH2* in APC defective cells worsened the already short replicative and chronological lifespans [31], and mutation of a single, conserved lysine in Fkh1 (K_{373}) mimicked the null *FKH1* allele, reduced chronological lifespan, and increased genomic instability [65]. Thus, it appears that ubiquitination of Fkh1 at K_{373}, mediated by APC^{Cdc20} at the onset of mitosis, is required to maintain normal lifespan and genomic stability.

In addition to Fkh1, the APC also targets a second lifespan determinant, Fob1, for degradation [64]. Fob1 in yeast is an rDNA replication fork blocking protein [152,153]. Fob1 condenses rDNA and stalls replication fork progression during mitosis, creating free DNA ends that produce extra chromosomal circles [92,154]. Fob1 also sequesters the Cdc14 phosphatase within the nucleolus at the rDNA locus during early mitosis [91,92]. Cdc14 is released from Fob1 by the combined activity of the FEAR (Cdc14 early anaphase release) and MEN (mitotic exit network) complexes during late mitosis, enabling activation of Cdh1 via Cdc14 dephosphorylation of Cdc28-Clb2 [93]. Deletion of *FOB1* enhances yeast replicative lifespan [64,154], while increased *FOB1* expression reduces replicative lifespan [64]. We identified Fob1 as a binding partner for Apc5 in a yeast 2-hybrid screen. Mutation of an amino acid required for Fob1-Apc5 interactions ($E_{420}V$) stabilized Fob1, increased rDNA instability, and abolished the accumulation of modified Fob1 species. We observed that Fob1 was specifically unstable during G1 and targeted for degradation by APC^{Cdh1} [64]. Deletion of *FOB1*, like that of *FKH1*, rescued the lifespan defect observed in APC mutants [64,65]. Taken together, the APC target substrates we have identified (Fkh1, Fob1, and Gcn5) function during mitosis and G1 to elicit wide-ranging effects on genomic stability and longevity (Figure 2).

13. The APC Triggers the End of Nutrient Signaling in the Presence of Stress

In order to fully maximize longevity, from the beginning to the end, coupling the stress and nutrient sensing pathways may be critical. The APC may be in a position to recognize both stress and nutrients. The APC is activated by phosphorylation to promote cell cycle progression. Using mouse fibroblast NIH/3T3 cells, it was shown that the Polo-like kinase, Plk, activates the APC by phosphorylating CDC16, CDC27, and APC1 [81] (Figure 1). Plk in yeast (Cdc5) also phosphorylates the APC, as does the cyclin-dependent kinase Cdc28 on Cdc16, Cdc23, and Cdc27 to activate APC^{Cdc20} function [80]. Conversely, mammalian protein kinase A (PKA) phosphorylates CDC27 and APC1 to inhibit APC function [81] (Figure 3). It is known in yeast that nutrients, such as glucose, and nutrient signaling networks involving Ras/PKA inhibit the APC [101–103,155]. The cell cycle proceeds in the presence of nutrients, so it remains unresolved how the positive and negative phosphorylation events on APC subunits using the nutrient response and cell cycle promoting kinases are coordinated. It remains possible that the APC's role in cell cycle progression and stress response are controlled via different mechanisms. If this were the case, PKA inhibition of the APC may be specific to its stress response activity, whereas activation by the cyclin-dependent and Polo-like kinases may be more geared towards the APC's cell cycle role. These observations suggest that the nutrient-sensing pathway plays a pivotal role in shutting down the APC and its stress-sensing functions.

The yeast nutrient-sensing kinases Sch9 (similar to the AKT/S6K homologues in humans [156]) and PKA also control APC activity in the presence of nutrients by phosphorylating the ubiquitin conjugating enzyme, Cdc34, the E2 component of the ubiquitin-ligase (E3) SCF [104]. Work in mammalian cells shows that the two E3 enzymes, the APC and the SCF, work to counterbalance one another during G1, with the SCF targeting the CDH1 for degradation [58,105], and the APC targeting the SCF F-box subunit SKP2 for degradation [111,112]. Thus, the nutrient response kinases inhibit APC activity in the presence of nutrients. Furthermore, our preliminary results indicate that the long life observed in *sch9*Δ and *tor1*Δ mutants requires functional Fkh1 or Fkh2, suggesting that Sch9 and/or Tor1 inhibit Fkh function (Postnikoff and Harkness, unpublished; Figure 3), leading to further inactivation of the APC.

However, how does the nutrient sensing pathway shut down when nutrients are limited? A recent report described the turnover of the nutrient sensing kinase Sch9 in yeast [157]. Deletion of *SCH9* in yeast increases yeast replicative and chronological lifespan [28,158], and, as mentioned above, deletion of both *FKH1* and *FKH2* in either the *sch9*Δ or *tor1*Δ background eliminates the observed long life (Postnikoff and Harkness, unpublished). As cells entered stationary phase, it was observed that total ubiquitinated protein decreased, as did total Sch9 protein levels [157]. In the presence of the proteasome poison MG132, it was observed that Sch9 protein levels increased [157], supporting the idea that Sch9 is ubiquitinated and degraded as nutrient levels decrease. We therefore asked whether Sch9 is targeted for ubiquitination by the APC, as a means to inactivate this arm of the nutrient response network when nutrient levels decline. Our preliminary experiments show that deletion of *SCH9* in APC mutants suppressed the chronological lifespan and oxidative stress sensitive defects in APC mutants (Postnikoff and Harkness, unpublished). We also confirmed that Sch9 turnover occurs as cells enter stationary phase, and that this is blocked in APC mutants (Malo and Harkness, unpublished). Taken as a whole, the published and unpublished literature supports the idea that the APC sits at the apex of the stress and nutrient-sensing pathways, controlling cell cycle progression, DNA repair, and chromosome maintenance (Figure 3).

14. Conclusions

The positioning of the APC at the intersection point of the stress and nutrient sensing pathways confers importance upon this complex, as it may have the potential to protect the cells that come together to form the zygote from the aging process. The potential for aging likely begins for an individual as soon as the germ cells responsible for them are born. For the oocyte, that means during the mother's in utero development. It will be many years before that oocyte is fertilized; therefore, plenty of time exists for damaging side effects of cell metabolism to rear their ugly heads. It is critical that the repair mechanisms within these cells are functioning optimally. As long as the APC is at its peak function, protection against cellular damage should be high. With continued proper function of the APC through the life of the germ cells and the subsequent offspring, increased healthspan may be possible.

Acknowledgments: Franco Vizeacoumar and Frederick Vizeacoumar generated the data displayed in Figure 4. Christopher Eskiw edited drafts of this manuscript, and Terra Arnason provided fruitful discussions during the writing of this manuscript.

References

1. Sobel, H. When does human aging start? *Gerontologist* **1966**, *6*, 17–22. [CrossRef] [PubMed]
2. Lakatta, E.G. So! What's aging? Is cardiovascular aging a disease? *J. Mol. Cell. Cardiol.* **2015**, *83*, 1–13. [CrossRef] [PubMed]
3. Paashuis-Lew, Y.R.; Heddle, J.A. Spontaneous mutation during fetal development and post-natal growth. *Mutagenesis* **1998**, *13*, 613–617. [CrossRef] [PubMed]
4. Relton, C.L.; Daniel, C.P.; Hammal, D.M.; Parker, L.; Janet Tawn, E.; Burn, J. DNA repair gene polymorphisms, pre-natal factors and the frequency of somatic mutations in the glycophorin-A gene among healthy newborns. *Mutat. Res.* **2004**, *545*, 49–57. [CrossRef] [PubMed]
5. Milne, E.M. When does human ageing begin? *Mech. Ageing Dev.* **2006**, *127*, 290–297. [CrossRef] [PubMed]
6. Kubben, N.; Misteli, T. Shared molecular and cellular mechanisms of premature ageing and ageing-associated diseases. *Nat. Rev. Mol. Cell Biol.* **2017**, *18*, 595–609. [CrossRef] [PubMed]
7. Hayflick, L. When does aging begin? *Res. Aging* **1984**, *6*, 99–103. [CrossRef] [PubMed]
8. Hayflick, L. The future of ageing. *Nature* **2000**, *408*, 267–269. [CrossRef] [PubMed]
9. Hayflick, L. The not-so-close relationship between biological aging and age-associated pathologies in humans. *J. Gerontol. A Biol. Sci. Med. Sci.* **2004**, *59*, B547–B550. [CrossRef] [PubMed]
10. Kirkwood, T.B.; Austad, S.N. Why do we age? *Nature* **2000**, *408*, 233–238. [CrossRef] [PubMed]
11. Nemoto, S.; Finkel, T. Ageing and the mystery at Arles. *Nature* **2004**, *429*, 149–152. [CrossRef] [PubMed]
12. Harman, D. Aging: A theory based on free radical and radiation chemistry. *J. Gerontol.* **1956**, *11*, 298–300. [CrossRef] [PubMed]
13. Hayflick, L. Entropy explains aging, genetic determination explains longevity, and undefined terminology explains misunderstanding both. *PLoS Genet.* **2007**, *3*, e220. [CrossRef] [PubMed]
14. Labbadia, J.; Morimoto, R.I. Proteostasis and longevity: When does aging really begin? *F1000Prime Rep.* **2014**, *6*, 7. [CrossRef] [PubMed]
15. Kirkwood, T.B.; Holliday, R. The evolution of ageing and longevity. *Proc. R. Soc. Lond. B Biol. Sci.* **1979**, *205*, 531–546. [CrossRef] [PubMed]
16. Kenyon, C.J. The genetics of ageing. *Nature* **2010**, *464*, 504–512. [CrossRef] [PubMed]
17. Salminen, A.; Kaarniranta, K. ER stress and hormetic regulation of the aging process. *Ageing Res. Rev.* **2010**, *9*, 211–217. [CrossRef] [PubMed]
18. Martins, I.; Galluzzi, L.; Kroemer, G. Hormesis, cell death and aging. *Aging* **2011**, *3*, 821–828. [CrossRef] [PubMed]
19. Williams, G.C. Pleiotrophy, natural selection and the evolution of senescence. *Evolution* **1957**, *22*, 406–421.
20. Kirkwood, T.B.; Rose, M.R. Evolution of senescence: Late survival sacrificed for reproduction. *Philos. Trans. R Soc. Lond. B Biol. Sci.* **1991**, *332*, 15–24. [CrossRef] [PubMed]
21. Nesse, R.M.; Williams, G.C. Evolution and the origins of disease. *Sci. Am.* **1998**, *279*, 86–93. [CrossRef] [PubMed]
22. Wick, G.; Berger, P.; Jansen-Dürr, P.; Grubeck-Loebenstein, B.A. Darwinian-evolutionary concept of age-related diseases. *Exp. Gerontol.* **2003**, *38*, 13–25. [CrossRef]

23. Artandi, S.E.; DePinho, R.A. A critical role for telomeres in suppressing and facilitating carcinogenesis. *Curr. Opin. Genet. Dev.* **2000**, *10*, 39–46. [CrossRef]
24. Shay, J.W.; Wright, W.E. Ageing and cancer: The telomere and telomerase connection. *Novartis Found. Symp.* **2001**, *235*, 116–125. [PubMed]
25. López-Otín, C.; Blasco, M.A.; Partridge, L.; Serrano, M.; Kroemer, G. The hallmarks of aging. *Cell* **2013**, *153*, 1194–1217. [CrossRef] [PubMed]
26. Aunan, J.R.; Watson, M.M.; Hagland, H.R.; Søreide, K. Molecular and biological hallmarks of ageing. *Br. J. Surg.* **2016**, *103*, e29–e46. [CrossRef] [PubMed]
27. Kaeberlein, M.; McVey, M.; Guarente, L. The SIR2/3/4 complex and SIR2 alone promote longevity in *Saccharomyces cerevisiae* by two different mechanisms. *Genes Dev.* **1999**, *13*, 2570–2580. [CrossRef] [PubMed]
28. Fabrizio, P.; Pozza, F.; Pletcher, S.D.; Gendron, C.M.; Longo, V.D. Regulation of longevity and stress resistance by Sch9 in yeast. *Science* **2001**, *292*, 288–290. [CrossRef] [PubMed]
29. Wei, M.; Fabrizio, P.; Hu, J.; Ge, H.; Cheng, C.; Li, L.; Longo, V.D. Life span extension by calorie restriction depends on Rim15 and transcription factors downstream of Ras/PKA, Tor, and Sch9. *PLoS Genet.* **2008**, *4*, e13. [CrossRef] [PubMed]
30. Lu, J.Y.; Lin, Y.Y.; Sheu, J.C.; Wu, J.T.; Lee, F.J.; Chen, Y.; Lin, M.I.; Chiang, F.T.; Tai, T.Y.; Berger, S.L.; et al. Acetylation of yeast AMPK controls intrinsic aging independently of caloric restriction. *Cell* **2011**, *146*, 969–979. [CrossRef] [PubMed]
31. Postnikoff, S.D.; Malo, M.M.; Wong, B.; Harkness, T.A. The yeast forkhead transcription factors fkh1 and fkh2 regulate lifespan and stress response together with the anaphase-promoting complex. *PLoS Genet.* **2012**, *8*, e1002583. [CrossRef] [PubMed]
32. Jiao, R.; Postnikoff, S.; Harkness, T.A.; Arnason, T.G. The SNF1 Kinase Ubiquitin-associated Domain Restrains Its Activation, Activity, and the Yeast Life Span. *J. Biol. Chem.* **2015**, *290*, 15393–15404. [CrossRef] [PubMed]
33. Mirisola, M.G.; Taormina, G.; Fabrizio, P.; Wei, M.; Hu, J.; Longo, V.D. Serine- and threonine/valine-dependent activation of PDK and Tor orthologs converge on Sch9 to promote aging. *PLoS Genet.* **2014**, *10*, e1004113. [CrossRef] [PubMed]
34. Dong, X.; Milholland, B.; Vijg, J. Evidence for a limit to human lifespan. *Nature* **2016**, *538*, 257–259. [CrossRef] [PubMed]
35. Robine, J.M.; Allard, M. The oldest human. *Science* **1998**, *279*, 1834–1835. [CrossRef] [PubMed]
36. Weon, B.M.; Je, J.H. Theoretical estimation of maximum human lifespan. *Biogerontology* **2009**, *10*, 65–71. [CrossRef] [PubMed]
37. Modig, K.; Andersson, T.; Vaupel, J.; Rau, R.; Ahlbom, A. How long do centenarians survive? Life expectancy and maximum lifespan. *J. Intern. Med.* **2017**, *282*, 156–163. [CrossRef] [PubMed]
38. Gerontology Research Group. Available online: http://supercentenarian-research-foundation.org/TableE.aspx (accessed on 30 April 2018).
39. De Grey, A. A strategy for postponing aging indefinitely. *Stud. Health Technol. Inform.* **2005**, *118*, 209–219. [PubMed]
40. Lenart, A.; Vaupel, J.W. Questionable evidence for a limit to human lifespan. *Nature* **2017**, *546*, E13–E14. [CrossRef] [PubMed]
41. Hughes, B.G.; Hekimi, S. Many possible maximum lifespan trajectories. *Nature* **2017**, *546*, E8–E9. [CrossRef] [PubMed]
42. Takahashi, Y.; Kuro-o, M.; Ishikawa, F. Aging mechanisms. *Proc. Natl. Acad. Sci. USA* **2000**, *97*, 12407–12408. [CrossRef] [PubMed]
43. Lucke, J.C.; Hall, W. Who wants to live forever? *EMBO Rep.* **2005**, *6*, 98–102. [CrossRef] [PubMed]
44. Tacutu, R.; Thornton, D.; Johnson, E.; Budovsky, A.; Barardo, D.; Craig, T.; Diana, E.; Lehmann, G.; Toren, D.; Wang, J.; et al. Human Ageing Genomic Resources: New and updated databases. *Nucleic Acids Res.* **2018**, *46*, D1083–D1090. [CrossRef] [PubMed]
45. Lindahl, T. Instability and decay of the primary structure of DNA. *Nature* **1993**, *362*, 709–715. [CrossRef] [PubMed]
46. Hoeijmakers, J.H. DNA damage, aging, and cancer. *N. Engl. J. Med.* **2009**, *361*, 1475–1485. [CrossRef] [PubMed]
47. Cervelli, T.; Borghini, A.; Galli, A.; Andreassi, M.G. DNA damage and repair in atherosclerosis: Current insights and future perspectives. *Int. J. Mol. Sci.* **2012**, *13*, 16929–16944. [CrossRef] [PubMed]

48. Vijg, J.; Suh, Y. Genome instability and aging. *Annu. Rev. Physiol.* **2013**, *75*, 645–668. [CrossRef] [PubMed]
49. Grindel, A.; Brath, H.; Nersesyan, A.; Knasmueller, S.; Wagner, K.H. Association of genomic instability with HbA1c levels and medication in diabetic patients. *Sci. Rep.* **2017**, *7*, 41985. [CrossRef] [PubMed]
50. Yuza, K.; Nagahashi, M.; Watanabe, S.; Takabe, K.; Wakai, T. Hypermutation and microsatellite instability in gastrointestinal cancers. *Oncotarget* **2017**, *8*, 112103–112115. [CrossRef] [PubMed]
51. Barzilai, A.; Schumacher, B.; Shiloh, Y. Genome instability: Linking ageing and brain degeneration. *Mech. Ageing Dev.* **2017**, *161*, 4–18. [CrossRef] [PubMed]
52. Henderson, K.A.; Gottschling, D.E. A mother's sacrifice: what is she keeping for herself? *Curr. Opin. Cell Biol.* **2008**, *20*, 723–728. [CrossRef] [PubMed]
53. Gottschling, D.E.; Nyström, T. The Upsides and Downsides of Organelle Interconnectivity. *Cell* **2017**, *169*, 24–34. [CrossRef] [PubMed]
54. Sun, Y.C.; Sun, X.F.; Dyce, P.W.; Shen, W.; Chen, H. The role of germ cell loss during primordial follicle assembly: A review of current advances. *Int. J. Biol. Sci.* **2017**, *13*, 449–457. [CrossRef] [PubMed]
55. Sivakumar, S.; Gorbsky, G.J. Spatiotemporal regulation of the anaphase-promoting complex in mitosis. *Nat. Rev. Mol. Cell Biol.* **2015**, *16*, 82–94. [CrossRef] [PubMed]
56. Zhang, S.; Chang, L.; Alfieri, C.; Zhang, Z.; Yang, J.; Maslen, S.; Skehel, M.; Barford, D. Molecular mechanism of APC/C activation by mitotic phosphorylation. *Nature* **2016**, *533*, 260–264. [CrossRef] [PubMed]
57. Zhou, Z.; He, M.; Shah, A.A.; Wan, Y. Insights into APC/C: From cellular function to diseases and therapeutics. *Cell Div.* **2016**, *11*, 9. [CrossRef] [PubMed]
58. Fukushima, H.; Ogura, K.; Wan, L.; Lu, Y.; Li, V.; Gao, D.; Liu, P.; Lau, A.W.; Wu, T.; Kirschner, M.W.; et al. SCF-mediated Cdh1 degradation defines a negative feedback system that coordinates cell-cycle progression. *Cell Rep.* **2013**, *4*, 803–816. [CrossRef] [PubMed]
59. Simpson-Lavy, K.J.; Sajman, J.; Zenvirth, D.; Brandeis, M. APC/CCdh1 specific degradation of Hsl1 and Clb2 is required for proper stress responses of *S. cerevisiae*. *Cell Cycle* **2009**, *8*, 3003–3009. [CrossRef] [PubMed]
60. Harkness, T.A.; Davies, G.F.; Ramaswamy, V.; Arnason, T.G. The ubiquitin-dependent targeting pathway in Saccharomyces cerevisiae plays a critical role in multiple chromatin assembly regulatory steps. *Genetics* **2002**, *162*, 615–632. [PubMed]
61. Harkness, T.A.; Shea, K.A.; Legrand, C.; Brahmania, M.; Davies, G.F. A functional analysis reveals dependence on the Anaphase Promoting Complex for prolonged life span in yeast. *Genetics* **2004**, *168*, 759–774. [CrossRef] [PubMed]
62. Lindsay, D.L.; Bonham-Smith, P.C.; Postnikoff, S.; Gray, G.R.; Harkness, T.A. A role for the anaphase promoting complex in hormone regulation. *Planta* **2011**, *233*, 1223–1235. [CrossRef] [PubMed]
63. Postnikoff, S.D.; Harkness, T.A. Mechanistic insights into aging, cell-cycle progression, and stress response. *Front. Physiol.* **2012**, *3*, 183. [CrossRef] [PubMed]
64. Menzel, J.; Malo, M.E.; Chan, C.; Prusinkiewicz, M.; Arnason, T.G.; Harkness, T.A. The anaphase promoting complex regulates yeast lifespan and rDNA stability by targeting Fob1 for degradation. *Genetics* **2014**, *196*, 693–709. [CrossRef] [PubMed]
65. Malo, M.E.; Postnikoff, S.D.; Arnason, T.G.; Harkness, T.A. Mitotic degradation of yeast Fkh1 by the Anaphase Promoting Complex is required for normal longevity, genomic stability and stress resistance. *Aging* **2016**, *8*, 810–830. [CrossRef] [PubMed]
66. Ganem, N.J.; Pellman, D. Linking abnormal mitosis to the acquisition of DNA damage. *J. Cell Biol.* **2012**, *199*, 871–881. [CrossRef] [PubMed]
67. Harkness, T.A.; Arnason, T.G.; Legrand, C.; Pisclevich, M.G.; Davies, G.F.; Turner, E.L. Contribution of CAF-I to anaphase-promoting-complex-mediated mitotic chromatin assembly in *Saccharomyces cerevisiae*. *Eukaryot Cell* **2005**, *4*, 673–684. [CrossRef] [PubMed]
68. Arnason, T.G.; Pisclevich, M.G.; Dash, M.D.; Davies, G.F.; Harkness, T.A. Novel interaction between Apc5p and Rsp5p in an intracellular signaling pathway in *Saccharomyces cerevisiae*. *Eukaryot Cell* **2005**, *4*, 134–146. [CrossRef] [PubMed]
69. Turner, E.L.; Malo, M.E.; Pisclevich, M.G.; Dash, M.D.; Davies, G.F.; Arnason, T.G.; Harkness, T.A. The *Saccharomyces cerevisiae* Anaphase Promoting Complex interacts with multiple histone-modifying enzymes to regulate cell cycle progression. *Eukaryot Cell* **2010**, *9*, 1418–1431. [CrossRef] [PubMed]
70. Islam, A.; Turner, E.L.; Menzel, J.; Malo, M.E.; Harkness, T.A. Antagonistic Gcn5-Hda1 interactions revealed by mutations to the Anaphase Promoting Complex in yeast. *Cell Div.* **2011**, *6*, 13. [CrossRef] [PubMed]

71. Linger, J.G.; Tyler, J.K. Chromatin Disassembly and Reassembly during DNA Repair. *Mutat. Res.* **2007**, *618*, 52–64. [CrossRef] [PubMed]
72. Li, X.; Tyler, J.K. Nucleosome disassembly during human non-homologous end joining followed by concerted HIRA- and CAF-1-dependent reassembly. *eLife* **2016**, *5*, e15129. [CrossRef] [PubMed]
73. Mello, J.A.; Sillјé, H.H.W.; Roche, D.M.J.; Kirschner, D.B.; Nigg, E.A.; Almouzni, G. Human Asf1 and CAF-1 interact and synergize in a repair-coupled nucleosome assembly pathway. *EMBO Rep.* **2002**, *3*, 329–334. [CrossRef] [PubMed]
74. Chen, C.C.; Tyler, J. Chromatin reassembly signals the end of DNA repair. *Cell Cycle* **2008**, *7*, 3792–3797. [CrossRef] [PubMed]
75. Kim, J.A.; Haber, J.E. Chromatin assembly factors Asf1 and CAF-1 have overlapping roles in deactivating the DNA damage checkpoint when DNA repair is complete. *Proc. Natl. Acad. Sci. USA* **2009**, *106*, 1151–1156. [CrossRef] [PubMed]
76. Rodriges Blanko, E.; Kadyrova, L.Y.; Kadyrov, F.A. DNA Mismatch Repair Interacts with CAF-1- and ASF1A-H3-H4-dependent Histone $(H3\text{-}H4)_2$ Tetramer Deposition. *J. Biol. Chem.* **2016**, *291*, 9203–9217. [CrossRef] [PubMed]
77. Izawa, D.; Pines, J. The mitotic checkpoint complex binds a second CDC20 to inhibit active APC/C. *Nature* **2015**, *517*, 631–634. [CrossRef] [PubMed]
78. Alfieri, C.; Chang, L.; Zhang, Z.; Yang, J.; Maslen, S.; Skehel, M.; Barford, D. Molecular basis of APC/C regulation by the spindle assembly checkpoint. *Nature* **2016**, *536*, 431–436. [CrossRef] [PubMed]
79. Zhu, G.; Spellman, P.T.; Volpe, T.; Brown, P.O.; Botstein, D.; Davis, T.N.; Futcher, B. Two yeast forkhead genes regulate the cell cycle and pseudohyphal growth. *Nature* **2000**, *406*, 90–94. [CrossRef] [PubMed]
80. Rudner, A.D.; Murray, A.W. Phosphorylation by Cdc28 activates the Cdc20-dependent activity of the anaphase-promoting complex. *J. Cell Biol.* **2000**, *149*, 1377–1390. [CrossRef] [PubMed]
81. Kotani, S.; Tugendreich, S.; Fujii, M.; Jorgensen, P.M.; Watanabe, N.; Hoog, C.; Hieter, P.; Todokoro, K. PKA and MPF-activated polo-like kinase regulate anaphase-promoting complex activity and mitosis progression. *Mol. Cell* **1998**, *1*, 371–380. [CrossRef]
82. Crasta, K.; Lim, H.H.; Giddings, T.H., Jr.; Winey, M.; Surana, U. Inactivation of Cdh1 by synergistic action of Cdk1 and polo kinase is necessary for proper assembly of the mitotic spindle. *Nat. Cell Biol.* **2008**, *10*, 665–675. [CrossRef] [PubMed]
83. Kim, H.S.; Vassilopoulos, A.; Wang, R.H.; Lahusen, T.; Xiao, Z. SIRT2 maintains genome integrity and suppresses tumorigenesis through regulating APC/C activity. *Cancer Cell* **2011**, *20*, 487–499. [CrossRef] [PubMed]
84. Zhang, J.; Wan, L.; Dai, X.; Sun, Y.; Wei, W. Functional characterization of Anaphase Promoting Complex/Cyclosome (APC/C) E3 ubiquitin ligases in tumorigenesis. *Biochim. Biophys. Acta* **2014**, *1845*, 277–293. [PubMed]
85. Peters, J.M. The anaphase promoting complex/cyclosome: A machine designed to destroy. *Nat. Rev. Mol. Cell Biol.* **2006**, *7*, 644–656. [CrossRef] [PubMed]
86. Sackton, K.L.; Dimova, N.; Zeng, X.; Tian, W.; Zhang, M.; Sackton, T.B.; Meaders, J.; Pfaff, K.L.; Sigoillot, F.; Yu, H.; et al. Synergistic blockade of mitotic exit by two chemical inhibitors of the APC/C. *Nature* **2014**, *514*, 646–649. [CrossRef] [PubMed]
87. Wang, L.; Zhang, J.; Wan, L.; Zhou, X.; Wang, Z.; Wei, W. Targeting Cdc20 as a novel cancer therapeutic strategy. *Pharmacol. Ther.* **2015**, *151*, 141–151. [CrossRef] [PubMed]
88. Sansregret, L.; Patterson, J.O.; Dewhurst, S.; López-García, C.; Koch, A.; McGranahan, N.; Chao, W.C.H.; Barry, D.J.; Rowan, A.; Instrell, R.; et al. APC/C Dysfunction Limits Excessive Cancer Chromosomal Instability. *Cancer Discov.* **2017**, *7*, 218–233. [CrossRef] [PubMed]
89. Thu, K.L.; Silvester, J.; Elliott, M.J.; Ba-Alawi, W.; Duncan, M.H.; Elia, A.C.; Mer, A.S.; Smirnov, P.; Safikhani, Z.; Haibe-Kains, B.; et al. Disruption of the anaphase-promoting complex confers resistance to TTK inhibitors in triple-negative breast cancer. *Proc. Natl. Acad. Sci. USA* **2018**, *115*, E1570–E1577. [CrossRef] [PubMed]
90. Kastl, J.; Braun, J.; Prestel, A.; Möller, H.M.; Huhn, T.; Mayer, T.U. Mad2 Inhibitor-1 (M2I-1): A Small Molecule Protein-Protein Interaction Inhibitor Targeting the Mitotic Spindle Assembly Checkpoint. *ACS Chem. Biol.* **2015**, *10*, 1661–1666. [CrossRef] [PubMed]

91. Stegmeier, F.; Huang, J.; Rahal, R.; Zmolik, J.; Moazed, D.; Amon, A. The replication fork block protein Fob1 functions as a negative regulator of the FEAR network. *Curr. Biol.* **2004**, *14*, 467–480. [CrossRef] [PubMed]
92. Waples, W.G.; Chahwan, C.; Ciechonska, M.; Lavoie, B.D. Putting the brake on FEAR: Tof2 promotes the biphasic release of Cdc14 phosphatase during mitotic exit. *Mol. Biol. Cell* **2009**, *20*, 245–255. [CrossRef] [PubMed]
93. Visintin, R.; Craig, K.; Hwang, E.S.; Prinz, S.; Tyers, M.; Amon, A. The phosphatase Cdc14 triggers mitotic exit by reversal of Cdk-dependent phosphorylation. *Mol. Cell* **1998**, *2*, 709–718. [CrossRef]
94. Karra, H.; Repo, H.; Ahonen, I.; Löyttyniemi, E.; Pitkänen, R.; Lintunen, M.; Kuopio, T.; Söderström, M.; Kronqvist, P. Cdc20 and securin overexpression predict short-term breast cancer survival. *Br. J. Cancer* **2014**, *110*, 2905–2913. [CrossRef] [PubMed]
95. Schmit, T.L.; Ledesma, M.C.; Ahmad, N. Modulating polo-like kinase 1 as a means for cancer chemoprevention. *Pharm. Res.* **2010**, *27*, 989–998. [CrossRef] [PubMed]
96. Staff, S.; Isola, J.; Jumppanen, M.; Tanner, M. Aurora-A gene is frequently amplified in basal-like breast cancer. *Oncol. Rep.* **2010**, *23*, 307–312. [CrossRef] [PubMed]
97. Heredia, F.F.; de Sousa, J.C.; Ribeiro Junior, H.L.; Carvalho, A.F.; Magalhaes, S.M.; Pinheiro, R.F. Proteins related to the spindle and checkpoint mitotic emphasize the different pathogenesis of hypoplastic MDS. *Leuk. Res.* **2014**, *38*, 218–224. [CrossRef] [PubMed]
98. Kuo, T.C.; Lu, H.P.; Chao, C.C. The tyrosine kinase inhibitor sorafenib sensitizes hepatocellular carcinoma cells to taxol by suppressing the HURP protein. *Biochem. Pharmacol.* **2011**, *82*, 184–194. [CrossRef] [PubMed]
99. Xiang, W.; Wu, X.; Huang, C.; Wang, M.; Zhao, X.; Luo, G.; Li, Y.; Jiang, G.; Xiao, X.; Zeng, F. PTTG1 regulated by miR-146a-3p promotes bladder cancer migration, invasion, metastasis and growth. *Oncotarget* **2017**, *8*, 664–678. [CrossRef] [PubMed]
100. Zhang, L.; Cai, M.; Gong, Z.; Zhang, B.; Li, Y.; Guan, L.; Hou, X.; Li, Q.; Liu, G.; Xue, Z.; et al. Geminin facilitates FoxO3 deacetylation to promote breast cancer cell metastasis. *J. Clin. Investig.* **2017**, *127*, 2159–2175. [CrossRef] [PubMed]
101. Irniger, S.; Bäumer, M.; Braus, G.H. Glucose and ras activity influence the ubiquitin ligases APC/C and SCF in *Saccharomyces cerevisiae*. *Genetics* **2000**, *154*, 1509–1521. [PubMed]
102. Bolte, M.; Dieckhoff, P.; Krause, C.; Braus, G.H.; Irniger, S. Synergistic inhibition of APC/C by glucose and activated Ras proteins can be mediated by each of the Tpk1-3 proteins in *Saccharomyces cerevisiae*. *Microbiology* **2003**, *149*, 1205–1216. [CrossRef] [PubMed]
103. Searle, J.S.; Schollaert, K.L.; Wilkins, B.J.; Sanchez, Y. The DNA damage checkpoint and PKA pathways converge on APC substrates and Cdc20 to regulate mitotic progression. *Nat. Cell Biol.* **2004**, *6*, 138–145. [CrossRef] [PubMed]
104. Cocklin, R.; Goebl, M. Nutrient sensing kinases PKA and Sch9 phosphorylate the catalytic domain of the ubiquitin-conjugating enzyme Cdc34. *PLoS ONE* **2011**, *6*, e27099. [CrossRef] [PubMed]
105. Choudhury, R.; Bonacci, T.; Arceci, A.; Lahiri, D.; Mills, C.A.; Kernan, J.L.; Branigan, T.B.; DeCaprio, J.A.; Burke, D.J.; Emanuele, M.J. APC/C and SCF(cyclin F) constitute a reciprocal feedback circuit controlling S-phase entry. *Cell Rep.* **2016**, *16*, 3359–3372. [CrossRef] [PubMed]
106. Wang, F.; Nguyen, M.; Qin, F.X.; Tong, Q. SIRT2 deacetylates FOXO3a in response to oxidative stress and caloric restriction. *Aging Cell* **2007**, *6*, 505–514. [CrossRef] [PubMed]
107. Linke, C.; Klipp, E.; Lehrach, H.; Barberis, M.; Krobitsch, S. Fkh1 and Fkh2 associate with Sir2 to control CLB2 transcription under normal and oxidative stress conditions. *Front. Physiol.* **2013**, *4*, 173. [CrossRef] [PubMed]
108. Jiao, R.; Lobanova, L.; Waldner, A.; Fu, A.; Xiao, L.; Harkness, T.A.; Arnason, T.G. The ubiquitin-conjugating enzyme, Ubc1, indirectly regulates SNF1 kinase activity via Forkhead-dependent transcription. *Microb. Cell* **2016**, *3*, 540–553. [CrossRef] [PubMed]
109. Chiacchiera, F.; Simone, C. The AMPK-FoxO3A axis as a target for cancer treatment. *Cell Cycle* **2010**, *9*, 1091–1096. [CrossRef] [PubMed]
110. Salminen, A.; Kaarniranta, K. AMP-activated protein kinase (AMPK) controls the aging process via an integrated signaling network. *Ageing Res. Rev.* **2012**, *11*, 230–241. [CrossRef] [PubMed]
111. Wei, W.; Ayad, N.G.; Wan, Y.; Zhang, G.J.; Kirschner, M.W.; Kaelin, W.G., Jr. Degradation of the SCF component Skp2 in cell-cycle phase G1 by the anaphase-promoting complex. *Nature* **2004**, *428*, 194–198. [CrossRef] [PubMed]

112. Bashir, T.; Dorrello, N.V.; Amador, V.; Guardavaccaro, D.; Pagano, M. Control of the SCF(Skp2-Cks1) ubiquitin ligase by the APC/C(Cdh1) ubiquitin ligase. *Nature* **2004**, *428*, 190–193. [CrossRef] [PubMed]
113. Wang, F.; Higgins, J.M. Histone modifications and mitosis: countermarks, landmarks, and bookmarks. *Trends Cell Biol.* **2013**, *23*, 175–184. [CrossRef] [PubMed]
114. Guppy, B.J.; McManus, K.J. Mitotic accumulation of dimethylated lysine 79 of histone H3 is important for maintaining genome integrity during mitosis in human cells. *Genetics* **2015**, *199*, 423–433. [CrossRef] [PubMed]
115. Recht, J.; Tsubota, T.; Tanny, J.C.; Diaz, R.L.; Berger, J.M.; Zhang, X.; Garcia, B.A.; Shabanowitz, J.; Burlingame, A.L.; Hunt, D.F.; et al. Histone chaperone Asf1 is required for histone H3 lysine 56 acetylation, a modification associated with S phase in mitosis and meiosis. *Proc. Natl. Acad. Sci. USA* **2006**, *103*, 6988–6993. [CrossRef] [PubMed]
116. Jeong, Y.S.; Cho, S.; Park, J.S.; Ko, Y.; Kang, Y.K. Phosphorylation of serine-10 of histone H3 shields modified lysine-9 selectively during mitosis. *Genes Cells* **2010**, *15*, 181–192. [CrossRef] [PubMed]
117. Karmodiya, K.; Krebs, A.R.; Oulad-Abdelghani, M.; Kimura, H.; Tora, L.H. 3K9 and H3K14 acetylation co-occur at many gene regulatory elements, while H3K14ac marks a subset of inactive inducible promoters in mouse embryonic stem cells. *BMC Genom.* **2012**, *13*, 424. [CrossRef] [PubMed]
118. Gates, L.A.; Shi, J.; Rohira, A.D.; Feng, Q.; Zhu, B.; Bedford, M.T.; Sagum, C.A.; Jung, S.Y.; Qin, J.; Tsai, M.J.; et al. Acetylation on histone H3 lysine 9 mediates a switch from transcription initiation to elongation. *J. Biol. Chem.* **2017**, *292*, 14456–14472. [CrossRef] [PubMed]
119. Downs, J.A. Histone H3 K56 acetylation, chromatin assembly, and the DNA damage checkpoint. *DNA Repair* **2008**, *7*, 2020–2024. [CrossRef] [PubMed]
120. Farooq, Z.; Banday, S.; Pandita, T.K.; Altaf, M. The many faces of histone H3K79 methylation. *Mutat. Res. Rev. Mutat. Res.* **2016**, *768*, 46–52. [CrossRef] [PubMed]
121. Wood, K.; Tellier, M.; Murphy, S. DOT1L and H3K79 Methylation in Transcription and Genomic Stability. *Biomolecules* **2018**, *8*, E11. [CrossRef] [PubMed]
122. Cea, M.; Cagnetta, A.; Adamia, S.; Acharya, C.; Tai, Y.T.; Fulciniti, M.; Ohguchi, H.; Munshi, A.; Acharya, P.; Bhasin, M.K.; et al. Evidence for a role of the histone deacetylase SIRT6 in DNA damage response of multiple myeloma cells. *Blood* **2016**, *127*, 1138–1150. [CrossRef] [PubMed]
123. Ercilla, A.; Llopis, A.; Feu, S.; Aranda, S.; Ernfors, P. New origin firing is inhibited by APC/CCdh1 activation in S-phase after severe replication stress. *Nucleic Acids Res.* **2016**, *44*, 4745–4762. [CrossRef] [PubMed]
124. Garzón, J.; Rodríguez, R.; Kong, Z.; Chabes, A.; Rodríguez-Acebes, S.; Méndez, J.; Moreno, S.; García-Higuera, I. Shortage of dNTPs underlies altered replication dynamics and DNA breakage in the absence of the APC/C cofactor Cdh1. *Oncogene* **2017**, *36*, 5808–5818. [CrossRef] [PubMed]
125. Wäsch, R.; Engelbert, D. Anaphase-promoting complex-dependent proteolysis of cell cycle regulators and genomic instability of cancer cells. *Oncogene* **2005**, *24*, 1–10. [CrossRef] [PubMed]
126. Cardozo, T.; Pagano, M. Wrenches in the works: Drug discovery targeting the SCF ubiquitin ligase and APC/C complexes. *BMC Biochem.* **2007**, *8* (Suppl. 1), S9. [CrossRef] [PubMed]
127. Bolanos-Garcia, V.M. Assessment of the mitotic spindle assembly checkpoint (SAC) as the target of anticancer therapies. *Curr. Cancer Drug Targets* **2009**, *9*, 131–141. [CrossRef] [PubMed]
128. Taniguchi, K.; Momiyama, N.; Ueda, M.; Matsuyama, R.; Mori, R.; Fujii, Y.; Ichikawa, Y.; Endo, I.; Togo, S.; Shimada, H. Targeting of CDC20 via Small Interfering RNA Causes Enhancement of the Cytotoxicity of Chemoradiation. *Anticancer Res.* **2008**, *28*, 1559–1563. [PubMed]
129. Chang, D.Z.; Ma, Y.; Ji, B.; Liu, Y.; Hwu, P.; Abbruzzese, J.L.; Logsdon, C.; Wang, H. Increased CDC20 expression is associated with pancreatic ductal adenocarcinoma differentiation and progression. *J. Hematol. Oncol.* **2012**, *5*, 15. [CrossRef] [PubMed]
130. Lub, S.; Maes, A.; Maes, K.; De Veirman, K.; De Bruyne, E.; Menu, E.; Fostier, K.; Kassambara, A.; Moreaux, J.; Hose, D.; et al. Inhibiting the anaphase promoting complex/cyclosome induces a metaphase arrest and cell death in multiple myeloma cells. *Oncotarget* **2016**, *7*, 4062–4076. [CrossRef] [PubMed]
131. Mortensen, E.M.; Haas, W.; Gygi, M.; Gygi, S.P.; Kellogg, D.R. Cdc28-dependent regulation of the Cdc5/Polo kinase. *Curr. Biol.* **2005**, *15*, 2033–2037. [CrossRef] [PubMed]
132. Visintin, C.; Tomson, B.N.; Rahal, R.; Paulson, J.; Cohen, M.; Taunton, J.; Amon, A.; Visintin, R. APC/C-Cdh1-mediated degradation of the Polo kinase Cdc5 promotes the return of Cdc14 into the nucleolus. *Genes Dev.* **2008**, *22*, 79–90. [CrossRef] [PubMed]

133. Pramila, T.; Wu, W.; Miles, S.; Noble, W.S.; Breeden, L.L. The Forkhead transcription factor Hcm1 regulates chromosome segregation genes and fills the S-phase gap in the transcriptional circuitry of the cell cycle. *Genes Dev.* **2006**, *20*, 2266–2278. [CrossRef] [PubMed]
134. Lamb, J.R.; Michaud, W.A.; Sikorski, R.S.; Hieter, P.A. Cdc16p, Cdc23p and Cdc27p form a complex essential for mitosis. *EMBO J.* **1994**, *13*, 4321–4328. [PubMed]
135. Irniger, S.; Nasmyth, K. The anaphase-promoting complex is required in G1 arrested yeast cells to inhibit B-type cyclin accumulation and to prevent uncontrolled entry into S-phase. *J. Cell Sci.* **1997**, *110*, 1523–1531. [PubMed]
136. Li, M.; York, J.P.; Zhang, P. Loss of Cdc20 causes a securin-dependent metaphase arrest in two-cell mouse embryos. *Mol. Cell. Biol.* **2007**, *27*, 3481–3488. [CrossRef] [PubMed]
137. TCGA. Available online: https://portal.gdc.cancer.gov (accessed on 1 January 2018).
138. Ishizawa, J.; Sugihara, E.; Kuninaka, S.; Mogushi, K.; Kojima, K.; Benton, C.B.; Zhao, R.; Chachad, D.; Hashimoto, N.; Jacamo, R.O.; et al. FZR1 loss increases sensitivity to DNA damage and consequently promotes murine and human B-cell acute leukemia. *Blood* **2017**, *129*, 1958–1968. [CrossRef] [PubMed]
139. Villa-Hernández, S.; Bueno, A.; Bermejo, R. The Multiple Roles of Ubiquitylation in Regulating Challenged DNA Replication. *Adv. Exp. Med. Biol.* **2017**, *1042*, 395–419. [PubMed]
140. Kitao, H.; Iimori, M.; Kataoka, Y.; Wakasa, T.; Tokunaga, E. DNA replication stress and cancer chemotherapy. *Cancer Sci.* **2018**, *109*, 264–271. [CrossRef] [PubMed]
141. Wang, Q.; Moyret-Lalle, C.; Couzon, F.; Surbiguet-Clippe, C.; Saurin, J.C.; Lorca, T.; Navarro, C.; Puisieux, A. Alterations of anaphase-promoting complex genes in human colon cancer cells. *Oncogene* **2003**, *22*, 1486–1490. [CrossRef] [PubMed]
142. Park, K.H.; Choi, S.E.; Eom, M.; Kang, Y. Downregulation of the anaphase-promoting complex (APC)7 in invasive ductal carcinomas of the breast and its clinicopathologic relationships. *Breast Cancer Res.* **2005**, *7*, R238–R247. [CrossRef] [PubMed]
143. Kim, I.Y.; Kwon, H.Y.; Park, K.H.; Kim, D.S. Anaphase-Promoting Complex 7 is a Prognostic Factor in Human Colorectal Cancer. *Ann. Coloproctol.* **2017**, *33*, 139–145. [CrossRef] [PubMed]
144. Tsuda, Y.; Iimori, M.; Nakashima, Y.; Nakanishi, R.; Ando, K.; Ohgaki, K.; Kitao, H.; Saeki, H.; Oki, E.; Maehara, Y. Mitotic slippage and the subsequent cell fates after inhibition of Aurora B during tubulin-binding agent-induced mitotic arrest. *Sci. Rep.* **2017**, *7*, 16762. [CrossRef] [PubMed]
145. Haschka, M.; Karbon, G.; Fava, L.L.; Villunger, A. Perturbing mitosis for anti-cancer therapy: Is cell death the only answer? *EMBO Rep.* **2018**, *19*, e45440. [CrossRef] [PubMed]
146. Kops, G.J.; Foltz, D.R.; Cleveland, D.W. Lethality to human cancer cells through massive chromosome loss by inhibition of the mitotic checkpoint. *Proc. Natl. Acad. Sci. USA* **2004**, *101*, 8699–8704. [CrossRef] [PubMed]
147. Bharadwaj, R.; Yu, H. The spindle checkpoint, aneuploidy, and cancer. *Oncogene* **2004**, *23*, 2016–2027. [CrossRef] [PubMed]
148. Lee, M.; Rivera-Rivera, Y.; Moreno, C.S.; Saavedra, H.I. The E2F activators control multiple mitotic regulators and maintain genomic integrity through Sgo1 and BubR1. *Oncotarget* **2017**, *8*, 77649–77672. [CrossRef] [PubMed]
149. Hollenhorst, P.C.; Bose, M.E.; Mielke, M.R.; Müller, U.; Fox, C.A. Forkhead genes in transcriptional silencing, cell morphology and the cell cycle. Overlapping and distinct functions for FKH1 and FKH2 in *Saccharomyces cerevisiae*. *Genetics* **2000**, *154*, 1533–1548. [PubMed]
150. Rodríguez-Colman, M.J.; Sorolla, M.A.; Vall-Llaura, N.; Tamarit, J.; Ros, J.; Cabiscol, E. The FOX transcription factor Hcm1 regulates oxidative metabolism in response to early nutrient limitation in yeast. Role of Snf1 and Tor1/Sch9 kinases. *Biochim. Biophys. Acta* **2013**, *1833*, 2004–2015. [CrossRef] [PubMed]
151. Rodrigo-Brenni, M.C.; Morgan, D.O. Sequential E2s drive polyubiquitin chain assembly on APC targets. *Cell* **2007**, *130*, 127–139. [CrossRef] [PubMed]
152. Kobayashi, T.; Horiuchi, T. A yeast gene product, Fob1 protein, required for both replication fork blocking and recombinational hotspot activities. *Genes Cells* **1996**, *1*, 465–474. [CrossRef] [PubMed]
153. Kobayashi, T.; Heck, D.J.; Nomura, M.; Horiuchi, T. Expansion and contraction of ribosomal DNA repeats in *Saccharomyces cerevisiae*: Requirement of replication fork blocking (Fob1) protein and the role of RNA polymerase I. *Genes Dev.* **1998**, *12*, 3821–3830. [CrossRef] [PubMed]

154. Defossez, P.A.; Prusty, R.; Kaeberlein, M.; Lin, S.J.; Ferrigno, P.; Silver, P.A.; Keil, R.L.; Guarente, L. Elimination of replication block protein Fob1 extends the life span of yeast mother cells. *Mol. Cell* **1999**, *3*, 447–455. [CrossRef]
155. Yamashita, Y.M.; Nakaseko, Y.; Samejima, I.; Kumada, K.; Yamada, H.; Michaelson, D.; Yanagida, M. 20S cyclosome complex formation and proteolytic activity inhibited by the cAMP/PKA pathway. *Nature* **1996**, *384*, 276–279. [CrossRef] [PubMed]
156. Madia, F.; Gattazzo, C.; Wei, M.; Fabrizio, P.; Burhans, W.C.; Weinberger, M.; Galbani, A.; Smith, J.R.; Nguyen, C.; Huey, S.; et al. Longevity mutation in SCH9 prevents recombination errors and premature genomic instability in a Werner/Bloom model system. *J. Cell Biol.* **2008**, *180*, 67–81. [CrossRef] [PubMed]
157. Qie, B.; Lyu, Z.; Lyu, L.; Liu, J.; Gao, X.; Liu, Y.; Duan, W.; Zhang, N.; Du, L.; Liu, K. Sch9 regulates intracellular protein ubiquitination by controlling stress responses. *Redox Biol.* **2015**, *5*, 290–300. [CrossRef] [PubMed]
158. Kaeberlein, M.; Powers, R.W., 3rd; Steffen, K.K.; Westman, E.A.; Hu, D.; Dang, N.; Kerr, E.O.; Kirkland, K.T.; Fields, S.; Kennedy, B.K. Regulation of yeast replicative life span by TOR and Sch9 in response to nutrients. *Science* **2005**, *310*, 1193–1196. [CrossRef] [PubMed]

5

Disordered Expression of *shaggy*, the *Drosophila* Gene Encoding a Serine-Threonine Protein Kinase GSK3, Affects the Lifespan in a Transcript-, Stage-, and Tissue-Specific Manner

Mikhail V. Trostnikov [1,2], Natalia V. Roshina [1,2], Stepan V. Boldyrev [1,2], Ekaterina R. Veselkina [1], Andrey A. Zhuikov [1], Anna V. Krementsova [1,3] and Elena G. Pasyukova [1,*]

1 Institute of Molecular Genetics of RAS, Kurchatov Sq. 2, 123182 Moscow, Russia; mikhail.trostnikov@gmail.com (M.V.T.); nwumr@yandex.ru (N.V.R.); beibaraban34@gmail.com (S.V.B.); veselkinaer@gmail.com (E.R.V.); homkabrut@gmail.com (A.A.Z.); akrementsova@mail.ru (A.V.K.)

2 Vavilov Institute of General Genetics, Russian Academy of Sciences, Gubkin 3, 119991 Moscow, Russia

3 Emmanuel Institute of Biochemical Physics, Russian Academy of Sciences, Kosygin St. 4, 119334 Moscow, Russia

* Correspondence: egpas@rambler.ru

Abstract: GSK3 (glycogen synthase kinase 3) is a conserved protein kinase governing numerous regulatory pathways. In *Drosophila melanogaster*, GSK3 is encoded by *shaggy* (*sgg*), which forms 17 annotated transcripts corresponding to 10 protein isoforms. Our goal was to demonstrate how differential *sgg* transcription affects lifespan, which GSK3 isoforms are important for the nervous system, and which changes in the nervous system accompany accelerated aging. Overexpression of three *sgg* transcripts affected the lifespan in a stage- and tissue-specific way: *sgg-RA* and *sgg-RO* affected the lifespan only when overexpressed in muscles and in embryos, respectively; the essential *sgg-RB* transcript affected lifespan when overexpressed in all tissues tested. In the nervous system, only *sgg-RB* overexpression affected lifespan, causing accelerated aging in a neuron-specific way, with the strongest effects in dopaminergic neurons and the weakest effects in GABAergic neurons. Pan-neuronal *sgg-RB* overexpression violated the properties of the nervous system, including the integrity of neuron bodies; the number, distribution, and structure of mitochondria; cytoskeletal characteristics; and synaptic activity. Such changes observed in young individuals indicated premature aging of their nervous system, which paralleled a decline in survival. Our findings demonstrated the key role of GSK3 in ensuring the link between the pathology of neurons and lifespan.

Keywords: GSK3 (glycogen synthase kinase 3); protein kinases; transcription; lifespan; the nervous system; *Drosophila melanogaster*

---

1. Introduction

GSK3 (glycogen synthase kinase 3) is an actively studied, highly conserved serine–threonine protein kinase that is primarily regulated by inhibition and is involved in multiple signaling pathways that regulate embryogenesis and differentiation; cell renewal, migration, and apoptosis; gene transcription; metabolism; and survival via more than 50 target proteins with phosphorylation sites for GSK3 [1,2]. In humans, there are two main forms of GSK3, α and β, encoded by the two highly homologous genes; in *Drosophila*, only one form exists, which is closer to GSK3β.

In *D. melanogaster*, GSK3 plays multiple roles in the development and function of the nervous system, starting from the early development stages. GSK3 directly phosphorylates aPKC (atypical protein kinase C) [3,4], a key component ensuring asymmetric neuroblast division during *D. melanogaster* early development. GSK3 participates in the development of neural precursor cells [5] and, via InR/TOR (Insulin Receptor/Target of Rapamycin) signaling, in the control of dendrite pruning during larval-pupal transition [6]. Moreover, GSK3 controls synapse formation, growth, and morphological structure by controlling the dynamics of the microtubule cytoskeleton [7–9] and regulates axonal stability and neural circuit integrity via the Wnt pathway [10]. GSK3 also regulates neurotransmitter release into NMJs (neuromuscular junctions) [8]. GSK3 directly phosphorylates microtubule-associated protein tau [11,12]. Overexpression of human tau in *D. melanogaster* disrupts axonal transport causing vesicle aggregation, and co-overexpression of constitutively active GSK3 enhances the effects [13]. Two functions of GSK3 specifically attracted our attention to this protein.

First, GSK3 participates in the control of asymmetric neuroblast division. Earlier, we demonstrated that functional changes in several genes involved in the regulation of this developmental process, namely, *aPKC* encoding the GSK3 target, aPKC, *escargot* and *inscutable*, affect the lifespan of adult flies [14,15]. Moreover, our previous studies suggest that changes in gene expression at the embryonic stage can be responsible for an increase in adult lifespan due to yet unknown mechanisms that provide this carry-over effect [16]. Therefore, we were interested in understanding whether GSK3 function, especially during the embryonic stage, also affects lifespan.

Second, GSK3 severely affects the functionality of the tau protein, which leads to the development of various age-dependent neurodegenerative diseases and significantly reduces life expectancy [11,17]. We were interested in understanding whether changes in GSK3 expression in the nervous system directly affect lifespan and, if yes, we aimed to identify which structural and functional properties of the nervous system accompany alterations in lifespan and rate of aging.

In *Drosophila melanogaster*, GSK3 is encoded by the gene, *shaggy* (*sgg*), which forms 17 annotated transcripts corresponding to 10 annotated protein isoforms (Available online: http://flybase.org/reports/FBgn0003371). To address the questions raised, first, it was necessary to understand which transcripts and protein isoforms encoded by *sgg* are functional. Ten *sgg* transcripts and at least five Sgg proteins of different primary structure were initially demonstrated [18]. The major Sgg isoform that is detected at essentially all stages of the life cycle and in different tissues [18,19] is encoded by six transcripts annotated in FlyBase (Available online: http://flybase.org/reports/FBgn0003371), including *sgg-RB* (GenBank #AY122193.1). Only a few other *sgg* transcripts were reported as full-size cDNAs: *sgg-RA* (GenBank #X70863.1); *sgg-RD* (GenBank #BT133153.1); *sgg-RG* (GenBank #AY119664.1 and #BT050474.1); and *sgg-RO* (GenBank #BT072831.1). Analysis of the proteome revealed three Sgg isoforms, namely, Sgg-PA, Sgg-PB, and Sgg-PD, in the embryonic cell line, Kc167; no isoforms were found in fly tissues [20–22]. Two isoforms, Sgg-PA and Sgg-PB, corresponding to sgg39 and sgg10 isoforms of Ruel and coauthors [18], were detected in recent functional studies; however, the functionality of alterations in Sgg-PA expression was not revealed [9,23].

In this paper, we described the effects of the misexpression of four *sgg* transcripts (*sgg-RA*, *sgg-RB*, *sgg-RG*, and *sgg-RO*) on *Drosophila* lifespan and aging. Different *sgg* transcripts demonstrated stage- and tissue-specificity; for example, *sgg-RA* affected lifespan only when overexpressed in muscles, and *sgg-RO* affected lifespan only when overexpressed in embryos. The sex-specific increase in adult lifespan was observed due to increased *sgg-RO* expression in embryos. Altering *sgg-RO* expression in embryos was enough to affect adult lifespan, which suggested the existence of some carry-over mechanisms of an epigenetic or other nature. The essential *sgg-RB* transcript was functional in all tissues tested, and in the nervous system, only *sgg-RB* overexpression affected lifespan, causing severe shortening. If overexpression took place in middle-aged adult flies, detrimental effects were alleviated compared to those of lifelong overexpression. Overexpression of *sgg-RB* in different types of neurons accelerated the aging of flies in a neuron-specific manner, with the most pronounced effects in dopaminergic neurons and the least pronounced effects in GABAergic neurons. Pan-neuronal *sgg-RB* overexpression severely violated the structural and functional properties of the nervous system: The integrity of neuron bodies, the number, distribution, and structure of mitochondria, cytoskeletal properties in the presynaptic zones, and synaptic activity. Overall, our data demonstrated a wide variety of effects of GSK3 on survival and proved its causal role in the aging of the nervous system.

2. Results and Discussion

2.1. *Differential Expression of Sgg Affects Lifespan*

According to the annotation given in FlyBase (Available online: https://flybase.org/reports/FBgn0003371), *sgg*, like many other genes, can potentially form many transcripts. Questions about what set of transcripts exist in a living organism, whether each transcript has specific functions that are different from those of other transcripts—in particular, whether the transcripts are specific for a given stage of development, age, and tissue—remain open. Our primary goal was to understand what *sgg* transcripts that are functional in the nervous system affect lifespan. However, to obtain a broader view, we tested the effects of some *sgg* transcripts in a restricted set of other tissues and at different stages. Our choice of transcripts was based on their presence in GenBank as full-size cDNAs, which indicated that these variants are actually formed when the gene is expressed. Our choice of additional tissues was based on the fact that the fat body was repeatedly shown to play an important role in lifespan control [24–26], whereas the role of muscles, on the contrary, is not broadly known [27]. Finally, to test the functionality of *sgg* transcripts, we used a complex phenotypic trait—lifespan.

A transgenic line providing overexpression of the essential *sgg* transcript *sgg-RB*, sggB, constructed by [19], was obtained from the Bloomington *Drosophila* Stock Center, USA (Available online: http://flystocks.bio.indiana.edu/) together with the corresponding control line (Control B). To assess the functionality of *sgg-RA*, *sgg-RG*, and *sgg-RO*, we obtained three transgenic lines providing overexpression of these transcripts: sggA, sggG, and sggO; the line initially used for transformations was used as a control line (Control AGO). We also acquired two lines with transgenic constructs providing *sgg* knockdown (sggKD1 and sggKD2), together with the control lines (Control KD1 and Control KD2) provided by the same manufacturer (Available online: http://flystocks.bio.indiana.edu/Browse/TRiPtb.htm).

Overexpression of *sgg-RA*, *sgg-RB*, *sgg-RG*, or *sgg-RO* induced by GAL4 drivers should specifically increase the amount of the corresponding transcripts, while knockdown induced by GAL4 drivers should decrease the amount of all *sgg* transcripts. The level of decrease was expected to depend on the effectiveness of the knockdown provided by different lines. sggKD1 was expected to provide a stronger level of knockdown and sggKD2 the weaker level of knockdown, according to the manufacturer's description (https://bdsc.indiana.edu/stocks/rnai/rnai_n_z.html). A detailed description of all the lines is given in the Materials and Methods section.

To roughly characterize *sgg* effects on lifespan, we induced transcript-specific *sgg* overexpression and overall *sgg* knockdown in embryos (the D1 driver line) and in three tissues: The fat body (the D2 driver line), muscles (the D3 driver line), and the nervous system (the D4 driver line), using the GAL4-UAS binary system [28].

Overexpression of *sgg-RB* in embryos was lethal, and overexpression of *sgg-RA* and *sgg-RG* had no effect on the lifespan of both males and females (Table S1, Figure 1A,B). Overexpression of *sgg-RO* affected male and female lifespans in opposite directions: In males, lifespan was significantly increased, while in females, lifespan was decreased (Table S1, Figure 1A,B). In the second experiment aimed to verify this result, the effects were reproduced, although the level of the effects was somewhat lower in both males and females (Table S1, Figure 1C,D). As expected, the effect of the overall *sgg* knockdown was lethal when the stronger sggKD1 line was used, while the weaker knockdown decreased the lifespans of both males and females (Table S1, Figure 1E,F).

Overexpression of *sgg-RB* in the fat body was lethal, and overexpression of *sgg-RA*, *sgg-RG*, and *sgg-RO* had no effect on the lifespans of both males and females (Table S2, Figure 2A,B). Strong *sgg* knockdown in the fat body caused lethality, while weak knockdown decreased the male lifespan and did not affect the female lifespan (Table S2, Figure 2C,D). In females, the survival curve indicated a possible positive effect of the reduced *sgg* function on lifespan.

Overexpression of *sgg-RA* and *sgg-RB* in muscles decreased both male and female lifespans, and overexpression of *sgg-RG* and *sgg-RO* had no effect on the lifespans of both males and females (Table S3, Figure 3A–D). A negative effect of *sgg-RA* overexpression was confirmed in the second experiment (Table S3). Both strong and weak knockdown in muscles decreased male and female lifespans to varying degrees (Table S3, Figure 3E,F).

Overexpression of *sgg-RB* in the nervous system severely reduced male and female lifespans (Table S4, Figure 4A,B), and overexpression of *sgg-RA*, *sgg-RG*, and *sgg-RO* had no effect on the lifespan of both males and females (Table S4, Figure 4C,D). Strong *sgg* knockdown in the nervous system caused lethality, while weak knockdown decreased both male and female lifespans (Table S4, Figure 4E,F). Of note, weak knockdown in the nervous system affected the lifespan to a lesser degree than in muscles and in embryos, where the effect was most pronounced.

Overall, a set of lifespan assays produced several noteworthy results (Figure 5). First, the effects of *sgg* misexpression on lifespan were mostly detrimental. The most adverse results, that is, lethality, were observed when either overexpression or knockdown were induced in embryos or in the fat body. However, increased *sgg-RO* expression in embryos increased the adult lifespan in a sex-dependent manner. Detailed research aimed at analyzing the molecular mechanisms underlying this positive effect is currently under way. The effects of gene expression early in life on lifespan are of particular interest for us because we have previously shown that changes in gene expression in embryos can lead to a sex-specific increase in longevity [16]. The sex-dependent effects of alterations in gene transcription on lifespan have often been observed by others, although the nature of this dependence remains unclear [29].

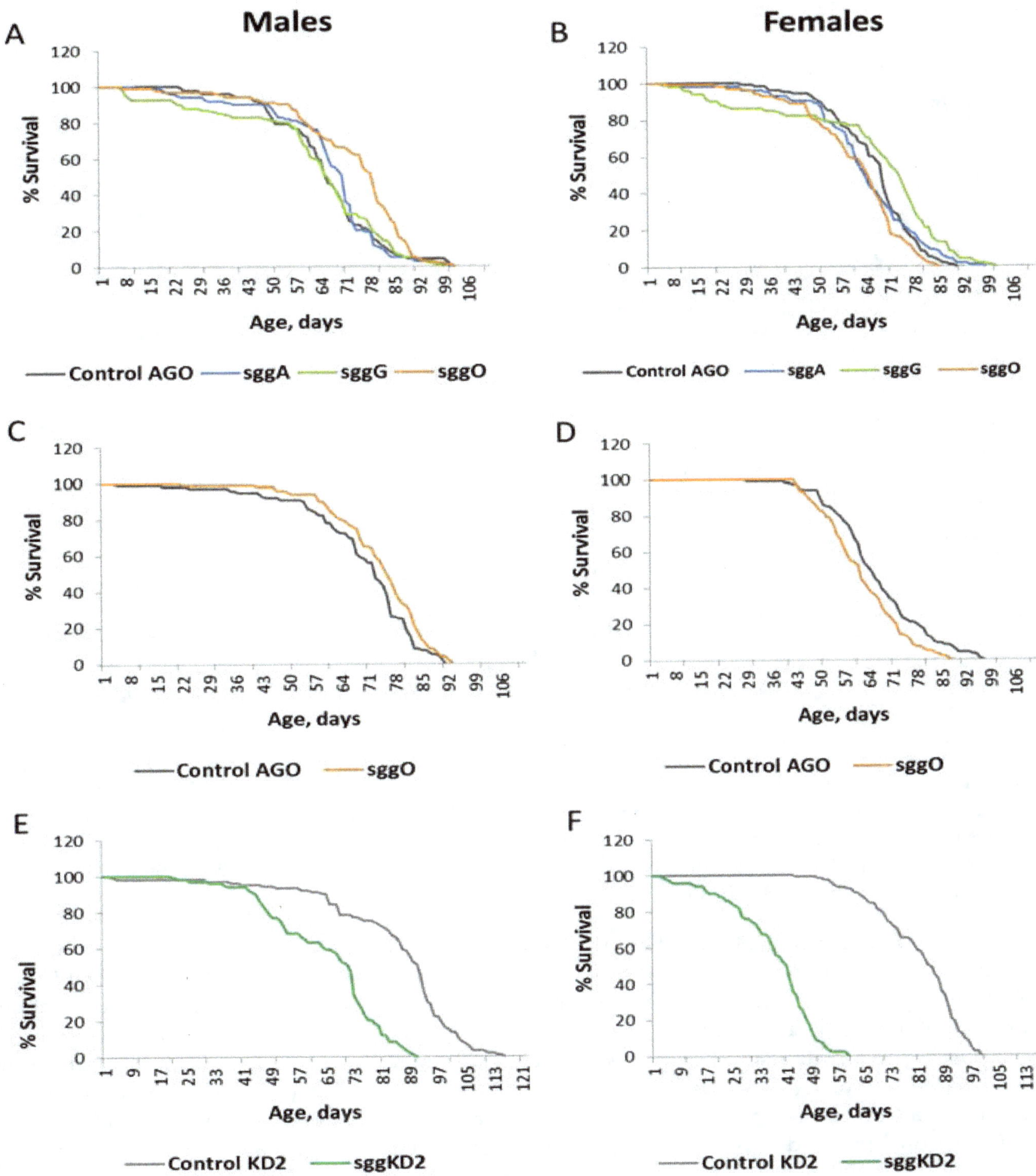

Figure 1. Effects of disordered *sgg* expression in embryos on male (**A**,**C**,**E**) and female (**B**,**D**,**F**) lifespans. Control AGO, sggA, sggG, sggO, Control KD2, and sggKD2 denote hybrid genotypes obtained as a result of crossing the corresponding lines with the driver line D1 inducing the expression of transgenic constructs in embryos. A full description of the genotypes is given in the Materials and Methods section.

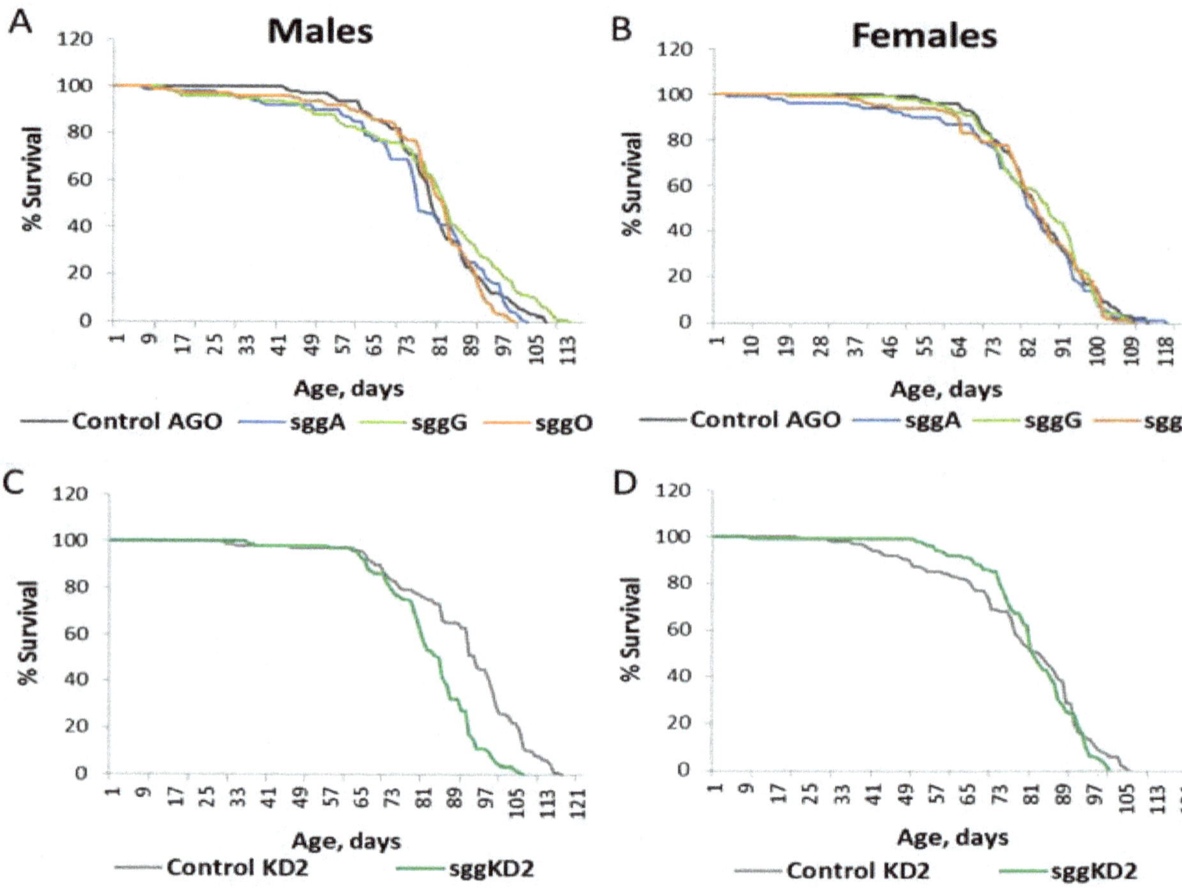

Figure 2. Effects of disordered *sgg* expression in the fat body on male (**A**,**C**) and female (**B**,**D**) lifespans. Control AGO, sggA, sggG, sggO, Control KD2, sggKD2, Control B, and sggA81T denote hybrid genotypes obtained as a result of crossing the corresponding lines with the driver line D2 inducing the expression of transgenic constructs in the fat body. A full description of genotypes is given in the Materials and Methods section. In panels **E** and **F**, the results of the two independent experiments are represented by solid and dotted lines.

Second, different transcripts had their own patterns of effects on lifespan. This fact confirmed that *sgg* functions in a cell-autonomous mode [19]. As expected, the previously well described [7,13,18,19] *sgg-RB* transcript affected lifespan when overexpressed in all tissues and at all stages tested, although the strength of the effect varied depending on the stage, age, and tissue. In the nervous system, *sgg-RB* appeared to be the only transcript with effects on lifespan. In embryos, of all minor transcripts tested, only the expression of *sgg-RO* affected the lifespan. As its effects were not detected in other tissues, we assume that this transcript may be specific for embryos and have a function that complements *sgg-RB* functions during development. Similarly, the *sgg-RA* transcript appeared to be functionally specific for muscles, where it also may complement *sgg-RB* functions. Transcripts that are specific for or preferred at certain developmental stages and particular tissues and organs have long been known (for example, [30–32]). The peculiarity of our data is that they allowed us to show in which tissues these transcripts are functional, judging by the integral phenotype used in our tests. Only one transcript, *sgg-RG*, did not show functionality in our tests, which, however, does not mean that it is generally deprived of any function, given the limited scope of our tests. Of note, we were able to overexpress individual transcripts, but knockdown reduced the expression of *sgg* transcripts all together; it would be interesting to evaluate the effects of decreased expression of individual transcripts on lifespan and other traits. We have already demonstrated that reduced transcription of a gene causes lifespan extension, whereas overexpression has detrimental effects [27].

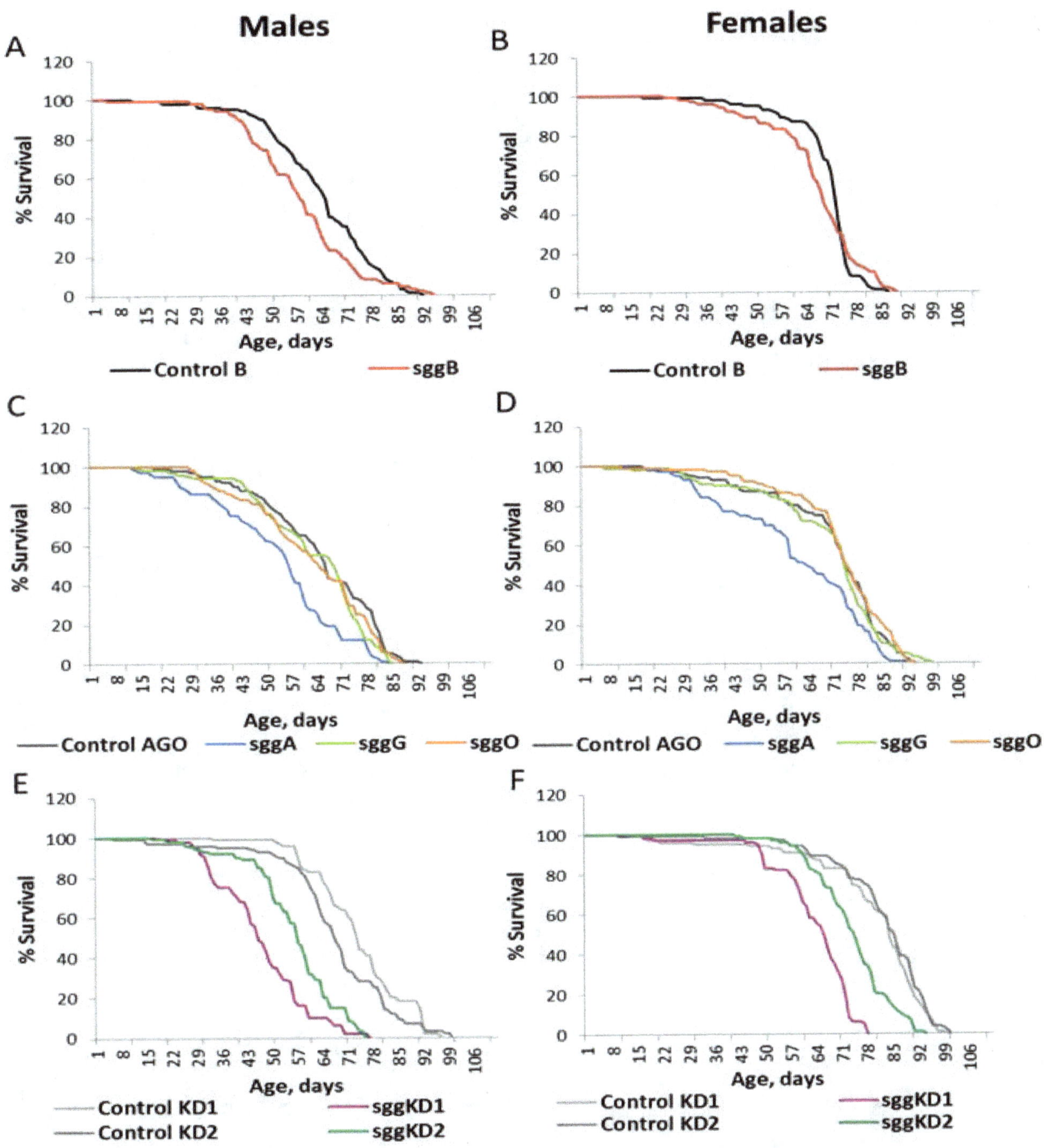

Figure 3. Effects of disordered *sgg* expression in muscles on male (**A**,**C**,**E**) and female (**B**,**D**,**F**) lifespans. Control B, sggB, Control AGO, sggA, sggG, sggO, Control KD1, sggKD1, Control KD2, and sggKD2 denote hybrid genotypes obtained as a result of crossing the corresponding lines with the driver line D3 inducing the expression of transgenic constructs in muscles. A full description of the genotypes is given in the Materials and Methods section.

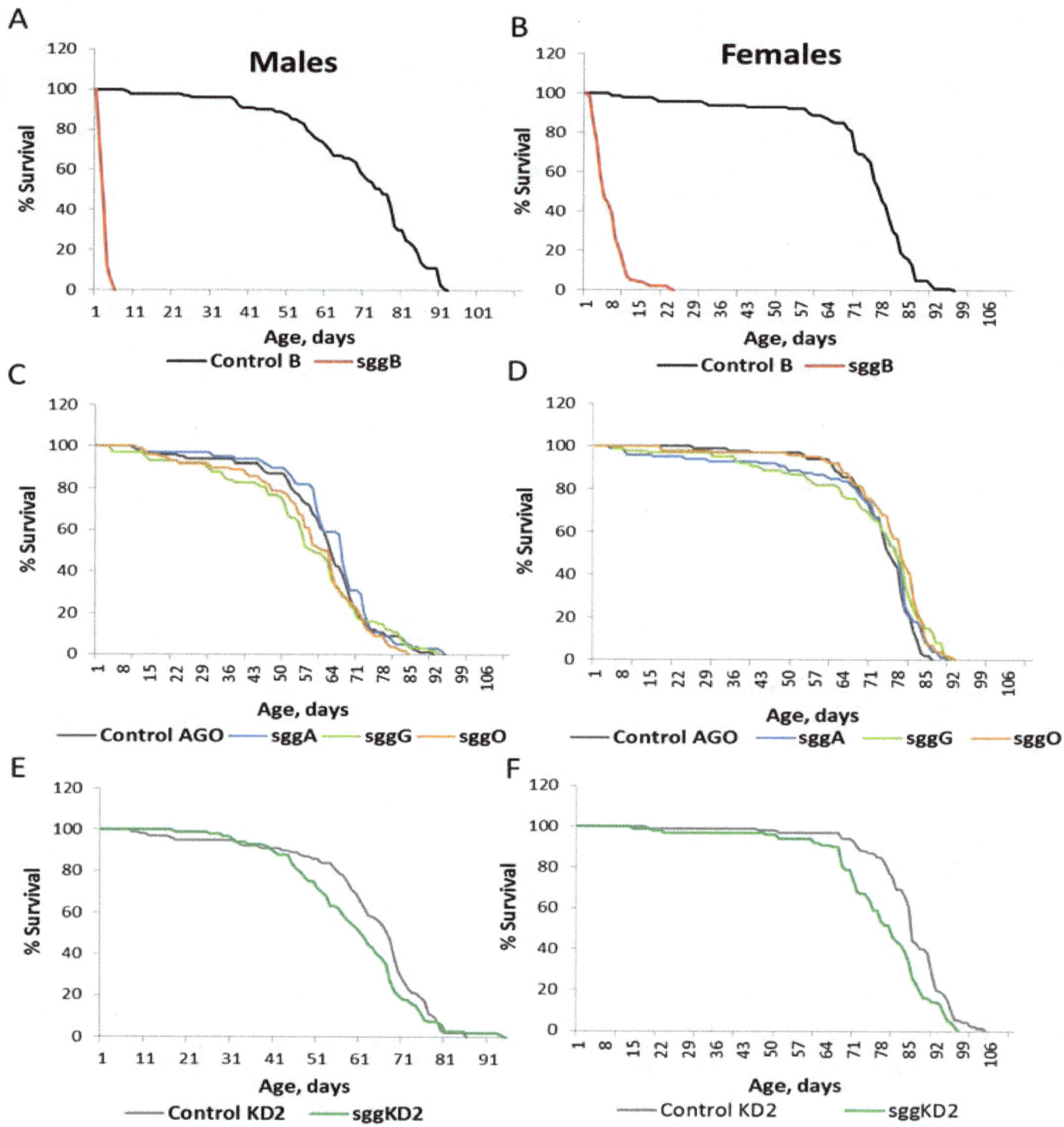

Figure 4. Effects of disordered *sgg* expression in the nervous system on male (**A**,**C**,**E**) and female (**B**,**D**,**F**) lifespans. Control B, sggB, Control AGO, sggA, sggG, sggO, Control KD2, and sggKD2 denote hybrid genotypes obtained as a result of crossing the corresponding lines with the driver line D4 inducing the lifelong expression of transgenic constructs in the nervous system. A full description of genotypes is given in the Materials and Methods section.

Tissues	**Embryo (D1 driver)**		**Fat body (D2 driver)**		**Muscles (D3 driver)**		**Nervous system (D4 driver)**	
Sex	♂	♀	♂	♀	♂	♀	♂	♀
***sgg* RA overexpression**	-	-	-	-	V-	VV	-	-
***sgg* RB overexpression**	L	L	L	L	V	V	VV	VV
***sgg* RG overexpression**	-	-	-	-	-	-	-	-
***sgg* RO overexpression**	ΛΛ	VV	-	-	-	-	-	-
Strong *sgg* knockdown	L	L	L	L	V	V	L	L
Weak *sgg* knockdown	V	V	V	-	V	V	V	V

Figure 5. Effects of disordered *sgg* expression in different tissues on male and female lifespans. Dark-red cells, L: lethal effects; red cells, V: lifespan significantly decreased; gray cells, -: no effect; green cells, Λ: lifespan significantly increased. The number of V or Λ characters in a cell denotes the number of independent experiments.

The fact that in the nervous system, only *sgg-RB* appeared to be functional gave us the necessary grounds for further analysis of the effects of *sgg* misexpression in the nervous system on the lifespan and structural and functional properties of neurons.

2.2. *Overexpression of sgg-RB in the Nervous System Affects Lifespan in a Stage/Age- and Neuron-Specific Manner*

We focused our efforts on the study of *sgg* overexpression in the nervous system because increased GSK3 function is thought to be associated with the development of several age-dependent pathological conditions, such as Alzheimer's disease and Parkinson's disease [12,33,34]. The increase in the number of *sgg-RB* transcripts and amount of GSK3 protein induced by the D4 panneuronal driver line was confirmed using real-time RT-qPCR and Western blotting, respectively ($p < 0.0001$ for comparisons between control and overexpressing individuals in both cases). Typical results of real-time RT-qPCR and Western blotting are illustrated in Figure S1.

Severe effects of *sgg-RB* overexpression in the nervous system on male and female lifespans were confirmed in the independent experiment, which was performed approximately a year after the first experiment (Table S4, Figure 6A,B). In both replicate experiments, the effects in males were more pronounced (Figure 4A,B and Figure 6A,B); however, flies of both sexes lived only several days.

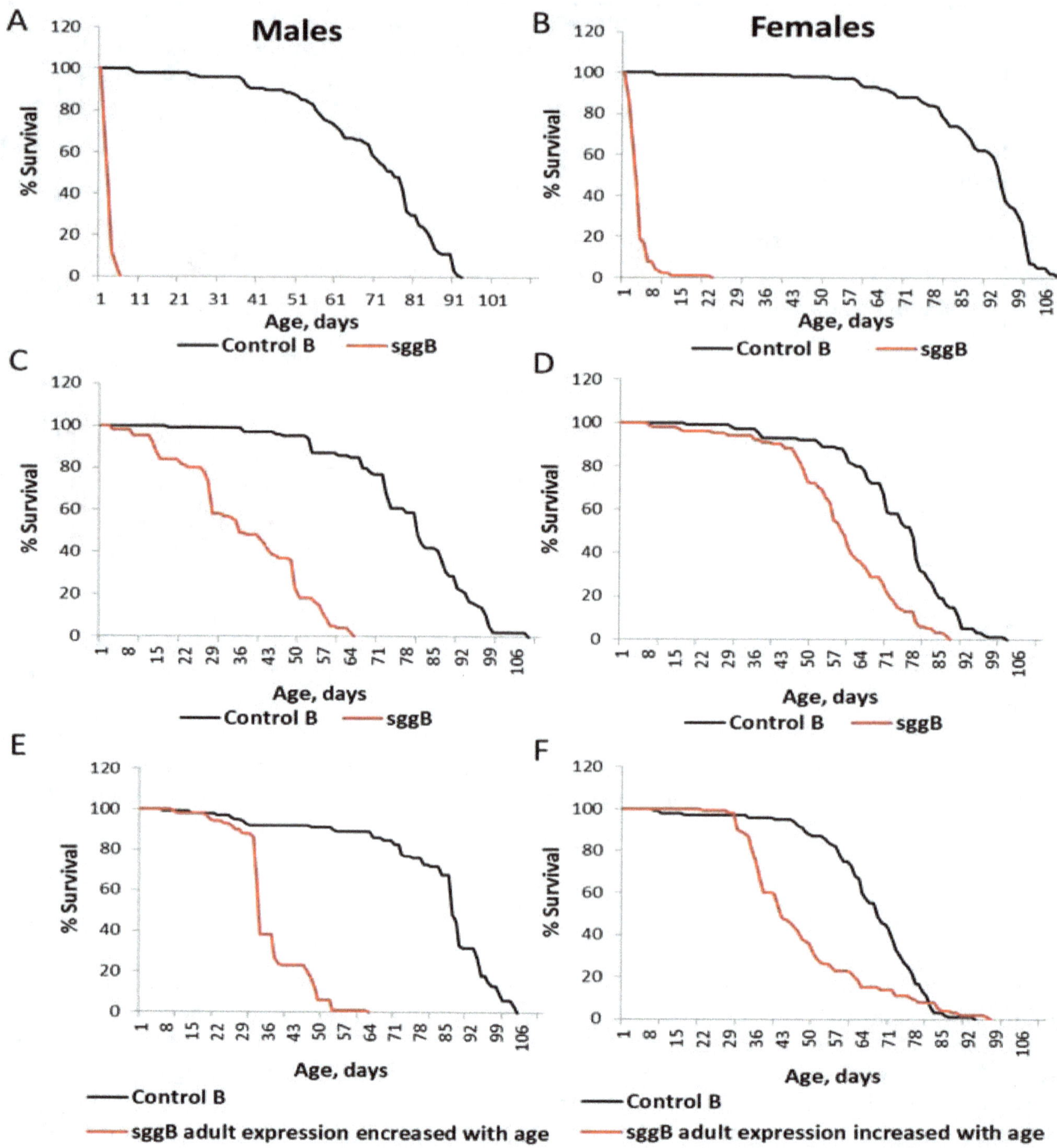

Figure 6. Effects of *sgg-RB* overexpression in the nervous system on male (**A**,**C**,**E**) and female (**B**,**D**,**F**) lifespans. Control B, sggB denote hybrid genotypes obtained as a result of crossing the corresponding lines with the driver line D4 inducing the lifelong expression of the transgenic construct in the nervous system (**A**,**B**), with the driver line D5 inducing the expression of the transgenic construct in the embryonic CNS (central nervous system) (**C**,**D**), and with the driver line D6 inducing the increasing expression of the transgenic construct in the adult nervous system with age (**E**,**F**). A full description of genotypes is given in the Materials and Methods section.

The *elav* driver (D4) used in the experiments described above provides lifelong expression in the nervous system, starting from the embryonic stage (see references at http://flybase.org/reports/FBti0002575.html).; therefore, we were not able to discriminate at which stage/age *sgg-RB* overexpression was significant for lifespan effects. To address this question, we used two additional drivers that induce the expression of transgenic constructs in the embryonic CNS (central nervous system) (D5; see references at http://flybase.org/reports/FBti0001255.html). and the increased with age expression of transgenic constructs in the adult nervous system (D6; see references at http://flybase.org/reports/FBti0040381.html). *sgg-RB* overexpression in the embryonic CNS decreased male and female lifespans, though to a lesser degree than lifelong panneuronal overexpression (Table S4, Figure 6C,D). This result indicated that normal *sgg-RB* expression in the CNS at the embryonic stage is important for lifespan determination; however, it does not fully account for the effects of lifelong panneuronal *sgg-RB* overexpression. According to the description given in FlyBase, the D6 driver should be switched on starting from the 50th day of life. However, survival curves obtained in our experiments (Table S4, Figure 6E,F) indicated that both control flies and flies with the *sgg-RB* transgene lived the same way until approximately the 30th day of life, but after that, the lifespans of both males and females with the *sgg-RB* transgene declined significantly faster compared to the control. These data clearly indicate that the D6 driver was switched on starting from the 30th day of life and that *sgg-RB* overexpression starting in the nervous system of middle-aged flies was sufficient to decrease their lifespans, though to a lesser degree than lifelong overexpression: The slope of survival curves in the latter case was much steeper both in males and females.

Overall, *sgg-RB* overexpression in the nervous system at different stages of development and aging negatively affected lifespan. Altering *sgg-RB* expression in the embryonic CNS was enough to affect the adult lifespan, which could be explained by epigenetic inheritance in cell lines or other yet unknown mechanisms. Based on our results, it is tempting to conclude that in the nervous system, embryonic *sgg-RB* overexpression is less detrimental than lifelong *sgg-RB* overexpression and *sgg-RB* overexpression in adults and that if overexpression took place in older adults, detrimental effects were alleviated. One of the theories of aging suggests that aging is caused by hyperfunction, that is, overactivity during adulthood of processes that are primarily important during development. Such hyperfunction can lead to hypertrophy-associated pathologies, which cause accelerated aging [35]. In the most general terms, smaller effects of overexpression in embryos would be in accordance with this theory. However, the strength of overexpression induced by different drivers in our experiments may be different and bias the comparisons. Experiments with a conditional tissue-specific transgene expression system using the elav-geneswitch driver could allow overexpression in larvae and adults at different ages and provide adequate comparison of the stage- and age-specific effects of altered *sgg-RB* expression. To compare the effects of overexpression in embryos and in adult flies, more sophisticated methods are needed, for example, combinations of GAL4 and GAL80 or split GAL4 drivers with different stage-specific patterns of expression, in accordance with the logic proposed in [36]. One cannot exclude the possibility that *sgg-RB* overexpression in old flies could become beneficial. Future experiments can shed light on these issues.

The *elav* driver (D4) provides panneuronal expression (see references at http://flybase.org/reports/FBti0002575.html); therefore, we were not able to discriminate which neurons are most sensitive to *sgg-RB* overexpression and are predominantly responsible for effects on lifespan. To address this question, we used several drivers (D7–D13) that induce the expression of transgenic constructs in neurons secreting different transmitters and in motor neurons. Two different drivers were used to induce *sgg-RB* overexpression in dopaminergic neurons, and in both cases, the effect was lethal. These neurons demonstrated maximum sensitivity to the level of *sgg-RB* expression. It remained unclear why in this case the panneuronal *sgg-RB* overexpression was not lethal; one mechanistic suggestion would be that in some neurons, *sgg-RB* overexpression had a positive effect on lifespan and that opposite effects counterbalanced each other. However, *sgg-RB* overexpression in all tested types of neurons decreased both male and female lifespans to varying degrees (Table S5, Figure S2). Overall, peptidergic neurons appeared to be highly sensitive; glutamate and cholinergic neurons, less sensitive; and motor and GABAergic neurons, the least sensitive to *sgg-RB* overexpression among the types of neurons tested, judging by the effect on lifespan. However, the level of the effect also depended on sex

(Figure S2). Other types of differently classified neurons might be worth testing in the future to better understand the specific impact of neurons on lifespan control provided by Sgg-RB.

Our results demonstrated that, despite the individual nuances, lifelong panneuronal *sgg-RB* overexpression would be an appropriate model system for further analyses of GSK impact on structural and functional properties of neurons. To better understand the association between the extent of lifespan reduction and alterations in neuronal characteristics, for further analyses, we also selected overexpression of *sgg-RB* in motor neurons as a second model system demonstrating moderate effects on lifespan. The choice of this additional model was also justified by the fact that we used larval NMJs (neuromuscular junctions) as a model synapse.

2.3. *Overexpression of Sgg-RB in the Nervous System Affects Neuronal Structure and Function*

We suggest that the lifespan reduction caused by aberrations in GSK3 expression in the nervous system is based on pathological changes in neurons. It was previously shown that *sgg* overexpression results in decreased numbers of synaptic boutons [7] and synapses [9], small synapses [8], and degeneration of presynaptic terminals and axons [10]. We decided to complement these results by some other structural and functional characteristics of the nervous system in flies with a dramatically decreased lifespan due to *sgg-RB* panneuronal overexpression and in flies with a moderately decreased lifespan due to *sgg-RB* overexpression in motor neurons.

2.3.1. Locomotion

First, we demonstrated that locomotion was highly impaired in 3- to 5-day-old males and females with panneuronal overexpression of *sgg-RB* (Figure 7A), indicating severe lesions in the functional status of the nervous system. These flies did not live longer than 10 days (males) or 15 days (females), and most of them hardly moved at all in the second half of life, so we were not able to characterize the age-dependent dynamics of their locomotion. In 3- to 5-day-old males and females with *sgg-RB* overexpression in motor neurons, locomotion was not changed compared to that of control flies, and in 20-day-old flies, locomotion was significantly increased compared to that of control flies (Figure 7B,C). In 40-day-old control flies, locomotion was still high, while in flies with *sgg-RB* overexpression in motor neurons, a substantial decline in locomotion was observed (Figure 7B,C). Of note, the mean lifespan of control males and females was 64 ± 3 and 68 ± 2 days, respectively (Table S4), and at the age of 40 days, the flies were not truly aging. The mean lifespan of males with *sgg-RB* overexpression in motor neurons was 35 ± 2 days (Table S4), and 40-day-old males were intensively aging, which was reflected in the rapid decline in locomotion that decreased below the control level. The mean lifespan of females with *sgg-RB* overexpression in motor neurons was 58 ± 2 days (Table S4), and the biological age of 40-day-old females was younger than in males, which was reflected in a smaller decline in locomotion that stayed at the control level. Overall, in our experiments, locomotion, as reported by [37], appeared to be a good marker of aging.

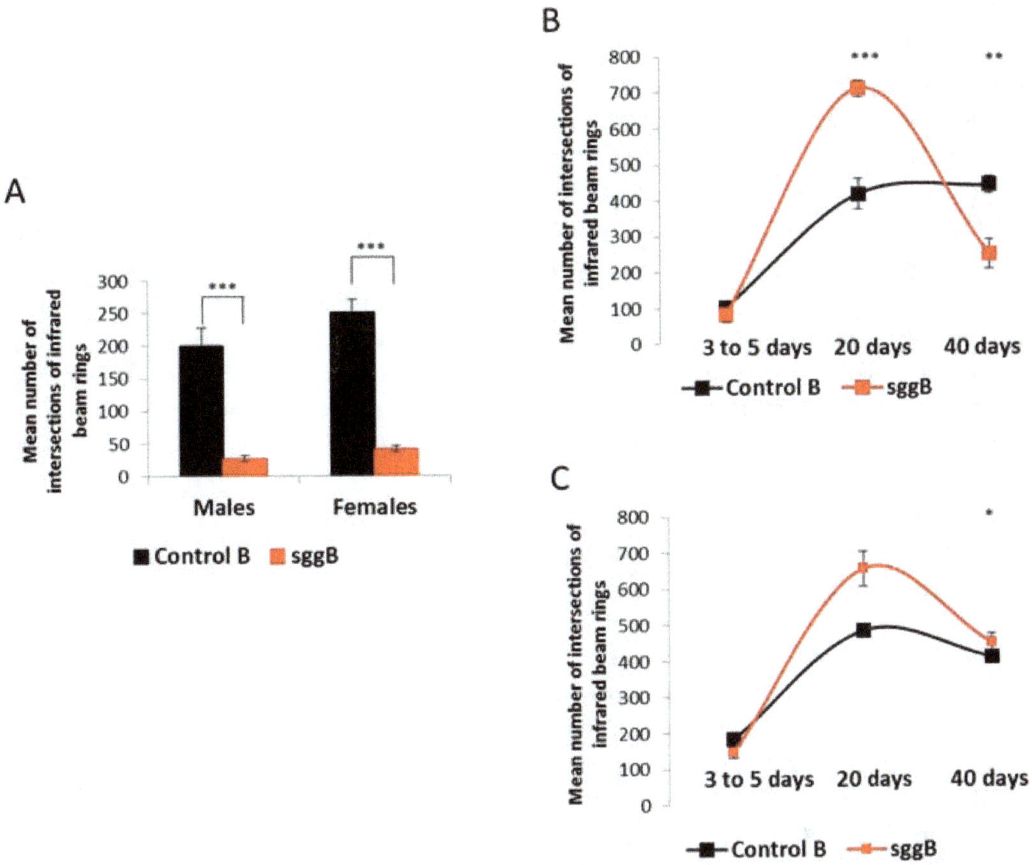

Figure 7. Effects of *sgg-RB* overexpression in the nervous system on locomotion of flies. Panneuronal *sgg-RB* overexpression in 1- to 3-day-old males and females (**A**). *sgg-RB* overexpression in motor neurons in males (**B**) and females (**C**). Control B, sggB denote hybrid genotypes obtained as a result of crossing the corresponding lines with the driver line D4 inducing the expression of transgenic constructs in the nervous system or the driver line D12 inducing the expression of transgenic constructs in motor neurons. A full description of genotypes is given in the Materials and Methods section. * denotes $p < 0.05$, ** denotes $p < 0.01$, *** denotes $p < 0.001$ determined by the Kruskal-Wallis test.

At the same time, an intriguing result of these experiments was that in 20-day-old flies with *sgg-RB* overexpression in motor neurons, the presumed decline in neuronal functions [7–10] and decreased lifespan were associated with elevated locomotion, indicating that the functional status of the nervous system necessary for ensuring motor functions was not only disturbed, but even improved. Simultaneous decreases in lifespan and increases in locomotion, both resulting from changes in the expression of a gene, have been reported previously [37]. It was suggested that mitochondrial function in neurons may change in such a way that the lifespan decreases due to the increased ROS (reactive oxygen species) production known to promote aging and shorten lifespan [38,39], whereas locomotion increases due to elevated mitochondrial activity and ATP levels. Indeed, the increase in mitochondrial function to a certain level should result in the increase of energy production accompanied by elevated levels of ROS. However, elevated ROS and ATP levels did not accompany a decrease in lifespan and an increase in locomotion described in [37], and the cellular mechanisms underlying an increase in locomotion remained obscure.

2.3.2. Mitochondria

The functionality of neurons critically depends on the energy supply, which is ensured by the work of mitochondria. Mitochondrial homeostasis, that is, precise control of mitochondrial number, integrity, and distribution, is especially critical to postmitotic cells, such as neurons. Violation of the fine-tuned interplay between mitochondrial function, energy metabolism, and neuronal activity is critical in the occurrence of various neurological pathologies [40]. We examined whether the number of mitochondria was affected by *sgg-RB* overexpression. For this purpose, we used larval NMJs, which are often used as a model system to study synapse development and function in *Drosophila* [41]. GSK3 is enriched in the presynaptic side of NMJs [7], so we focused on studying the presynaptic zone. Mitochondria are especially abundant at the presynaptic parts of axons. The number of GFP-labeled mitochondrial clusters was decreased in NMJs of individuals with panneuronal *sgg-RB* overexpression (Figure 8A,B) and *sgg-RB* overexpression in motor neurons (Figure 8C,D) to a similar extent. Thus, the decreased number of mitochondrial clusters was associated with both severe and moderate decreases in lifespan, but appeared to be not relevant to locomotion. Analysis of the brains of 3-day-old flies revealed swollen, dense mitochondria in all three individuals with pan-neuronal *sgg-RB* overexpression (Figure 9A–D). We failed to observe such mitochondria in control individuals (Figure 9E).

In individuals with *sgg-RB* overexpression, mitochondria were clustered predominantly in synaptic boutons, possibly to compensate for the overall decrease in number, whereas in control individuals, they were distributed more evenly along terminal ends of axons (Figure 8A,C). Mitochondria are produced in the neuronal soma and move to synapses, where they are needed for neuronal firing, along microtubules using kinesin motors; they can also move in the retrograde direction for reparation using dynein motors [42]. GSK3β is involved in the control of mitochondrial movement, both in increasing upon activation of the serotonin receptor [43] and in decreasing upon activation of the dopamine receptor [44,45]. GSK3β directly regulates dynein [46] and promotes anterograde movement [47]. We hypothesize that *sgg-RB* overexpression might affect mitochondrial movement and thus be responsible for disturbances in the distribution of mitochondria along axons.

2.3.3. Cytoskeleton

Not only mitochondrial movement, but also the overall functionality and architecture of neurons depend on the integrity of their cytoskeletons. We assessed the effects of *sgg-RB* overexpression in individuals with pan-neuronal *sgg-RB* overexpression and *sgg-RB* overexpression in motor neurons on the morphology of the microtubule network in NMJs, as visualized by antibodies to α-acetylated tubulin and to Futsch, a neuronal microtubule-associated protein [48]. Staining with antibodies to α-acetylated tubulin failed to reveal visual differences between the individuals with and without *sgg-RB* overexpression (Figure S3). Differences in the distribution of Futsch within the NMJs were found. In particular, in individuals with *sgg-RB* overexpression, only weak, diffuse Futsch staining in synaptic boutons of NMJs was observed compared to that in controls (Figure 10), indicating cytoskeletal abnormalities. In this case, the effect was more pronounced in individuals with pan-neuronal *sgg-RB* overexpression (Figure 10A) than in individuals with *sgg-RB* overexpression in motor neurons (Figure 10B), which correlates with the comparative effect on lifespan. It was shown that *sgg* interacts with Futsch, which functions downstream of *sgg* [7]; most likely, *sgg* controls synaptic growth through the direct phosphorylation of Futsch. Sgg is able to inhibit transcription factor AP-1 and the JNK (Jun-N-terminal kinase) cascade and, in this way, also affects synaptic growth [8]. Our data shed light on the cellular consequences of presumed increased phosphorylation of Futsch, which disappeared from synaptic boutons of NMJs, and demonstrated that Sgg-RB, when overexpressed, controlled the dynamics of the microtubule cytoskeleton.

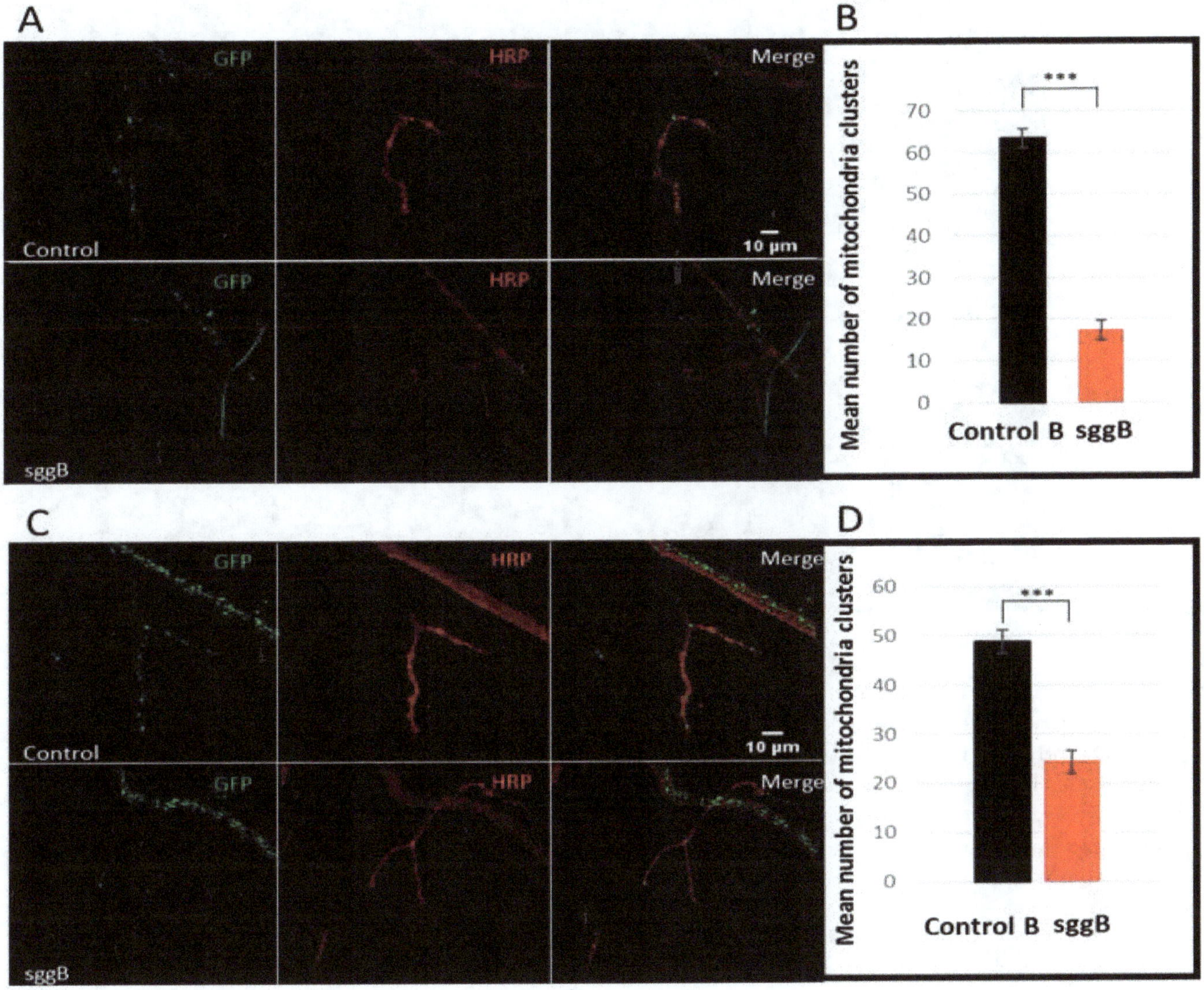

Figure 8. Mitochondrial clusters in NMJs of third-instar female larvae with panneuronal *sgg-RB* overexpression (**A**,**B**) and *sgg-RB* overexpression in motor neurons (**C**,**D**). Control B, sggB denote hybrid genotypes obtained as a result of crossing the corresponding lines with the driver line D4 inducing the expression of transgenic constructs in the nervous system or the driver line D12 inducing the expression of transgenic constructs in motor neurons. A full description of genotypes is given in the Materials and Methods section. Representative confocal images of NMJs (muscle 4, hemi-segment 34–) stained for mitochondria clusters (GFP, green) and neural membranes (HRP, horseradish peroxidase, red) (**A**,**C**). Bar = 10 µm. Quantification of the number of mitochondrial clusters (**B**,**D**). *** denotes $p < 0.001$ determined by the Kruskal-Wallis test.

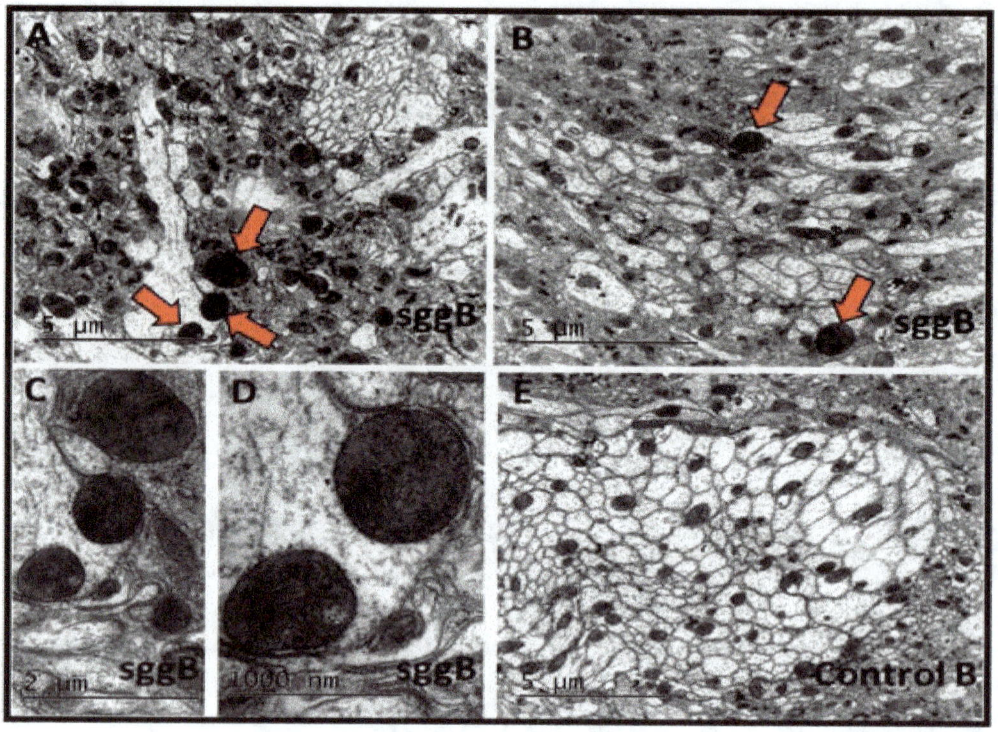

Figure 9. Fine structure of the adult brain in females with pan-neuronal *sgg-RB* overexpression. Control B, sggB denote hybrid genotypes obtained as a result of crossing the corresponding lines with the driver line D4 inducing the expression of transgenic constructs in the nervous system. A full description of genotypes is given in the Materials and Methods section. Three representative transmission electron microscopy images of the *Drosophila* inferior dorsofrontal protocerebrum at the age of 3 days (**A**,**B**,**E**); enlarged fragments of panel B (**C**,**D**). Mitochondria with violated structures are indicated by red arrows. Bar = 5 µm or 2 µm.

2.3.4. Active Synaptic Zones

Given that the number and size of synapses were shown to be affected by *sgg* function [7,8], we decided to evaluate the number of active synaptic zones in individuals with *sgg-RB* overexpression. The number of active zones in larval NMJs visualized by antibodies to BRP (Bruchpilot), a Drosophila homolog of vertebrate active zone protein ELKS [29], was significantly (approximately two-fold) decreased in individuals with pan-neuronal *sgg-RB* overexpression (Figure 11A,B) and *sgg-RB* overexpression in motor neurons (Figure 11C,D), indicating reduced synaptic activity. *sgg-RB* overexpression driven by both drivers had comparable effects on NMJs. These results supplemented the data on the role of Sgg in controlling the functionality of synapses, which demonstrated that it was involved in the regulation of neurotransmitter release [8]. Earlier, it was shown that the number of boutons was significantly decreased as a result of pan-neuronal GSK3 overexpression [7]. Importantly, although *sgg* overexpression has an inhibitory role on the quantity of boutons, it may not play an important role in bouton differentiation [7]. Overall, our data demonstrated that negative changes in lifespan caused by Sgg-RB overexpression in the nervous system were accompanied by negative changes in synaptic properties.

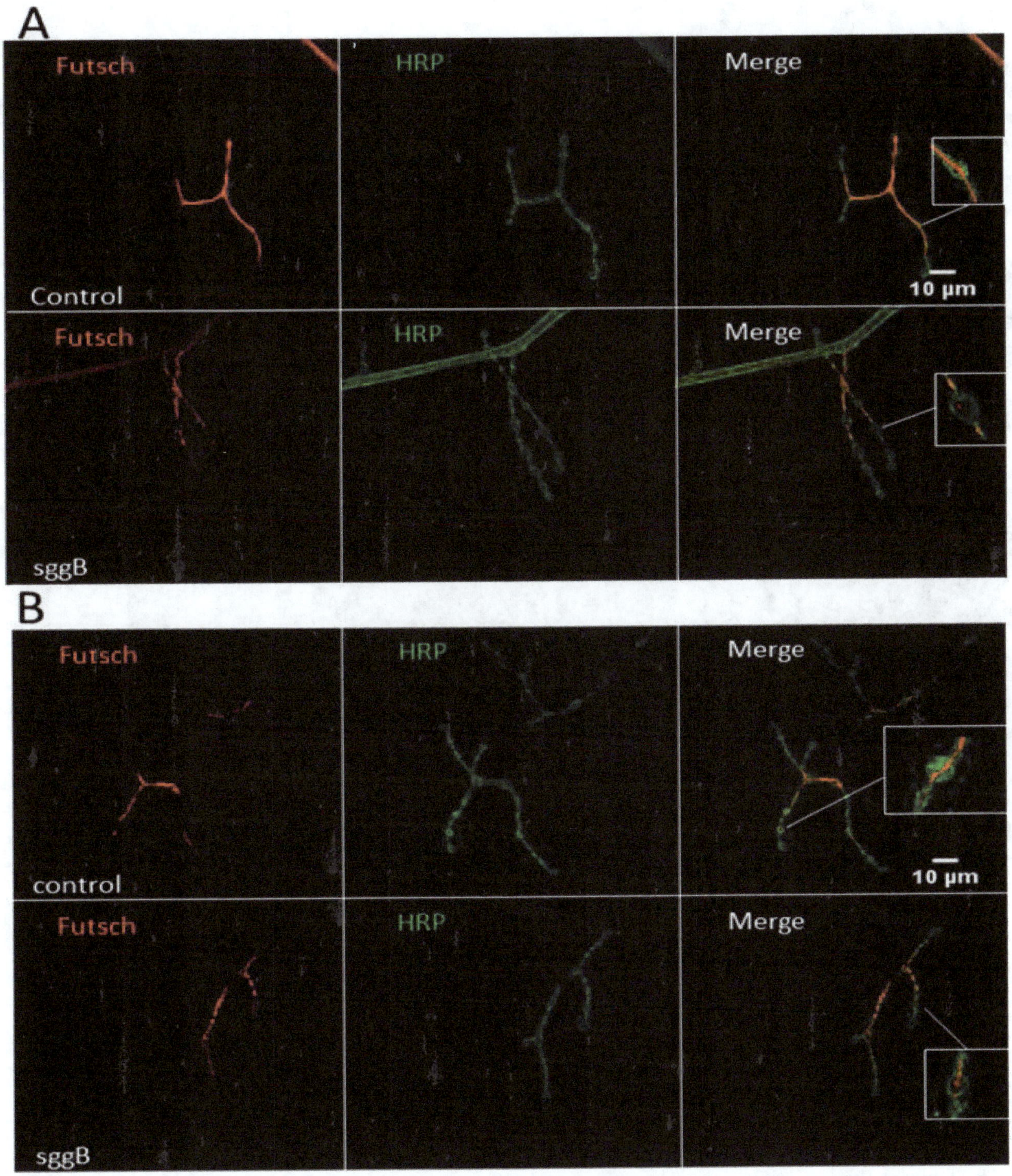

Figure 10. Distribution of Futsch in NMJs of third-instar female larvae with panneuronal *sgg-RB* overexpression (**A**) and *sgg-RB* overexpression in motor neurons (**B**). Control B, sggB denote hybrid genotypes obtained as a result of crossing the corresponding lines with the driver line D4 inducing the expression of transgenic constructs in the nervous system or the driver line D12 inducing the expression of transgenic constructs in motor neurons. A full description of genotypes is given in the Materials and Methods section. Representative confocal images of NMJs (muscle 4, hemi-segment 34–) stained for Futsch (red) and neural membranes (HRP, green). Bar = 10 μm.

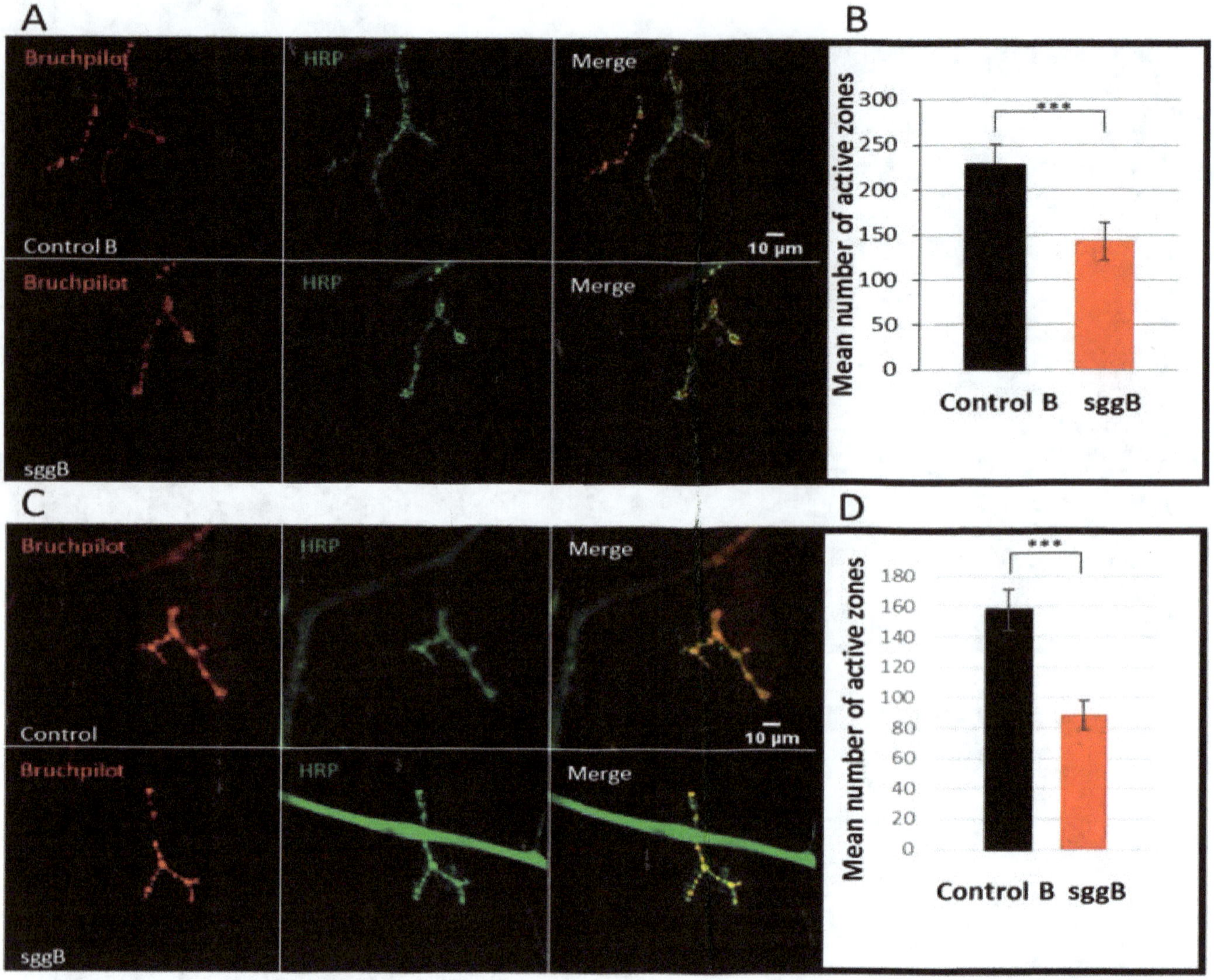

Figure 11. Active zones in NMJs of third-instar female larvae with panneuronal *sgg-RB* overexpression (**A**,**B**) and *sgg-RB* overexpression in motor neurons (**C**,**D**). Control B, sggB denote hybrid genotypes obtained as a result of crossing the corresponding lines with the driver line D4 inducing the expression of transgenic constructs in the nervous system or the driver line D12 inducing the expression of transgenic constructs in motor neurons. A full description of genotypes is given in the Materials and Methods section. Representative confocal images of NMJs (muscle 4, hemi-segment 34–) stained for active zones (BRP, red) and neural membranes (HRP, green) (**A**,**C**). Bar = 10 µm. Quantification of the number of active zones (**B**,**D**). *** denotes $p < 0.001$ determined by the Kruskal-Wallis test.

2.3.5. Neuronal Structure

We suggest that a significant decrease in the lifespan of individuals with pan-neuronal *sgg-RB* overexpression might be accompanied by pathological processes in the adult nervous system. Analysis of the brains of 3-day-old flies using transmission electron microscopy revealed a number of degenerative marks both in the bodies of the nerve cells and in the axonal structures in the neuropil region. The presence of "holes" surrounded by membranes and, in some cases, containing fragments of organelles apparently subjected to autophagy was demonstrated in the brains of all three individuals with pan-neuronal *sgg-RB* overexpression, whereas these structures were not found in the control brains (Figure 12A,B). These "holes" apparently represent destroyed areas of the neuron bodies and may indicate accelerated aging processes in the nervous system of individuals with pan-neuronal *sgg-RB* overexpression. In *Drosophila*, photosensitive structures, namely, rhabdomeres, are often used along with the brain to study neurodegenerative processes. We examined whether pathological changes occur in the rhabdomeres of individuals with pan-neuronal *sgg-RB* overexpression compared to those of controls. No changes were revealed in three control individuals, whereas in two out of three individuals with pan-neuronal *sgg-RB* overexpression, lacunae and irregular rhabdomere structures were found (Figure 12C,D), also indicating pathological processes in flies with pan-neuronal *sgg-RB* overexpression. Of note, in individuals with pan-neuronal *sgg-RB* overexpression, a high heterogeneity of external phenotypic manifestations was observed: For example, the wing shape varied fairly widely. In view of this fact, some difference in the level of degeneration of rhabdomeres was not surprising.

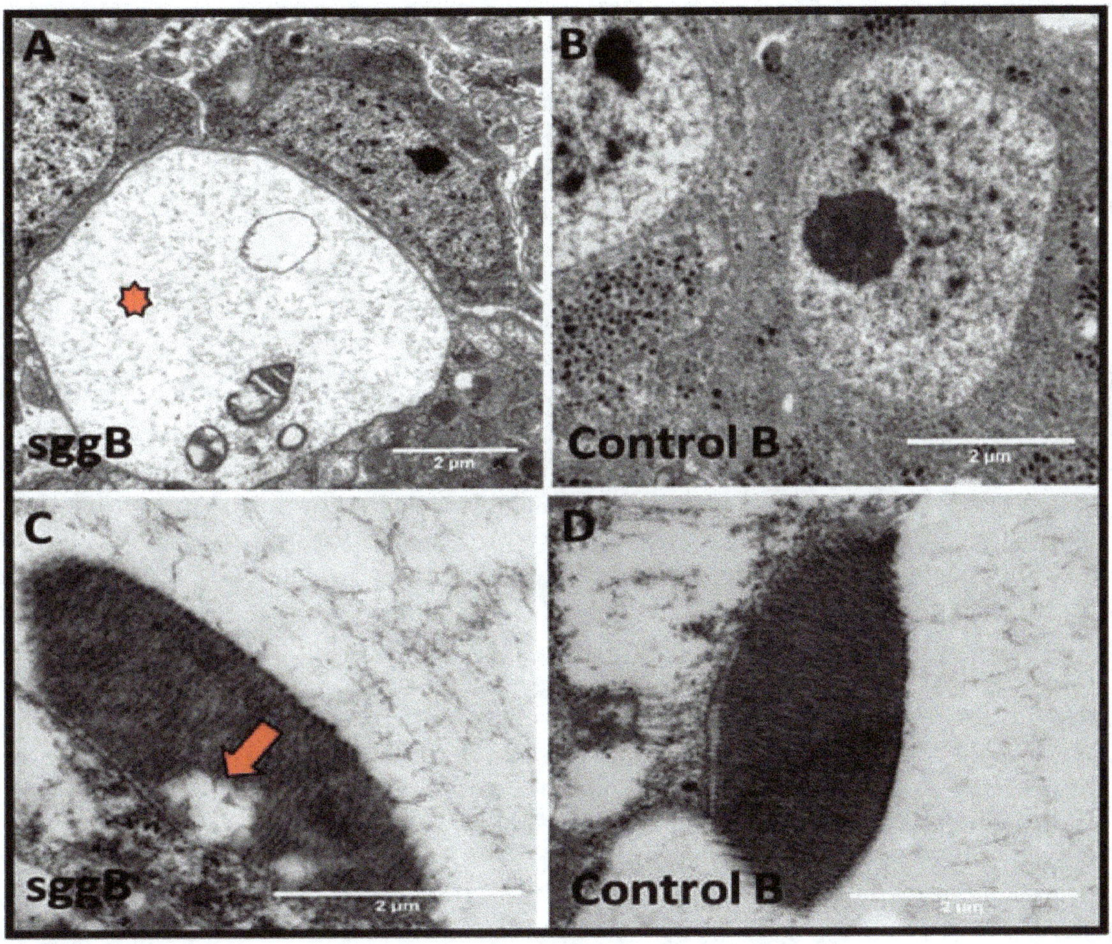

Figure 12. Signs of degeneration in the nervous system of females with pan-neuronal *sgg-RB* overexpression. Control B, sggB denote hybrid genotypes obtained as a result of crossing the corresponding lines with the driver line D4 inducing the expression of transgenic constructs in the nervous system. A full description of genotypes is given in the Materials and Methods section. Representative transmission electron microscopy images of the *Drosophila* brain (**A**,**B**) and rhabdomeres (**C**,**D**) at the age of 3 days. An example of a degeneration sign in the neuron body (**A**, indicated by the red star); rhabdomeres with violated structure (**C**, lacuna is indicated by the red arrow) compared to the respective controls (**B**,**D**). Bar = 1 μm or 2 μm.

Summing up the results presented in this chapter, we conclude that overexpression of the main Sgg-RB isoform in the nervous system had severe effects on its structural and functional properties. Overall, Sgg-RB overexpression in the nervous system affected the integrity of neuron bodies, the number, distribution, and structure of mitochondrial and cytoskeletal properties in the presynaptic zones, and synaptic activity. These changes indicated that Sgg-RB overexpression caused accelerated aging of the nervous system in young individuals. The accelerated aging led to a more or less sharp reduction in lifespan, depending on the cell types where Sgg-RB overexpression was induced. While pan-neuronal overexpression caused a severe lifespan decline and overexpression in motor neurons reduced the lifespan to a much lesser extent, and the effects of pan-neuronal overexpression and overexpression in motor neurons on the nervous system were mostly of similar scales. Thus, the rate of lifespan decline was not correlated with the rate of structural and functional changes in the nervous system. The only exception identified was a change in the structure of the cytoskeleton, namely, the Futsch protein distribution along the terminal parts of axons.

3. Materials and Methods

3.1. Fly Strains and Crosses

To provide *sgg* overexpression, several lines were used. The line providing *sgg-RB* overexpression w^{1118}; *P{*w^{+mC} *= UAS-sgg. B}MB5* (in short, sggB) with the transgenic construct encoding the normal PB form of GSK3 was obtained from the Bloomington *Drosophila* Stock Center (USA) (Available online: http://flystocks.bio.indiana.edu/); the w^{1118} (Control B) line without transgenic insertions was used as a control line [19].

To obtain lines providing *sgg-RA*, *sgg-RG*, and *sgg-RO* overexpression, cDNAs corresponding to these transcripts were cloned into the *pBID-UASC* vector (Addgene plasmid # 35200, Available online: https://www.addgene.org/35200/), which contains an attB site for *phi31* site-specific transformation of *Drosophila* embryos and UAS enhancer sequences [49]. Single clones with the unimpaired *sgg-RA*, *sgg-RG* and *sgg-RO* sequences and the line y^1 *M{vas-int.Dm}ZH-2A w*; M{3xP3-RFP.attP'}ZH-51C* with the second chromosome attP *phi31* integration site [50] were used for the transformation performed by BestGene, Inc. (Available online: https://www.thebestgene.com/HomePage.do). In the transgenic lines obtained, most of the auxiliary sequences were excised from the inserted transgenes due to induction of recombination between the *loxP* sites present in the *pBID-UASC* vector. One homozygous transgenic line of each genotype, namely, y^1 *M{vas-int.Dm}ZH-2A w*; M{3xP3-RFP.attP'}ZH-51C P{*w^{+mC} *= UAS-sgg.A}2M* (in short, sggA), y^1 *M{vas-int.Dm}ZH-2A w*; M{3xP3-RFP.attP'}ZH-51C P{*w^{+mC} *= UAS-sgg.G}1M* (in short, sggG), y^1 *M{vas-int.Dm}ZH-2A w**; and *M{3xP3-RFP.attP'}ZH-51C P{*w^{+mC} *= UAS-sgg.O}1M* (in short, sggO), were used in further experiments. The line y^1 *M{vas-int.Dm}ZH-2A w*; M{3xP3-RFP.attP'}ZH-51C* (Control AGO) initially used for transformations was used as a control line with the same genetic background.

To provide *sgg* RNAi knockdown, two lines were obtained from the Bloomington *Drosophila* Stock Center: y^1 *sc** v^1; *P{*$y^{+t7.7}$ $v^{+t1.8}$ *= TriP. HMS01751}attP40* (in short, sggKD1, with VALIUM20, hairpin size 21 bp, affects all *sgg* transcripts) and y^1 v^1; *P{*$y^{+t7.7}$ $v^{+t1.8}$ *= TriP. JF01255}attP2* (in short, sggKD2, with VALIUM1, hairpin size 400 bp, affects all *sgg* transcripts). Y^1 v^1; *P{*$y^{+t7.7}$ *= CaryP}attP40* (Control KD1) and y^1 v^1; *P{*$y^{+t7.7}$*=CaryP}attP2* (Control KD2) lines without transgenes providing RNAi were used as control lines for *sgg* RNAi knockdown, as suggested by the manufacturer (Available online: http://flystocks.bio.indiana.edu/Browse/TRiPtb.htm).

To induce *sgg* overexpression or knockdown, several driver lines were obtained from the Bloomington *Drosophila* Stock Center.

Y^1 *w*; P{*$w^{+mW.hs}$ *= en2.4-GAL4}e22c; P{*w^{+mC} *= tGPH}4/TM3, Ser*^{1} (D1) was used to induce the expression of transgenic constructs in embryos.

W; P{*w^{+mC} *= ppl-GAL4. P}2* (D2) was used to induce the expression of transgenic constructs in the fat body.

P{w^{+mC} *= UAS-Dcr-2. D}1,* w^{1118}; *P{*w^{+mC} *= GAL4-Mef2. R}R1* (D3) was used to induce the expression of transgenic constructs in somatic muscle cells.

P{$w^{+mW.hs}$ *= GawB}elavC155* w^{1118}; *P{*w^{+mC} *= UAS-Dcr-2. D}2* (D4) was used to induce the lifelong expression of transgenic constructs in the nervous system.

W; P{*$w^{+mW.hs}$ *= GawB}389* (D5) was used to induce the expression of transgenic constructs in the embryonic nervous system.

W^{1118}; *P{GawB}DJ695* (D6) was used to induce the increased expression of transgenic constructs in the adult nervous system with age.

W^{1118}; *P{w*$^{+mC}$ *= Ddc-GAL4.L}Lmpt*$^{4.36}$ (D7) and *w**; *P{w[+mC] = UAS-mCD8::GFP. L}LL5/Cy*; and *P{w*$^{+mC}$ *= ple-GAL4. F}3* (D8) were used to induce the expression of transgenic constructs in dopaminergic neurons.

*W**; *P{w*$^{+mW.hs}$ *= GawB}386Y* (D9) was used to induce the expression of transgenic constructs in peptidergic neurons.

W^{1118}; *P{w*$^{+mW.hs}$ *= GawB}Vglut*^{OK371} (D10) was used to induce the expression of transgenic constructs in glutamatergic neurons.

*W**; *P{w*$^{+mC}$ *= ChAT-GAL4.7.4}19B* (D11) was used to induce the expression of transgenic constructs in cholinergic neurons.

*W**; *P{GawB}D42* (D12) was used to induce the expression of transgenic constructs in motoneurons.

P{w^{+mC} *= Gad1-GAL4.3.098}2/CyO* (D13) was used to induce the expression of transgenic constructs in GABAergic neurons.

Additionally, the driver line w^{1118};*P{w*$^{+mC}$ *= UAS-mito- HA-GFP.AP}2/CyO* (D14) was used to induce GFP expression in mitochondria.

D1, D3, and D4 driver lines proved to be effective in our previous work, according to the real-time RT-qPCR data [27].

To induce the expression of transgenic constructs, females of each of the driver lines were crossed to males of sggB, sggY214F, sggA81T, sggA, sggG, sggO, KD1, KD2, Control B, Control AGO, Control KD1, and Control KD2 lines. In all experiments, flies were kept at 25 °C on a standard medium of semolina, sugar, raisins, yeast, and agar with nipagin, propionic acid, and streptomycin.

3.2. Tests for Wolbachia

Prior to the experiments, all the lines were checked for the presence of *Wolbachia*, a *Drosophila* symbiont known to affect life history traits [51], via quantitative PCR (MiniOpticon real-time PCR detection system, Bio-Rad, Hercules, CA, USA) with primers for the 16S rRNA gene, 5′-CATACCTATTCGAAGGGATAG-3′ and 5′-AGCTTCGAGTGAAACCAATTC-3′ [52]. Negative results were obtained for all lines except sggA, D3, and D12. These lines were treated with tetracycline (0.25 mg/mL, [53]) for three generations followed by at least three generations of recovery before they were used in experiments.

3.3. Lifespan Assay

Lifespan was measured as described in [16]. Five virgin flies of the same genotype and sex, all collected on the same day from cultures with moderate density, were placed in replicate vials. Flies were transferred to vials with fresh food containing approximately 5 mL of standard medium without live yeast on the surface weekly. The number of dead flies was recorded daily. Experiments comparing fly lifespans were conducted simultaneously. Sample sizes were 50 to 100 flies per sex per genotype. The experiments that showed noteworthy results were repeated two to three times with an interval of approximately six months. The lifespan for each fly was estimated as the number of days alive from the day of eclosion to the day of death. Mean lifespans and survival curves were primarily used to characterize lifespan.

3.4. Locomotion Assay

Locomotion was measured as described in [16]. Flies were collected and maintained by the same procedures as for the lifespan assays, but without recording the deaths. Locomotion was measured at the same time each day in unmated males and females at age 3 to 5 days, 20 days and 40 days. Experiments comparing locomotion were conducted simultaneously. Sample sizes were 65 to 75 flies (13 to 15 vials) per sex per genotype. To measure locomotor activity, the vials were placed horizontally in a *Drosophila* Population Monitor (TriKinetics Inc, Waltham, MA, USA). Fly movement along the walls or in the middle of the vial crossed the infrared beam rings along the length of the vial. Beam interruptions were detected, and totals were reported every five minutes to the host computer. Two measurements for five minutes were made for each vial. Locomotion was characterized as the mean number of beam interruptions per vial.

3.5. Real-Time RT-qPCR

Transcript levels were measured as described in [15,16]. Total RNA for real-time reverse transcription quantitative PCR (RT-qPCR) was extracted from batches of 30 whole bodies of 3- to 5-day-old males and females using TRIzol reagent (Invitrogen, Carlsbad, CA, USA) and DNase I (Sigma-Aldrich, St. Louis, MO, USA) according to the manufacturers' instructions.

First-strand cDNA was synthesized using SuperScript II Reverse Transcriptase (Invitrogen) with oligo(dT)$_{15}$ primers according to the manufacturer's instructions. Amounts of cDNA were determined by RT-qPCR using SYBR Green I in a MiniOpticon real-time PCR detection system (Bio-Rad).

Gdh and *Adh* housekeeping genes, characterized by relatively low expression comparable to *sgg* expression, were used as reference genes to normalize for differences in total cDNA between the samples. The forward and reverse primer sequences used were as follows: For *sggB*, shaggyPB1 5′-ATATACAGATCTTTTGTTTGGCAA-3′ and shaggyPB2 5′-AGGAGGAAGTTCTTGGACGA-3′; for *Gdh*, Gdh1 5′-TATGCCACCGAGCACCAGATTCC-3′ and Gdh2 5′-GGATGCCCTTCACCTTCTGCTT CTT-3′; for *Adh*, Adhd3: 5′-CGGCATCTAAGAAGTGATACTCCCAAAA-3′ and Adhr3: 5′-TGAGTGT GCATCGAATCAGCCTTATT-3′.

CFX Manager 3.1 software (Bio-Rad, 2012) was used to evaluate the relative gene expression. Inter-run calibrations were used for each panel of experiments since the experiments were conducted for several years. Three independent RNA extractions (biological replicates) per sex per genotype and three technical repeats for each RNA extraction were made.

3.6. Immunostaining and Microscopy

Immunostaining and microscopy were performed according to [27]. Male and female third-stage larvae and brains of 3- to 5-day-old unmated males and females were dissected in phosphate-buffered saline (PBS), fixed in 4% paraformaldehyde (Sigma-Aldrich, St. Louis, MO, USA) at room temperature for 20 min, and washed in PBS (3 × 15 min). For immunostaining, preparations were blocked in blocking buffer (BlockPRO, Visual Protein Biotechnology Corporation, Taiwan) for one hour at room temperature, incubated in primary antibodies (diluted in BlockPRO) overnight at 4 °C, washed in PBS (3 × 15 min), incubated in secondary antibodies (diluted in BlockPRO) for two hours, washed in PBS (3 × 15 min), and placed in a medium for immunofluorescence (VectaShield, Vector Labs, Burlingame, CA, USA). NMJs were analyzed in the fourth muscle of the third and fourth abdominal segments of larvae. A confocal laser scanning microscope (LSM 510, Zeiss, Oberkochen, Germany), ImageJ (http://rsb.info.nih.gov/ij/index.html) and LSM Image Browser (Zeiss) were used. Sample sizes were 10 to 15 specimens per genotype per experiment. To estimate bouton numbers and numbers of synaptic active zones, the same preparations were used. Mean numbers of type 1b boutons and satellite boutons were used to characterize NMJ morphology. The mean number of synaptic active zones was used to characterize synapse activity. Mean numbers of mitochondria and dopaminergic neurons were calculated.

The following primary antibodies were used: Mouse anti-Brp (mAb NC82, 1:200; Developmental Studies Hybridoma Bank (DSHB)) against Bruchpilot (BRP), a protein specific to active synaptic zones [54]; mouse anti-Futsch (mAb 22C10, 1:200; DSHB) against the microtubule-associated protein, Futsch [48]; mouse anti-α-acetylated tubulin (1:200; Santa Cruz Biotechnology, Dallas, TX, USA) against a tubulin isoform, a marker of microtubule networks [55]; Alexa Fluor 647-conjugated goat anti-HRP (1:400, Jackson ImmunoResearch), against Horseradish Peroxidase (HRP), a widely used marker of presynaptic membranes [7]. The secondary antibodies used were goat anti-mouse Cy3 conjugated (1:400, Jackson ImmunoResearch). Antibodies obtained from the DSHB were developed under the auspices of the NICHD and maintained by The University of Iowa, Department of Biology, Iowa City, IA 52242. Mitochondria were visualized with GFP using the D13 driver line. Dopaminergic neuron neurons were visualized with GFP using the D8 driver line.

3.7. Electron Microscopy

Three heads of 3- to 5-day-old unmated males and females of each genotype were dissected and fixed in 2.5% glutaraldehyde in cacodylate buffer at room temperature for 2 h. Samples were washed in sodium cacodylate buffer, fixed in 2% OsO_4 for 2 h at 4 °C, washed and, dehydrated by transferring through solutions of increasing alcohol concentration (30%, 50%, 70%, 90%, and 100%) for 15 min at room temperature followed by acetone for 15 min. Resin (Epon 812 with DDSA and MNA) infiltration was carried out according to the following protocol: Resin-acetone (1:3), resin-acetone (1:1), resin-acetone (3:1) at room temperature for 1 h, and resin alone for 12 h; and resin with a DMP 30 catalysator at 37 °C for 24 h and at 60 °C for 48 h. Hardened blocks were cut on the Leica UC7 (Leica) microtome into 70 nm slices, contrasted by uranyl acetate (30 min) and lead citrate (5 min) and then analyzed using a transmission electron microscope (JEM-1011, Jeol, Akishima, Tokyo, Japan).

3.8. Western Blotting

Approximately 50 heads of 3- to 5-day-old adults of each genotype were dissected and homogenized in 8 M urea solution. Equal amounts of samples from the supernatants were preincubated with sample buffer (deionized water, 0.5 M Tris-HCl, glycerol, 10% SDS, 0.5% bromphenol blue, DTT) for 5 min at 95 °C and separated in a 4–12% (*w*/*v*) acrylamide Bis/Tris SDS-PAGE gel using the vertical electrophoretic chamber Mini-Protean Tetra (Bio-Rad). Proteins were transferred from the gel to the PVDF membrane (Immobilon-P Membrane,Millipore, Burlington, MA, USA) using electroblotting (Mini Trans-Blot Modul, Bio-Rad), blocked in BlockPro blocking buffer (Visual Protein Biotechnology Corporation, Taiwan), and incubated with anti–GSK3 beta primary antibodies (1:300; ab18893, Abcam, Cambridge, Great Britain) for one hour. Bound antibodies were detected with goat anti–rabbit secondary antibodies conjugated with alkaline phosphatase (1:20000; A3687, Sigma). Prior to visualization, the membranes were incubated in the alkaline CDP buffer for 5 min and then in the Immun-Star AP-Substrate (Bio-Rad) for 7 min. After scanning, the relative intensity quantification of each band was evaluated with Image Lab software (Bio-Rad). Three independent protein extractions (biological replicates) per genotype were made.

3.9. Statistical Analyses

To compare control and mutant genotypes, Student's *t*-test and the nonparametric, distribution-free Kruskal-Wallis test were used for analyses of *sgg* transcript amounts; locomotion; and numbers of large boutons, satellite boutons, active zones, and mitochondria in NMJs. These two tests gave consistent results, so only the results of the Kruskal-Wallis test are reported here. Standard descriptive statistical analysis of lifespan [56,57] was performed to determine the mean lifespan and its accompanying variances, standard deviations, and standard errors; the median, minimum, and maximum lifespans; and the lifespans of the lower and upper quartiles and the 10 and 90 percentiles (Tables S1–S5). Survival curves were estimated using the Kaplan–Meier procedure. The nonparametric, distribution-free Mann-Whitney test and Kolmogorov-Smirnov test were used to evaluate the statistical significance of the difference between the survival curves.

4. Conclusions

Understanding the genetic and molecular basis of pathological changes of the nervous system underlying accelerated aging and shortening of lifespan are important for the development of evidence-based recommendations for life extension. GSK3 is an important enzyme governing numerous regulatory pathways and metabolic processes via interaction with InR/TOR, Wnt, JNK, and other signaling cascades [1,2]. GSK3 is specifically important in the nervous system, where it is involved in the control of synaptic development, structure, and function due to regulation of axonal size, the microtubule cytoskeleton, and neurotransmitter release [7–10]. Here, we demonstrated GSK involvement in the regulation of mitochondria number, intracellular distribution and structure, and control of synaptic activity. We showed that GSK3 affected the axonal distribution of the microtubule-associated protein, Futsch, thus confirming the role of protein kinases in governing the architecture of the microtubule cytoskeleton. We also demonstrated that GSK3 overexpression caused signs of neurodegeneration in the brains of young individuals. All these findings certified that GSK3 misexpression is crucially important for the structural and functional integrity of the nervous system. The main GSK3 isoform is responsible for the normal operation of neurons.

It is generally clear that the structural and functional integrity of the nervous system, in turn, is important for ensuring a long life. Here, we showed that pathological changes in neurons caused by aberrations in GSK3 expression in the nervous system were paralleled by a rapid decline in survival and shortening lifespan. Our data also demonstrated that GSK3 misexpression in other tissues affected lifespan in a transcript-, stage-, and tissue-specific mode. We proved that some minor *shaggy* transcripts are functional and, moreover, may have the specificity required for a particular function. This result allowed us to lift the veil on the complexity of the gene structure and expression strategy. Most of the *Drosophila* genes have multiple annotated transcripts and proteins (https://flybase.org), and there are not many examples showing whether the alleged complexity of the structural organization of a gene is in line with reality and why such a sophisticated structure is needed. Of particular interest to us was the fact that the embryonic overexpression of one of the minor transcripts was enough to cause an increase in adult lifespan. This fact underscored the role of gene expression early in life for lifespan control and the existence of carry-over mechanisms of an epigenetic or other nature underlying this effect.

Altogether, our results demonstrated the key role of GSK3 in ensuring the link between the pathology of neurons and lifespan. The data presented in this article indicated how disentangling expression strategy and general gene biology might eventually provide a selective approach to the choice of potential drugs and therapies based on an understanding of the molecular mechanisms underlying the development of pathologies shortening lifespan. Obviously, treatment should be aimed at suppressing or enhancing the expression of certain gene transcripts in certain tissues. Our data allowed us to come closer to understanding the characteristics of *shaggy* gene expression, which are important for the search for potential drugs that specifically affect the pathologies of the nervous system and aging caused by the GSK3 malfunction.

Author Contributions: Conceptualization, M.V.T., N.V.R., and E.G.P.; methodology, M.V.T., N.V.R., S.V.B., A.A.Z., A.V.K.; formal analysis, M.V.T., N.V.R., A.V.K., E.G.P.; investigation, M.V.T., N.V.R., S.V.B., E.R.V., A.A.Z.; writing—original draft preparation, M.V.T. and E.G.P.; writing—review and editing, M.V.T., N.V.R., S.V.B., E.R.V., A.A.Z., A.V.K., E.G.P.; visualization, M.V.T. and A.V.K.; supervision, E.G.P.; funding acquisition, M.V.T., N.V.R. and E.R.V.

Acknowledgments: We thank Tatiana Morozova for invaluable assistance in handling and transferring fly cultures, Svetlana Sarantseva and Ludmila Olenina for help in acquiring new methods and inspiring discussions, and Natalia Biserova, Alfiya Mustafina and Vladimir Popenko for tips on analyzing electron microphotographs. The equipment of the Shared Research Center of the Institute of Molecular Genetics of the Russian Academy of Sciences was used for this work. Stocks obtained from the Bloomington Drosophila Stock Center (NIH P40OD018537) were used in this study, and we express our sincere gratitude to the Center and its personnel for their continuous support. We also thank Addgene for providing the pBID-UASC plasmid and BestGene, Inc., for creating transgenic flies. We are grateful to American Journal Experts for English editing services.

References

1. McCubrey, J.A.; Rakus, D.; Gizak, A.; Steelman, L.S.; Abrams, S.L.; Lertpiriyapong, K.; Fitzgerald, T.L.; Yang, L.V.; Montalto, G.; Cervello, M.; et al. Effects of mutations in Wnt/β-catenin, hedgehog, Notch and PI3K pathways on GSK-3 activity-Diverse effects on cell growth, metabolism and cancer. *Biochim. Biophys. Acta Mol. Cell Res.* **2016**, *1863*, 2942–2976. [CrossRef]

2. Patel, P.; Woodgett, J.R. Glycogen Synthase Kinase 3: A Kinase for All Pathways? *Curr. Top. Dev. Biol.* **2017**, *123*, 277–302. [CrossRef]
3. Colosimo, P.F.; Liu, X.; Kaplan, N.A.; Tolwinski, N.S. GSK3beta affects apical-basal polarity and cell-cell adhesion by regulating aPKC levels. *Dev. Dyn.* **2010**, *239*, 115–125. [CrossRef] [PubMed]
4. Kaplan, N.A.; Colosimo, P.F.; Liu, X.; Tolwinski, N.S. Complex interactions between GSK3 and aPKC in *Drosophila* embryonic epithelial morphogenesis. *PLoS ONE* **2011**, *6*, e18616. [CrossRef] [PubMed]
5. Kanuka, H.; Kuranaga, E.; Takemoto, K.; Hiratou, T.; Okano, H.; Miura, M. *Drosophila* caspase transduces Shaggy/GSK-3beta kinase activity in neural precursor development. *EMBO J.* **2005**, *24*, 3793–3806. [CrossRef]
6. Wong, J.J.L.; Li, S.; Lim, E.K.H.; Wang, Y.; Wang, C.; Zhang, H.; Kirilly, D.; Wu, C.; Liou, Y.-C.; Wang, H.; et al. A Cullin1-based SCF E3 ubiquitin ligase targets the InR/PI3K/TOR pathway to regulate neuronal pruning. *PLoS Biol.* **2013**, *11*, e1001657. [CrossRef]
7. Franco, B.; Bogdanik, L.; Bobinnec, Y.; Debec, A.; Bockaert, J.; Parmentier, M.-L.; Grau, Y. Shaggy, the homolog of glycogen synthase kinase 3, controls neuromuscular junction growth in *Drosoph. J. Neurosci.* **2004**, *24*, 6573–6577. [CrossRef] [PubMed]
8. Franciscovich, A.L.; Mortimer, A.D.V.; Freeman, A.A.; Gu, J.; Sanyal, S. Overexpression screen in *Drosophila* identifies neuronal roles of GSK-3β *shaggy* as a regulator of AP-1-dependent developmental plasticity. *Genetics* **2008**, *180*, 2057–2071. [CrossRef]
9. Cuesto, G.; Jordán-Álvarez, S.; Enriquez-Barreto, L.; Ferrús, A.; Morales, M.; Acebes, Á. GSK3β inhibition promotes synaptogenesis in *Drosophila* and mammalian neurons. *PLoS ONE* **2015**, *10*, e0118475. [CrossRef] [PubMed]
10. Chiang, A.; Priya, R.; Ramaswami, M.; Vijayraghavan, K.; Rodrigues, V. Neuronal activity and Wnt signaling act through Gsk3-beta to regulate axonal integrity in mature *Drosophila* olfactory sensory neurons. *Development* **2009**, *136*, 1273–1282. [CrossRef]
11. Noble, W.; Hanger, D.P.; Miller, C.C.J.; Lovestone, S. The importance of tau phosphorylation for neurodegenerative diseases. *Front Neurol.* **2013**, *4*, 83. [CrossRef]
12. Ma, T. GSK3 in Alzheimer's disease: Mind the isoforms. *J. Alzheimers Dis.* **2014**, *39*, 707–710. [CrossRef] [PubMed]
13. Mudher, A.; Shepherd, D.; Newman, T.A.; Mildren, P.; Jukes, J.P.; Squire, A.; Mears, A.; Drummond, J.A.; Berg, S.; MacKay, D.; et al. GSK-3beta inhibition reverses axonal transport defects and behavioural phenotypes in *Drosoph. Mol. Psychiatry* **2004**, *9*, 522–530. [CrossRef]
14. Pasyukova, E.G.; Symonenko, A.V.; Roshina, N.V.; Trostnikov, M.V.; Veselkina, E.R.; Rybina, O.Y. Neuronal genes and developmental neuronal pathways in *Drosophila* life span control. In *Life Extension: Lessons from Drosophila*; Vaiserman, A.M., Moskalev, A.A., Pasyukova, E.G., Eds.; Springer International Publishing: Cham, Switzerland, 2015; pp. 3–37.
15. Symonenko, A.V.; Roshina, N.V.; Krementsova, A.V.; Pasyukova, E.G. Reduced neuronal transcription of *escargot*, the *Drosophila* gene tncoding a Snail-type transcription factor, promotes longevity. *Front. Genet.* **2018**, *9*, 151. [CrossRef]
16. Roshina, N.V.; Symonenko, A.V.; Krementsova, A.V.; Trostnikov, M.V.; Pasyukova, E.G. Embryonic expression of shuttle craft, a *Drosophila* gene involved in neuron development, is associated with adult lifespan. *Aging (Albany NY)* **2014**, *6*, 1076–1093. [CrossRef]
17. Hernandez, F.; Lucas, J.J.; Avila, J. GSK3 and tau: Two convergence points in Alzheimer's disease. *J. Alzheimers Dis.* **2013**, *33*, S141–S144. [CrossRef]
18. Ruel, L.; Bourouis, M.; Heitzler, P.; Pantesco, V.; Simpson, P. *Drosophila shaggy* kinase and rat glycogen synthase kinase-3 have conserved activities and act downstream of Notch. *Nature* **1993**, *362*, 557–560. [CrossRef]
19. Bourouis, M. Targeted increase in *shaggy* activity levels blocks wingless signaling. *Genesis* **2002**, *34*, 99–102. [CrossRef]
20. Bodenmiller, B.; Mueller, L.N.; Pedrioli, P.G.A.; Pflieger, D.; Jünger, M.A.; Eng, J.K.; Aebersold, R.; Tao, W.A. An integrated chemical, mass spectrometric and computational strategy for (quantitative) phosphoproteomics: Application to *Drosophila melanogaster* Kc167 cells. *Mol. Biosyst.* **2007**, *3*, 275–286. [CrossRef] [PubMed]
21. Brunner, E.; Ahrens, C.H.; Mohanty, S.; Baetschmann, H.; Loevenich, S.; Potthast, F.; Deutsch, E.W.; Panse, C.; de Lichtenberg, U.; Rinner, O.; et al. A high-quality catalog of the *Drosophila melanogaster* proteome. *Nat. Biotechnol.* **2007**, *25*, 576–583. [CrossRef]

22. Tress, M.L.; Bodenmiller, B.; Aebersold, R.; Valencia, A. Proteomics studies confirm the presence of alternative protein isoforms on a large scale. *Genome Biol.* **2008**, *9*, R162. [CrossRef] [PubMed]
23. Wolf, F.W.; Eddison, M.; Lee, S.; Cho, W.; Heberlein, U. GSK-3/Shaggy regulates olfactory habituation in *Drosophila*. *Proc. Natl. Acad. Sci. USA* **2007**, *104*, 4653–4657. [CrossRef]
24. Giannakou, M.E.; Goss, M.; Jünger, M.A.; Hafen, E.; Leevers, S.J.; Partridge, L. Long-lived Drosophila with overexpressed dFOXO in adult fat body. *Science* **2004**, *305*, 361. [CrossRef] [PubMed]
25. Bai, H.; Kang, P.; Tatar, M. *Drosophila* insulin-like peptide-6 (dilp6) expression from fat body extends lifespan and represses secretion of *Drosophila* insulin-like peptide-2 from the brain. *Aging Cell* **2012**, *11*, 978–985. [CrossRef] [PubMed]
26. Hoffmann, J.; Romey, R.; Fink, C.; Yong, L.; Roeder, T. Overexpression of Sir2 in the adult fat body is sufficient to extend lifespan of male and female *Drosophila*. *Aging (Albany NY)* **2013**, *5*, 315–327. [CrossRef]
27. Rybina, O.Y.; Sarantseva, S.V.; Veselkina, E.R.; Bolschakova, O.I.; Symonenko, A.V.; Krementsova, A.V.; Ryabova, E.V.; Roshina, N.V.; Pasyukova, E.G. Tissue-specific transcription of the neuronal gene *Lim3* affects *Drosophila melanogaster* lifespan and locomotion. *Biogerontology* **2017**, *18*, 739–757. [CrossRef]
28. Brand, A.H.; Perrimon, N. Targeted gene expression as a means of altering cell fates and generating dominant phenotypes. *Development* **1993**, *118*, 401–415. [PubMed]
29. Tower, J. Sex-specific gene expression and life span regulation. *Trends Endocrinol. Metab.* **2017**, *28*, 735–747. [CrossRef] [PubMed]
30. Vigoreaux, J.O.; Tobin, S.L. Stage-specific selection of alternative transcriptional initiation sites from the 5C actin gene of *Drosophila melanogaster*. *Genes Dev.* **1987**, *1*, 1161–1171. [CrossRef] [PubMed]
31. Uv, A.E.; Harrison, E.J.; Bray, S.J. Tissue-specific splicing and functions of the *Drosophila* transcription factor Grainyhead. *Mol. Cell. Biol.* **1997**, *17*, 6727–6735. [CrossRef]
32. Jones, L.; Richardson, H.; Saint, R. Tissue-specific regulation of *cyclin E* transcription during *Drosophila melanogaster* embryogenesis. *Development* **2000**, *127*, 4619–4630.
33. Golpich, M.; Amini, E.; Hemmati, F.; Ibrahim, N.M.; Rahmani, B.; Mohamed, Z.; Raymond, A.A.; Dargahi, L.; Ghasemi, R.; Ahmadiani, A. Glycogen synthase kinase-3 beta (GSK-3β) signaling: Implications for Parkinson's disease. *Pharmacol. Res.* **2015**, *97*, 16–26. [CrossRef]
34. Choi, H.; Koh, S.-H. Understanding the role of glycogen synthase kinase-3 in L-DOPA-induced dyskinesia in Parkinson's disease. *Expert. Opin. Drug Metab. Toxicol.* **2018**, *14*, 83–90. [CrossRef]
35. Blagosklonny, M.V. MTOR-driven quasi-programmed aging as a disposable soma theory: Blind watchmaker vs. intelligent designer. *Cell Cycle* **2013**, *12*, 1842–1847. [CrossRef]
36. Xie, T.; Ho, M.C.W.; Liu, Q.; Horiuchi, W.; Lin, C.-C.; Task, D.; Luan, H.; White, B.H.; Potter, C.J.; Wu, M.N. A genetic toolkit for dissecting dopamine circuit function in *Drosophila*. *Cell Rep.* **2018**, *23*, 652–665. [CrossRef]
37. Ridgel, A.L.; Ritzmann, R.E. Insights into age-related locomotor declines from studies of insects. *Ageing Res. Rev.* **2005**, *4*, 23–39. [CrossRef]
38. Cui, H.; Kong, Y.; Zhang, H. Oxidative stress, mitochondrial dysfunction, and aging. *J. Signal Transduct.* **2012**, *2012*, 646354. [CrossRef] [PubMed]
39. Orr, W.C.; Radyuk, S.N.; Sohal, R.S. Involvement of redox state in the aging of *Drosophila melanogaster*. *Antioxid. Redox Signal.* **2013**, *19*, 788–803. [CrossRef] [PubMed]
40. Kann, O.; Kovács, R. Mitochondria and neuronal activity. *Am. J. Physiol. Cell Physiol.* **2007**, *292*, C641–C657. [CrossRef]
41. Ruiz-Cañada, C.; Budnik, V. Introduction on the use of the *Drosophila* embryonic/larval neuromuscular junction as a model system to study synapse development and function, and a brief summary of pathfinding and target recognition. *Int. Rev. Neurobiol.* **2006**, *75*, 1–31. [CrossRef]
42. Course, M.M.; Wang, X. Transporting mitochondria in neurons. *F1000Res* **2016**, *18*, 5. [CrossRef]
43. Chen, S.; Owens, G.C.; Crossin, K.L.; Edelman, D.B. Serotonin stimulates mitochondrial transport in hippocampal neurons. *Mol. Cell. Neurosci.* **2007**, *36*, 472–483. [CrossRef] [PubMed]
44. Morfini, G.; Szebenyi, G.; Elluru, R.; Ratner, N.; Brady, S.T. Glycogen synthase kinase 3 phosphorylates kinesin light chains and negatively regulates kinesin-based motility. *EMBO J.* **2002**, *21*, 281–293. [CrossRef]
45. Chen, S.; Owens, G.C.; Edelman, D.B. Dopamine inhibits mitochondrial motility in hippocampal neurons. *PLoS ONE* **2008**, *3*, e2804. [CrossRef]
46. Gao, F.J.; Hebbar, S.; Gao, X.A.; Alexander, M.; Pandey, J.P.; Walla, M.D.; Cotham, W.E.; King, S.J.; Smith, D.S.

GSK-3β phosphorylation of cytoplasmic dynein reduces Ndel1 binding to intermediate chains and alters dynein motility. *Traffic* **2015**, *16*, 941–961. [CrossRef]

47. Ogawa, F.; Murphy, L.C.; Malavasi, E.L.; O'Sullivan, S.T.; Torrance, H.S.; Porteous, D.J.; Millar, J.K. NDE1 and GSK3β associate with TRAK1 and regulate axonal mitochondrial motility: Identification of cyclic AMP as a novel modulator of axonal mitochondrial trafficking. *ACS Chem. Neurosci.* **2016**, *7*, 553–564. [CrossRef]
48. Roos, J.; Hummel, T.; Ng, N.; Klämbt, C.; Davis, G.W. *Drosophila* Futsch regulates synaptic microtubule organization and is necessary for synaptic growth. *Neuron* **2000**, *26*, 371–382. [CrossRef]
49. Wang, J.-W.; Beck, E.S.; McCabe, B.D. A modular toolset for recombination transgenesis and neurogenetic analysis of *Drosophila*. *PLoS ONE* **2012**, *7*, e42102. [CrossRef]
50. Bischof, J.; Maeda, R.K.; Hediger, M.; Karch, F.; Basler, K. An optimized transgenesis system for *Drosophila* using germ-line-specific phiC31 integrases. *Proc. Natl. Acad. Sci. USA* **2007**, *104*, 3312–3317. [CrossRef]
51. McGraw, E.A.; O'Neill, S.L. *Wolbachia pipientis*: Intracellular infection and pathogenesis in *Drosophila*. *Curr. Opin. Microbiol.* **2004**, *7*, 67–70. [CrossRef] [PubMed]
52. Werren, J.H.; Windsor, D.M. *Wolbachia* infection frequencies in insects: Evidence of a global equilibrium? *Proc. Biol. Sci.* **2000**, *267*, 1277–1285. [CrossRef] [PubMed]
53. Holden, P.R.; Jones, P.; Brookfield, J.F. Evidence for a *Wolbachia* symbiont in *Drosophila melanogaster*. *Genet. Res.* **1993**, *62*, 23–29.
54. Wagh, D.A.; Rasse, T.M.; Asan, E.; Hofbauer, A.; Schwenkert, I.; Dürrbeck, H.; Buchner, S.; Dabauvalle, M.-C.; Schmidt, M.; Qin, G.; et al. Bruchpilot, a protein with homology to ELKS/CAST, is required for structural integrity and function of synaptic active zones in *Drosophila*. *Neuron* **2006**, *49*, 833–844. [CrossRef]
55. Sherwood, N.T.; Sun, Q.; Xue, M.; Zhang, B.; Zinn, K. *Drosophila* spastin regulates synaptic microtubule networks and is required for normal motor function. *PLoS Biol.* **2004**, *2*, e429. [CrossRef]
56. Wilmoth, J.R.; Horiuchi, S. Rectangularization revisited: Variability of age at death within human populations. *Demography* **1999**, *36*, 475–495. [CrossRef] [PubMed]
57. Carey, J.R. *Longevity: The Biology and Demography of Life Span*; Princeton University Press: Princeton, NT, USA, 2003.

6

Thirty-Five Years of Computerized Cognitive Assessment of Aging—Where are we Now?

Avital Sternin [1,*], Alistair Burns [2] and Adrian M. Owen [1,3]

1 Brain and Mind Institute, Department of Psychology, University of Western Ontario, London, ON N6A 3K7, Canada
2 Division of Neuroscience & Experimental Psychology, Manchester Institute for Collaborative Research on Ageing, School of Social Sciences, University of Manchester, Manchester M13 9PL, UK
3 Department of Physiology and Pharmacology, University of Western Ontario, London, ON N6A 3K7, Canada
* Correspondence: avital.sternin@uwo.ca

Abstract: Over the past 35 years, the proliferation of technology and the advent of the internet have resulted in many reliable and easy to administer batteries for assessing cognitive function. These approaches have great potential for affecting how the health care system monitors and screens for cognitive changes in the aging population. Here, we review these new technologies with a specific emphasis on what they offer over and above traditional 'paper-and-pencil' approaches to assessing cognitive function. Key advantages include fully automated administration and scoring, the interpretation of individual scores within the context of thousands of normative data points, the inclusion of 'meaningful change' and 'validity' indices based on these large norms, more efficient testing, increased sensitivity, and the possibility of characterising cognition in samples drawn from the general population that may contain hundreds of thousands of test scores. The relationship between these new computerized platforms and existing (and commonly used) paper-and-pencil tests is explored, with a particular emphasis on why computerized tests are particularly advantageous for assessing the cognitive changes associated with aging.

Keywords: computerized cognitive assessment; aging; dementia; memory; executive function

---

1. Introduction

Cognitive assessment has been of interest to psychology, cognitive neuroscience, and general medicine for more than 150 years. In the earliest reports, such as the widely-discussed case of Phineas Gage [1], cognitive 'assessment' was based solely on observation and subjective reports of the behavioural changes that followed a serendipitous brain injury. By the early 20th century, there had been several attempts to standardize cognitive assessments by individuals such as James Cattell [2] and Alfred Binet [3], although these were few and far between, often based on subsets of cognitive processes, and designed with specific populations in mind (e.g., children). It was not until the 1950s, 60s and 70s that the field of cognitive assessment exploded, and dozens of batteries of tests were developed, 'normed', and made widely available for general use (e.g., the Wechsler Adult Intelligence Scale [4], the Wechsler Memory Scale [5], the Stroop task [6,7]).

In the 1980s, a shift in emphasis occurred, as portable computers became more accessible and existing 'paper and pencil' cognitive assessments began to be digitized. Finally, by the turn of the century, the emergence of the world wide web made 'internet based' testing a reality, resulting in the creation of more reliable and efficient tests that could be taken from anywhere in the world. In parallel with the development of computerized tests for cognitive assessment, computerized brain-training games have also become popular (e.g., Lumosity). In this paper, we will only be discussing batteries designed for assessment (rather than 'training') purposes. Despite the proliferation of both laboratory-based and internet-based computerized cognitive assessment platforms and the many advantages they offer, these systems are still not as widely used as many of the classic paper-and-pencil batteries, particularly in older adult populations. For example, a PsychInfo search for peer-reviewed journal articles published in the 10 years between 1 July 2009 and 1 July 2019 that used the Wechsler Adult Intelligence Scale [4] and the Mini-Mental State Examination [8] in participants over the age of 65 returned 983 and 2224 studies, respectively. By comparison, when the same parameters were used to search for 'computerized cognitive assessment' only 364 results were returned.

The goal of this paper is to provide an overview of how both laboratory-based and internet-based cognitive assessments have evolved since the 1980s when computerized approaches were first introduced to the present day when they routinely make use of small, ultra-portable technologies such as cell phones and tablets (e.g., iPads). We will focus our discussion on how these assessments are being applied to detect and track dementia. Key differences between these new computerized platforms and existing (and commonly used) paper-and-pencil tests will be discussed, with a particular emphasis on why computerized tests are particularly advantageous for assessing the cognitive changes associated with aging.

2. Computerized Cognitive Assessment—Historically

The computerization of cognitive assessment tools began in the 1980s with the development of personal computers. Although initial digitization efforts mainly focused on the straight conversion of paper-and-pencil tests to computerized formats, new methods of assessment soon began to be developed that capitalized on emerging technologies (such as touchscreens, response pads, computer mice, etc.). These new methods, when used alongside computers to collect data, led to the creation of tests that were more efficient at assessing an individual's abilities than their paper-and-pencil equivalents. For example, computerized tests are able to measure response latencies with millisecond accuracy and record and report on many aspects of performance simultaneously. Computers can calculate scores and modify test difficulty on the fly, as well as automate instructions, practice questions, and administration of the tests across large groups of people—something that is not so easy for a human test administrator to accomplish. Moreover, because test difficulty can be adjusted on-the-fly, assessments can be shorter and therefore less frustrating, or exhausting, for impaired individuals. In addition, predefined criteria can dictate the maximum number of successes or failures that each individual is exposed to, such that the subjective experience of being tested is equivalent across participants. The reporting of scores also becomes easier and more accurate because their interpretation can be made entirely objectively based on calculated statistics using information gleaned from large normative datasets.

Some of these advantages lead to greater test sensitivity [9] and as such, computerized cognitive assessments are valuable for investigating changes that may not be detected using conventional methods. This makes them ideal for assessing and following subtle cognitive changes in aging over the long term and increases the possibility that emerging mild cognitive impairments will be detected as early as possible [10].

An early example of a set of computerized cognitive tests was the Cambridge Neuropsychological Test Automated Battery (CANTAB). CANTAB was originally designed for the neuropsychological assessment of neurodegenerative diseases and was the first touch-screen based, comprehensive, computerized cognitive battery. CANTAB was standardized in nearly 800 older adult participants [11], and early studies indicated that specific tests, or combinations of tests, were sensitive to deficits and progressive decline in both Alzheimer's disease and Parkinson's disease [12–16]. Specific tests from the CANTAB battery also appear to be able to predict the development of dementia in preclinical populations, while also differentiating between different disorders such as Alzheimer's disease and Frontotemporal dementia [10,17,18]. This early example of a computerized neuropsychological battery paved the way for others, designed to assess similar, or different, types of cognitive function and dysfunction (e.g., Cambridge Brain Sciences [19], Automatic Neuropsychological Assessment

Metrics [20], Computerized Neuropsychological Test Battery [21], Touch Panel-Type Dementia Assessment Scale [22]).

Although the broad body of literature that has accumulated over the last 35 years indicates that computerized tests are adept at detecting and monitoring cognitive decline in neurodegenerative disorders, little consensus exists about which are the most effective and suitable for this task. Two recent reviews described 17 such batteries as being suitable for use in aging populations (see [23,24] for tables illustrating these batteries in detail). The consensus across both reviews was that, although broadly valid for testing aging populations, many of these batteries had serious shortcomings. For example, many batteries relied on normative data from small samples sizes or samples that lacked data specific to older adults. Ultimately, both reviews suggested that how useful any given battery was must be assessed on a case-by-case basis and that no one test, or battery of tests, could be singled out as being the most reliable for screening and monitoring cognitive impairment in the elderly. Without doubt, this general lack of consensus about computerized cognitive tests has contributed to their slow adoption into health care systems. Clinicians are rightly hesitant to adopt any new platform for screening or monitoring patients when normative population data are lacking [25], and this issue needs to be urgently resolved. The obvious way to accomplish this is to greatly increase the number of participants who have completed any given computerized test or battery, and generate norms based on these large databases that can be used to assess the performance of groups or individuals with known, or suspected, clinical disorders. For practical and economic reasons, this is not feasible when assessments need to be taken by a trained administrator in a laboratory testing environment. However, with the advent of the internet, mass 'self-administration' of computerized cognitive tests has become a reality, opening up many new and transformative opportunities in this domain.

3. Cognitive Assessment in the Internet Age

The internet and the proliferation of portable computers into every aspect of our lives (e.g., phones, TVs, tablets), has created many new opportunities, and challenges, for computerized cognitive assessment. For example, by making cognitive assessments available online, a much larger number of participants can be reached than would be possible when the tests are administered on paper and/or in a laboratory setting. With increasing numbers, demographic variables such as age, geographical location and socioeconomic status can also be fed into each assessment, and on-the-fly comparisons with large normative databases can be used to provide 'personalized' results that take these factors into account.

One example of such an online tool is the Cambridge Brain Sciences (CBS) platform. The tests in this battery are largely based on well validated neuropsychological tasks but have been adapted and designed to capitalize on the numerous advantages that internet and computer-based testing can offer. The CBS battery has been used to conduct several large-scale population-based studies involving tens of thousands of participants from all over the world [19,26], as well as more than 300 bespoke scientific studies (e.g., [27–29]). As testament to the 'power of the internet', in total, more than 8 million tests have been taken, and normative data from 75,000 healthy participants are available, including approximately 5000 adults over the age of 65.

Having access to such a large number of datapoints also makes it possible to investigate how demographic factors affect cognition in a way and on a scale that was never before feasible, shedding new light on the interplay between biology and environmental factors and their effects on cognitive function. For example, in one recent study of 45,000 individuals, the CBS battery was used to examine the influence of factors like gender differences, anxiety, depression, substance abuse, and socio-economic status on cognitive function, as well as how they interact during the aging process to uniquely affect different aspects of performance [30].

Other computerized assessment batteries that have been used in older adult populations include the Automatic Neuropsychological Assessment Metrics [20], Computerized Neuropsychological Test Battery [21], and the Touch Panel-Type Dementia Assessment Scale [22]. Each of these batteries consists of a series of tests designed to measure various aspects of cognitive functioning such as processing speed, memory retention, and working memory using tasks based on command following, object recognition, logical reasoning, mathematical processing, and symbol-digit coding.

3.1. Meaningful Change

When normative databases include tens of thousands of participants, it becomes possible to compute indices that are simply not possible with smaller (e.g., lab-based) data samples. Estimates of 'meaningful' or 'reliable' change are one such example that has particular relevance for monitoring cognitive decline or improvement on an individual basis. Estimates of meaningful or reliable change compare the difference in an individual's performance on a task between two time points (e.g., between a patient's current assessment results and previous baseline results) to the variability in repeated measurements that would occur in the absence of a meaningful change. The latter is estimated from a sample of healthy control subjects, and the larger that sample is, the better. Gathering data from a large number of individuals via online testing allows for a database of thousands of normative data points [19,31]. The meaningful change index used by the CBS platform, for example, uses the test-retest reliability and the standard deviation of scores (measured in the control sample) of each task to describe the range of possible differences that could occur with repeated task completion. If an individual's change in performance from one time point to another is much larger than expected by chance (i.e., larger than the fluctuations seen in the control sample), then one can conclude that there was a meaningful change. This may be crucial for evaluating a single aging patient and deciding whether or not a change in performance from one assessment to the next is 'meaningful' or simply a reflection of the day to day fluctuations that are characteristic of healthy cognitive functioning. The above method of calculating a meaningful change score is one example of how computerized cognitive testing can be used to monitor cognitive changes over time. Other methods that, for example, investigate the longitudinal measurement invariance can also be used [32,33] to determine whether the scores from a single metric collected over time are stable or changing in a meaningful way.

The increased size of the normative database to which individual scores are compared is one way in which modern internet-based assessment tools are able to address an issue raised by Zygouris and Tsolaki [24]; that is, physicians rarely have time to wade through the complicated data output of computerized testing batteries to interpret their meaning. When the meaning of test results can be determined through automated statistical algorithms that interrogate a large normative database, the task of interpreting test results is offloaded to the battery itself (something that is clearly not possible with traditional pencil-and-paper methods). When a meaningful change is detected, caregivers or health care providers can be alerted 'automatically' so that more in-depth testing can be initiated to assess the individual's cognitive status. This has relevance in home care, assisted living facilities, and in hospital settings for reducing the administrative burden of monitoring cognitive changes, while also increasing the sensitivity of testing to catch important changes early enough to be appropriately addressed. This in turn, increases the likelihood that physicians will be amenable to adopting these methods for monitoring and screening aging individuals because the logistic and economic overheads are low. In addition, the immediate delivery, objectivity, and interpretation of scores makes them straightforward for non-experts to understand and increases the probability that these methods will be adopted into the broader health care system because any health care provider or family member can, in principle, monitor an aging patient's cognitive changes over time, the effect of drugs, or even cognitive changes post-surgically [34].

3.2. Validity of At-Home Testing

As we have implied above, one of the main advantages of internet-based testing is that it can be conducted at home (or theoretically, anywhere), as long as a computer with an internet connection is available. One of the obvious questions, however, is its validity in comparison to in-lab testing. To assess this question, we had 19 healthy young adult control participants complete the full CBS battery (12 tests) both while unsupervised at home and while supervised in the laboratory (test order was counterbalanced across participants). The mean standardized scores for each of the tests showed no significant effect of at home versus in laboratory testing ($F = 1.71$, $p = 0.2$) and the tasks showed reliable correlations within participants across the two testing environments ($p < 0.05$) (See Figure 1A). A follow-up study explored whether the stability in scores across testing environments was applicable to patient groups as well as healthy controls. A total of 27 participants with Parkinson's disease were assessed on 4 of the 12 CBS tests at home and in-lab as well as tests of simple and choice reaction time similar to the ones included in the CANTAB battery (the order of tasks was counterbalanced across participants). Again, there was no significant effect of at home versus in-lab testing ($p > 0.1$), and the tasks showed reliable correlations across the two testing environments ($p < 0.05$) (See Figure 1B). Moreover, the results of the simple and choice reaction time tasks demonstrated that response time measures could be collected accurately over the internet, regardless of the testing platform used. Together, the results of these two studies indicate that computerized tests taken unsupervised at home produce results no different than those taken in a laboratory, both in healthy controls and in a patient population.

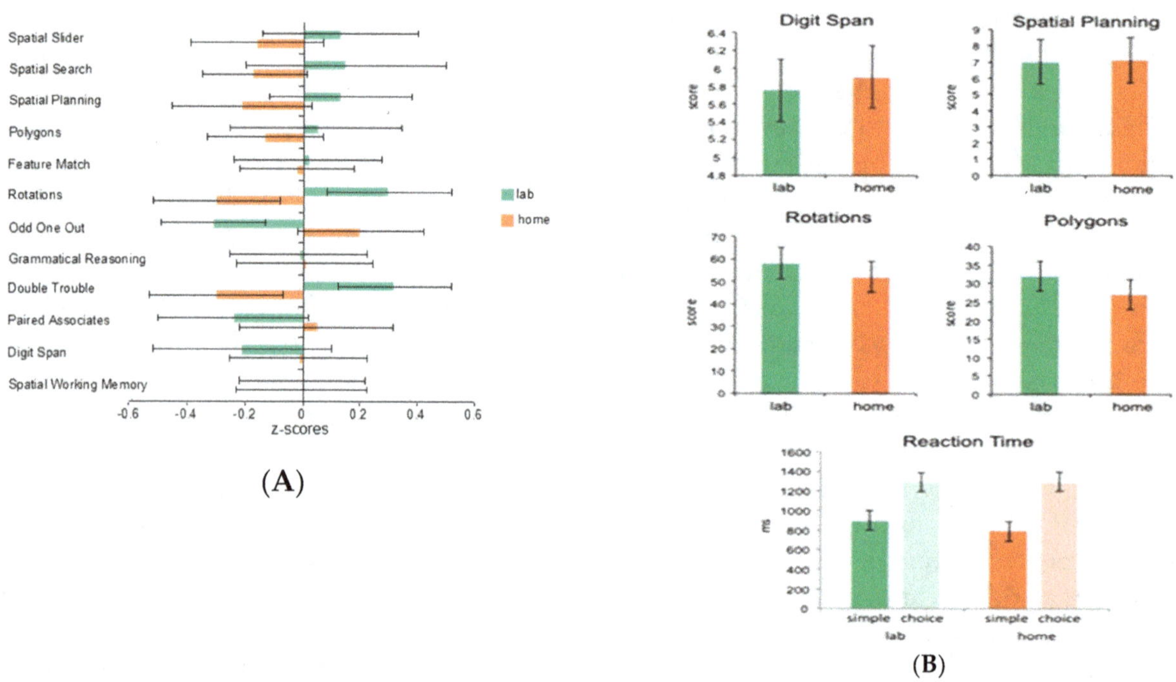

Figure 1. (**A**) average standardized scores on the 12 Cambridge Brain Sciences (CBS) tasks taken at home and in the lab by 19 healthy young adult controls. The results showed no significant effect of at home versus in laboratory testing ($F = 1.71$, $p = 0.2$); (**B**) average raw scores on 4 CBS tasks as well as simple and choice reaction time tasks taken at home and in the lab by 27 patients with Parkinson's Disease. Again, there was no significant effect of at home versus in-lab testing ($p > 0.1$) and the tasks showed reliable correlations across the two testing environments ($p < 0.05$).

In a third recently published study examining the relationship between unsupervised cognitive testing 'at home' and supervised lab-based assessment, the performance of more than 100 participants was compared on three of the CBS tests, Digit Span, Spatial Span and Token Search [35] There were no significant differences in performance between those participants who completed the tests online via Amazon's MTurk platform and those who completed the testing supervised within the laboratory (Figure 2). In the case of the Token Search test, this was even true after extensive training on the task over several weeks [35].

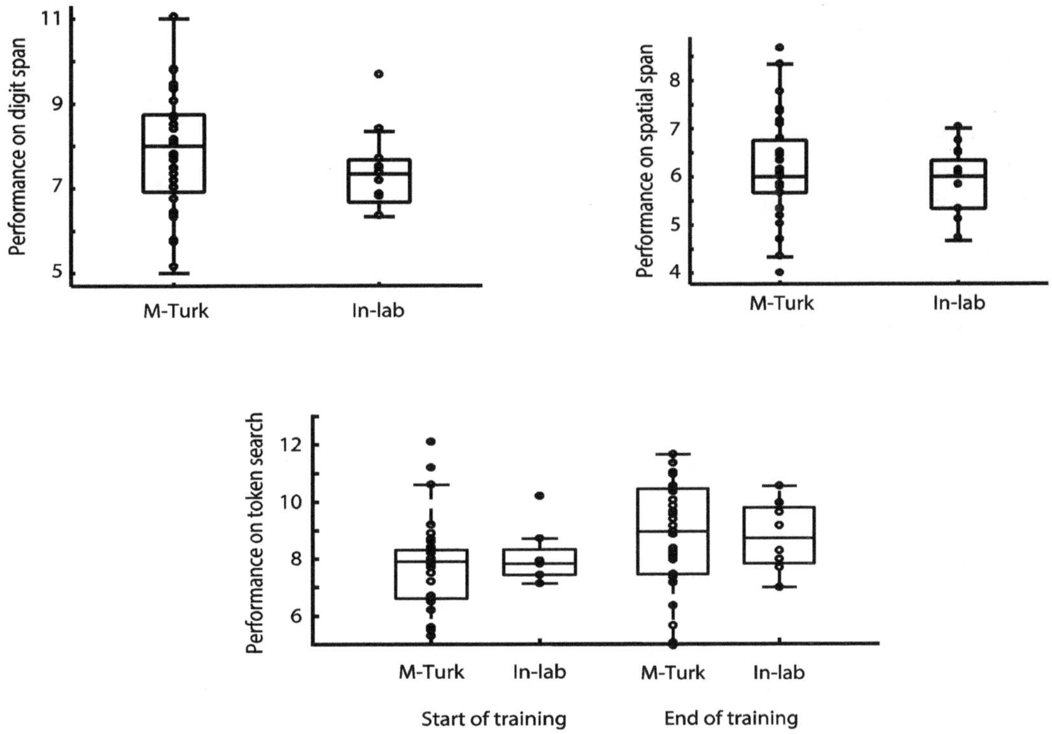

Figure 2. Average scores on 3 CBS tasks (Digit Span, Spatial Span and Token Search), taken at home and in the lab by more than 100 young adult controls. The results showed no significant effect of at home versus in laboratory testing [35]. In the case of Token Search (lower panel), the overlap in performance for participants tested at home using Amazon's MTurk and those tested in the laboratory persisted even after several weeks of intensive training on the task [35].

Another advantage of internet-based testing and large-scale normative databases is that it is relatively straightforward to calculate indicators of 'validity' on-the-fly which can then be used to 'flag' when testing has not been completed properly, or according to the instructions. By analyzing thousands of data points, a set of parameters can be defined that must be met for a score on a test to be considered valid. Including a simple and easy-to-read marker on a score report that conveys whether performance on a task is within reasonable bounds increases the usability and confidence in the test by health care providers.

Finally, there are other mechanisms that can be used to ensure reliable data are collected when tasks are self-administered at home in online settings. For example, interactive learning tutorials can guide participants through practice trials and objectively determine when an individual has understood task instructions before beginning a testing session. Such practice trials increase the validity of the tests, particularly when they are taken for the first time.

4. Online Testing vs. Existing Alternatives

The ability to quickly and accurately assess changes in cognitive functioning on a regular basis has implications for quality of life, level of independence, and degree of care in the aging adult population. Currently, assessments like the Mini-Mental Status Exam (MMSE) [8] and the Montreal Cognitive Assessment (MoCA) [36] are used by health care providers to monitor cognitive changes and screen for deficits. Although these tests are useful because they are short and easy to administer, there are some downsides to using these paper-and-pencil based methods of assessment. For example, they are not adaptive to an individual's ability level, which can lead to frustration in patients with deficits or unnecessary redundancy in individuals who are clearly completely unimpaired. In addition, the questions are not randomly generated with each administration (so opportunities for retesting are reduced). Third, these tests must be administered by a trained individual, which introduces testing bias and takes time and resources away from other health care duties. Fourth, rather than detecting fine grained changes in cognition, these paper-pencil tests assign patients to very broad categories (impaired or unimpaired)—binary classification of this sort is highly susceptible to error through day to day fluctuations in normal cognitive functioning. Finally, the cutoff scores used in these tests may not be appropriate for aging populations [37–39] and result in larger numbers of patients being labeled as 'impaired' than perhaps is necessary.

Several recent studies have investigated whether short computerized assessments can effectively monitor cognitive changes over time and better differentiate between older adult populations with differing abilities than the most widely used paper-and-pencil alternatives. When 45 older adults recruited from a geriatric psychiatry outpatient clinic were tested on five computerized tests from the CBS battery, results showed that some of these tests provided more information about each individual's cognitive abilities than the standard MoCA when administered on its own [40]. The addition of scores from just two of the computerized tests (total testing time of 6 min) to a MoCA, better sorted participants into impaired or unimpaired categories. Specifically, 81% of those patients who were classified as being borderline (between 'impaired' and 'not impaired') based on their MoCA scores alone were reclassified as one or the other when scores from two computerized tests were introduced. Additionally, this study demonstrated that some computerized tests provide more information than others when used in this context. That is to say, two of the five tests employed were not at all useful in classifying borderline patients and the fifth test was too difficult for the older adults to understand and complete.

To follow-up this study, we recently investigated whether other tests in the CBS battery, beyond the five used by Brenkel et al. [40], could provide more information about older adults' cognitive abilities, as well as whether traditional tests like the MoCA or the MMSE could be replaced entirely by an online computerized assessment battery.

A total of 52 older adults (average age = 81 years, 62–97 years) were asked to complete the 12 online tests from the CBS battery in random order. Each task was presented on a touchscreen tablet computer and was preceded by instructions and practice trials. Afterwards, the MoCA (version 7.1 English) and MMSE were administered in interview format, always by the same person (AS). Possibly because of the location of the retirement homes from which participants were recruited, the sample was highly educated. All but one earned high school diplomas, 24 earned postsecondary degrees, and 16 earned postgraduate degrees. Two participants did not complete all 12 tasks due to fatigue and loss of interest; thus 50 participants' scores were analysed. MoCA scores ranged from 12–30 (mean = 24.6) and MMSE scores ranged from 16–30 (mean = 27.7; see Supplementary Figure S1).

Participant scores were split into three categories based on the results of the MoCA test (See Figure 3): unimpaired (n = 25; MoCA score $\geq$ 26), borderline cognitive impairment (n = 14; MoCA score 23–25), and impaired (n = 12; MoCA score $\leq$ 22), based on thresholds from previous literature (e.g., [36–38]). Each participant in the borderline MoCA group was then reclassified to either the impaired or unimpaired groups based on their CBS test scores. A ceiling effect precluded such an analysis for the MMSE results.

Using the MoCA score alone, 72% of participants were classified as impaired or unimpaired. The addition of a single CBS task (Spatial Planning) improved this classification to 92% of the participants. This was not simply because Spatial Planning was the most difficult test, as the equally difficult Spatial Span test left 5 participants in the borderline group. Test difficulty was determined from an unrelated study with scores from 327 participants age 71–80 (see Supplementary Figure S2).

A second analysis using a step-wise multiple regression indicated that MoCA scores were best predicted by two additional CBS tests: Odd One Out and Feature Match (R^2 = 0.65). Age did not significantly predict any variance over and above these tests. Alone, age predicted 22% of the variance in MoCA scores (R^2 = 0.22). Another step-wise multiple regression showed that MMSE scores were best predicted by Feature Match and Grammatical Reasoning (R^2 = 0.38). Again, age did not explain a significant amount of variance over and above the task scores. Alone, age predicted 8% ($R^2 = 0.08$) of the variance in MMSE scores.

A third regression showed that level of education did not explain a significant amount of variance in MMSE or MoCA scores, although this may be due to overall high educational levels and the ceiling effect seen in MMSE scores (see Supplementary Figure S1).

Scores on the three CBS tasks identified in the two analyses (Feature Match, Odd One Out, Spatial Planning) were then combined to create a composite score. The composite score was highly correlated with MoCA scores and was better than the MoCA alone at differentiating impaired from unimpaired participants (84% versus 72% for the MoCA on its own; see Figure 3).

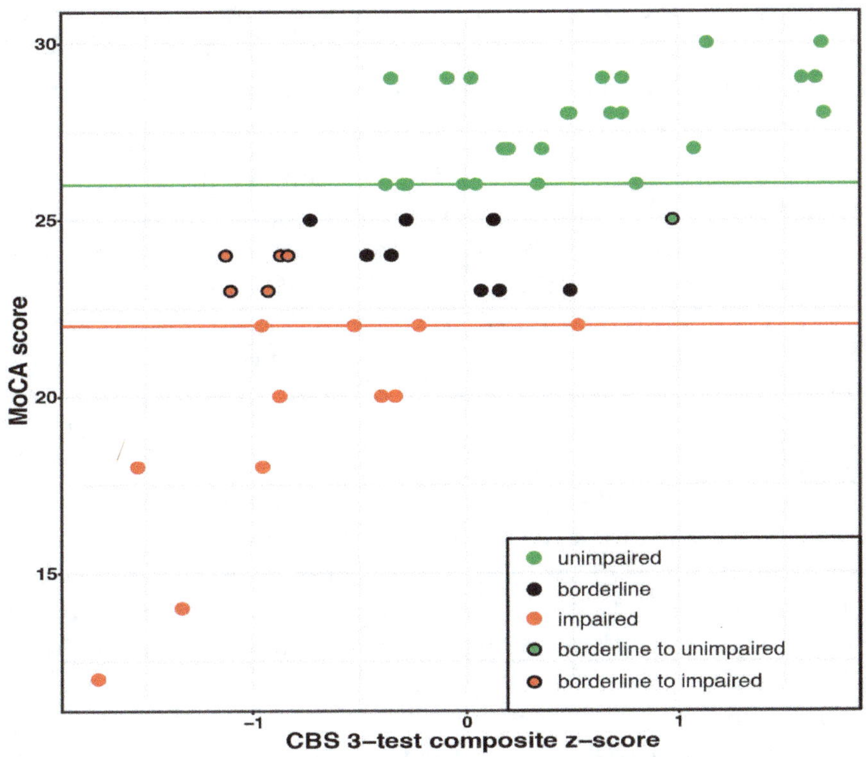

Figure 3. The CBS composite score was highly correlated with Montreal Cognitive Assessment (MoCA) scores and better differentiated impaired and unimpaired individuals. The border colour of each datapoint indicates the categorization of individuals based on MoCA scores alone. The fill colour indicates to which group borderline participants are categorized when the composite score of 3 CBS tests is used.

The results discussed above illustrate the potential that short computerized tests have as screening tools for efficiently monitoring cognitive changes over time. This study also suggests that minimal computer literacy is required when using a touchscreen tablet as technical limitations did not preclude individuals from participating. Another potential use for computerized testing is as a replacement for, or supplement to, neuropsychological assessments that are used for the diagnosis of various brain disorders. In one recent foray into this area, the relationship between a 30 min computerized testing battery and a standard 2–3 h neuropsychological assessment [41] was explored in 134 healthy adults (mean age was 47 years). Although the computerized testing battery could not account for significant variance in the assessments of verbal abilities (e.g., WASI Vocabulary subtest, Word List Generation), it did account for 61% of the variance in the remainder of the traditional neuropsychological battery. The results confirmed that a 30 min internet-based assessment of attention, memory, and executive functioning was comparable to a standard 2–3 h neuropsychological test battery and may even have some diagnostic capabilities.

In the sections above, we have sought to illustrate our arguments with just a few examples of how cognitive changes in older adults can be effectively monitored using self-administered, internet-based computerized testing batteries. Although further validation is required in some cases, there is already good reason to believe that a shift towards internet-based computerized cognitive testing in health care may be warranted.

5. Neural Validation

A key aspect to cognitive assessment is validating the areas of the brain that are involved in the cognitive functions in question. This has long been the domain of neuropsychologists who use results from neurally validated assessments to triangulate brain function from behavioural assessment results. Historically, cognitive assessments were validated using brain lesion studies, but the rise of imaging technologies has made the neural validation of newly developed cognitive assessments accessible and easier to complete.

Coincidentally, the computerization of cognitive assessments has grown alongside this increase in the availability of imaging tools. These parallel timelines have resulted in many examples of computerized cognitive tasks that have been validated from the get-go with neural information gleaned from neuroimaging studies [19,42]. Importantly, however, these imaging studies have underscored the fact that there is rarely a one-to-one mapping between cognitive functions and the brain areas, or networks, that underpin them. One approach to this issue is to examine the complex statistical relationships between performance on any one cognitive task (or group of tasks) and changes in brain activity to reveal how one is related to the other. In order to do this most effectively, large amounts of data need to be included because of the natural variance in cognitive performance (and brain activity) across tests and across individuals. In the age of computerized internet testing and so-called 'big data', this problem becomes much easier to solve. Thus, the sheer amount of data that can be collected allows statistical tests to be performed that were simply not possible when data were collected by hand. For example, Hampshire et al. [19] collected data on the 12 CBS tasks from 45,000 participants. These data were then subjected to a factor analysis, and 3 discrete factors relating to overall cognitive performance were identified. Each one of these factors represents an independent cognitive function that is best described by a combination of performance on multiple tests, something that no single test can assess, and were labeled as encapsulating aspects of short-term memory, reasoning, and verbal abilities, respectively. This technique allows an individual's performance to be compared to a very large normative database in terms of these descriptive factors rather than performance on a single test.

As an example of how this might be applied to a question related directly to aging, Wild et al. [31] recently used this same approach to investigate how sleeping patterns affect cognitive function across the lifespan in a global sample of more than 10,000 people. Using the same analysis of factor structure employed previously by Hampshire et al. [19], the results showed that the relationship between sleep and short-term memory, reasoning and verbal factors was invariant with respect to age, overturning the widely-held notion that the optimal amount of sleep is different in older age groups. Indeed, sleep-related impairments in these three aspects of cognition were shown to affect all ages equally, despite the fact that, as expected, older people tended to sleep less [31]. Put simply, the amount of sleep that resulted in optimal cognitive performance (7–8 h), and the impact of deviating from this amount, was the same for everyone—regardless of age. Somewhat counter-intuitively, this implies that older adults who slept more or less than the optimal amount were impacted no more than younger adults who had non-optimal sleep. If sleep is especially important for staving off dementia and age-related cognitive decline [43], then one might predict that a lack of sleep (or too much sleep) would be associated with more pronounced cognitive impairment in the elderly than in younger adults. Nonetheless, given that 7–8 h of sleep was associated with optimal cognition for all ages and that increasing age was associated with less sleep, the results suggest that older populations in general would likely benefit from more sleep.

Additionally, the neural networks responsible for cognitive factors that are derived from analysing data from multiple tests across large samples of participants can be assessed. For example, Hampshire et al. [19] described the neural correlates of each factor in a group of 16 healthy young participants who completed the testing battery in an fMRI scanner. The short-term memory factor was related to activation in the insula/frontal operculum, the superior frontal sulcus, and the ventral portion of the anterior cingulate cortex and pre-supplementary motor areas. The reasoning factor was related to activation in the inferior frontal sulcus, the inferior parietal cortex, and the dorsal portion of the anterior cingulate and pre-supplementary motor areas. The verbal factor was related to activation in the left inferior frontal gyrus and the bilateral temporal lobes. These data indicate that identifying the neural correlates of cognitive functions is possible with a very large database of participants allowing for complex statistical tests to be performed to interrogate their complex inter-relationships. Computerized assessments are particularly suited to the task of collecting thousands of datapoints and combined with imaging data can provide valuable insights into how a brain injury or neural degeneration as a result of aging affects the brain networks responsible for complex cognitive functions.

6. Conclusions

Computerized cognitive assessments have come a long way in the past 35 years. The proliferation of technology has resulted in reliable and easy to administer batteries that have great potential for affecting how the health care system monitors and screens for cognitive changes in the aging population. Importantly, modern computerized and internet-based cognitive tasks have been designed to capitalize on the many advantages that computers can offer to create more efficient and accurate assessments than existing paper-and-pencil options. One of the key advantages is the way in which these tasks are scored and interpreted. Computerized tests can use statistical measures to interpret one individual's score within the context of thousands of normative data points and provide an objective interpretation of that individual's performance 'on-the-fly'. This shift moves away from the traditional intuition-based approach that more typically required a highly trained individual to interpret a constellation of test scores.

The objective nature of computerized test scores has implications for the adoption of these test batteries into health care because they do not need to be administered or interpreted by a highly trained individual. These batteries can be used by physicians, family members, or other front-line health care workers to monitor for subtle changes in cognition. Catching these changes and flagging them for a more thorough follow-up with the appropriate health-care professional helps to improve quality of life in patients with declining cognitive abilities as well as moves the responsibility of monitoring cognitive changes from a few highly trained individuals to a large number of front-line health-care providers. In short, self-administered online cognitive testing batteries have the potential to help close the dementia diagnosis gap without adding undue burden to the existing health care system.

Author Contributions: Conceptualization; writing–reviewing and editing, A.S., A.B., and A.M.O.; writing–original draft preparation, A.S.; funding acquisition, A.M.O.

References

1. Harlow, J.M. Passage of an iron rod through the head. *Boston Med. Surg. J.* **1848**, *39*, 389–393. [CrossRef]
2. Cattell, J.M.; Farrand, L. Physical and mental measurements of the students of Columbia University. *Psychol. Rev.* **1896**, *3*, 618–648. [CrossRef]
3. Binet, A. *L'étude expérimentale de l'intelligence*; Schleicher frères & cie: Paris, France, 1903.
4. Wechsler, D. *Manual for the Wechsler Adult Intelligence Scale*; Psychological Corp.: Oxford, UK, 1955.
5. Wechsler, D. A standardized memory scale for clinical use. *J. Psychol.* **1945**, *19*, 87–95. [CrossRef]
6. Stroop, J.R. Studies of interference in serial verbal reactions. *J. Exp. Psychol.* **1935**, *18*, 643–662. [CrossRef]
7. Golden, C.J. *Stroop Color and Word Test: A Manual for Clinical and Experimental Uses*; Stoelting Co.: Wood Dale, IL, USA, 1978.

8. Folstein, M.F.; Folstein, S.E.; McHugh, P.R. "Mini-mental state". A practical method for grading the cognitive state of patients for the clinician. *J. Psychiatr. Res.* **1975**, *12*, 189–198. [CrossRef]
9. Bor, D.; Duncan, J.; Lee, A.C.H.; Parr, A.; Owen, A.M. Frontal lobe involvement in spatial span: Converging studies of normal and impaired function. *Neuropsychologia* **2006**, *44*, 229–237. [CrossRef]
10. Blackwell, A.D.; Sahakian, B.J.; Vesey, R.; Semple, J.M.; Robbins, T.W.; Hodges, J.R. Detecting Dementia: Novel Neuropsychological Markers of Preclinical Alzheimer's Disease. *Dement. Geriatr. Cogn. Disord.* **2003**, *17*, 42–48. [CrossRef]
11. Robbins, T.W.; James, M.; Owen, A.M.; Sahakian, B.J.; McInnes, L.; Rabbitt, P. Cambridge Neuropsychological Test Automated Battery (CANTAB): A Factor Analytic Study of a Large Sample of Normal Elderly Volunteers. *Dementia* **1994**, *5*, 266–281. [CrossRef]
12. Downes, J.J.; Roberts, A.C.; Sahakian, B.J.; Evenden, J.L.; Morris, R.G.; Robbins, T.W. Impaired extra-dimensional shift performance in medicated and unmedicated Parkinson's disease: Evidence for a specific attentional dysfunction. *Neuropsychologia* **1989**, *27*, 1329–1343. [CrossRef]
13. Morris, R.G.; Downes, J.J.; Sahakian, B.J.; Evenden, J.L.; Heald, A.; Robbins, T.W. Planning and spatial working memory in Parkinson's disease. *J. Neurol. Neurosurg. Psychiatry* **1988**, *51*, 757–766. [CrossRef]
14. Sahakian, B.J.; Owen, A.M. Computerized assessment in neuropsychiatry using CANTAB: discussion paper. *J. R. Soc. Med.* **1992**, *85*, 399–402.
15. Sahakian, B.J.; Morris, R.G.; Evenden, J.L.; Heald, A.; Levy, R.; Philpot, M.; Robbins, T.W. A comparative study of visuospatial memory and learning in Alzheimer-type dementia and Parkinson's Disease. *Brain* **1988**, *111*, 695–718. [CrossRef]
16. Sahakian, B.J.; Downes, J.J.; Eagger, S.; Everden, J.L.; Levy, R.; Philpot, M.P.; Roberts, A.C.; Robbins, T.W. Sparing of attentional relative to mnemonic function in a subgroup of patients with dementia of the Alzheimer type. *Neuropsychologia* **1990**, *28*, 1197–1213. [CrossRef]
17. Swainson, R.; Hodges, J.R.; Galton, C.J.; Semple, J.; Michael, A.; Dunn, B.D.; Iddon, J.L.; Robbins, T.W.; Sahakian, B.J. Early detection and differential diagnosis of Alzheimer's disease and depression with neuropsychological tasks. *Dement. Geriatr. Cogn. Disord.* **2001**, *12*, 265–280. [CrossRef]
18. Lee, A.C.H.; Rahman, S.; Hodges, J.R.; Sahakian, B.J.; Graham, K.S. Associative and recognition memory for novel objects in dementia: implications for diagnosis. *Eur. J. Neurosci.* **2003**, *18*, 1660–1670. [CrossRef]
19. Hampshire, A.; Highfield, R.R.; Parkin, B.L.; Owen, A.M. Fractionating Human Intelligence. *Neuron* **2012**, *76*, 1225–1237. [CrossRef]
20. Kane, R.; Roebuckspencer, T.; Short, P.; Kabat, M.; Wilken, J. Identifying and monitoring cognitive deficits in clinical populations using Automated Neuropsychological Assessment Metrics (ANAM) tests. *Arch. Clin. Neuropsychol.* **2007**, *22*, 115–126. [CrossRef]
21. Veroff, A.E.; Cutler, N.R.; Sramek, J.J.; Prior, P.L.; Mickelson, W.; Hartman, J.K. A new assessment tool for neuropsychopharmacologic research: the Computerized Neuropsychological Test Battery. *Top. Geriatr.* **1991**, *4*, 211–217. [CrossRef]
22. Inoue, M.; Jimbo, D.; Taniguchi, M.; Urakami, K. Touch Panel-type Dementia Assessment Scale: A new computer-based rating scale for Alzheimer's disease: A new computer-based rating scale for AD. *Psychogeriatrics* **2011**, *11*, 28–33. [CrossRef]
23. Wild, K.; Howieson, D.; Webbe, F.; Seelye, A.; Kaye, J. The status of computerized cognitive testing in aging: A systematic review. *Alzheimers Dement.* **2008**, *4*, 428–437. [CrossRef]
24. Zygouris, S.; Tsolaki, M. Computerized Cognitive Testing for Older Adults: A Review. *Am. J. Alzheimer's Dis. Other Dement.* **2015**, *30*, 13–28. [CrossRef]
25. Barnett, J.H.; Blackwell, A.D.; Sahakian, B.J.; Robbins, T.W. The Paired Associates Learning (PAL) Test: 30 Years of CANTAB Translational Neuroscience from Laboratory to Bedside in Dementia Research. *Curr. Top. Behav. Neurosci.* **2016**, *28*, 449–474.
26. Owen, A.M.; Hampshire, A.; Grahn, J.A.; Stenton, R.; Dajani, S.; Burns, A.S.; Howard, R.J.; Ballard, C.G. Putting brain training to the test. *Nature* **2010**, *465*, 775–778. [CrossRef]
27. Metzler-Baddeley, C.; Caeyenberghs, K.; Foley, S.; Jones, D.K. Task complexity and location specific changes of cortical thickness in executive and salience networks after working memory training. *NeuroImage* **2016**, *130*, 48–62. [CrossRef]

28. Pausova, Z.; Paus, T.; Abrahamowicz, M.; Bernard, M.; Gaudet, D.; Leonard, G.; Peron, M.; Pike, G.B.; Richer, L.; Séguin, J.R.; et al. Cohort Profile: The Saguenay Youth Study (SYS). *Int. J. Epidemiol.* **2017**, *46*, e19. [CrossRef]
29. Esopenko, C.; Chow, T.W.P.; Tartaglia, M.C.; Bacopulos, A.; Kumar, P.; Binns, M.A.; Kennedy, J.L.; Müller, D.J.; Levine, B. Cognitive and psychosocial function in retired professional hockey players. *J. Neurol. Neurosurg. Psychiatry* **2017**, *88*, 512–519. [CrossRef]
30. Nichols, E.S.; Wild, C.J.; Owen, A.M.; Soddu, A. Cognition across the lifespan: Aging and gender differences. *Cognition.* in submission.
31. Wild, C.J.; Nichols, E.S.; Battista, M.E.; Stojanoski, B.; Owen, A.M. Dissociable effects of self-reported daily sleep duration on high-level cognitive abilities. *Sleep* **2018**, *41*, 1–11. [CrossRef]
32. Schaie, K.; Maitland, S.B.; Willis, S.L.; Intrieri, R. Longitudinal invariance of adult psychometric ability factor structures across 7 years. *Psychol. Aging* **1998**, *13*, 8–20. [CrossRef]
33. Widaman, K.F.; Ferrer, E.; Conger, R.D. Factorial Invariance within Longitudinal Structural Equation Models: Measuring the Same Construct across Time. *Child. Dev. Perspect.* **2010**, *4*, 10–18. [CrossRef]
34. Honarmand, K.; Malik, S.; Wild, C.; Gonzalez-Lara, L.E.; McIntyre, C.W.; Owen, A.M.; Slessarev, M. Feasibility of a web-based neurocognitive battery for assessing cognitive function in critical illness survivors. *PLoS ONE* **2019**, *14*, e0215203. [CrossRef]
35. Stojanoski, B.; Lyons, K.M.; Pearce, A.A.A.; Owen, A.M. Targeted training: Converging evidence against the transferable benefits of online brain training on cognitive function. *Neuropsychologia* **2018**, *117*, 541–550. [CrossRef]
36. Nasreddine, Z.S.; Phillips, N.A.; Bédirian, V.; Charbonneau, S.; Whitehead, V.; Collin, I.; Cummings, J.L.; Chertkow, H. The Montreal Cognitive Assessment, MoCA: A brief screening tool for mild cognitive impairment. *J. Am. Geriatr. Soc.* **2005**, *53*, 695–699. [CrossRef]
37. Gluhm, S.; Goldstein, J.; Loc, K.; Colt, A.; Liew, C.V.; Corey-Bloom, J. Cognitive Performance on the Mini-Mental State Examination and the Montreal Cognitive Assessment Across the Healthy Adult Lifespan. *Cogn. Behav. Neurol.* **2013**, *26*, 1–5. [CrossRef]
38. Damian, A.M.; Jacobson, S.A.; Hentz, J.G.; Belden, C.M.; Shill, H.A.; Sabbagh, M.N.; Caviness, J.N.; Adler, C.H. The montreal cognitive assessment and the mini-mental state examination as screening instruments for cognitive impairment: Item analyses and threshold scores. *Dement. Geriatr. Cogn. Disord.* **2011**, *31*, 126–131. [CrossRef]
39. Malek-Ahmadi, M.; Powell, J.J.; Belden, C.M.; O'Connor, K.; Evans, L.; Coon, D.W.; Nieri, W. Age- and education-adjusted normative data for the Montreal Cognitive Assessment (MoCA) in older adults age 70–99. *Aging Neuropsychol. Cogn.* **2015**, *22*, 755–761. [CrossRef]
40. Brenkel, M.; Shulman, K.; Hazan, E.; Herrmann, N.; Owen, A.M. Assessing Capacity in the Elderly: Comparing the MoCA with a Novel Computerized Battery of Executive Function. *Dement. Geriatr. Cogn. Disord. Extra.* **2017**, *7*, 249–256. [CrossRef]
41. Levine, B.; Bacopulous, A.; Anderson, N.; Black, S.; Davidson, P.; Fitneva, S.; McAndrews, M.; Spaniol, J.; Jeyakumar, N.; Abdi, H.; et al. Validation of a Novel Computerized Test Battery for Automated Testing. In *Stroke*; Lippincott Williams & Wilkins: Philadelphia, PA, USA, 2013; Volume 44, p. 196.
42. Robbins, T.W.; James, M.; Owen, A.M.; Sahakian, B.J.; McInnes, L.; Rabbitt, P.; James, M.; Owen, A.M.; Sahakian, B.J.; McInnes, L.; et al. A Neural Systems Approach to the Cognitive Psychology of Ageing Using the CANTAB Battery. In *Methodology of Frontal and Executive Function*; Routledge: London, UK, 2004; pp. 216–239.
43. Yaffe, K.; Falvey, C.M.; Hoang, T. Connections between sleep and cognition in older adults. *Lancet Neurol.* **2014**, *13*, 1017–1028. [CrossRef]

7

Characterization of Ageing- and Diet-Related Swine Models of Sarcopenia and Sarcopenic Obesity

Consolacion Garcia-Contreras [1,†], Marta Vazquez-Gomez [2,†], Laura Torres-Rovira [1], Jorge Gonzalez [3], Esteban Porrini [4], Magali Gonzalez-Colaço [5], Beatriz Isabel [2], Susana Astiz [1] and Antonio Gonzalez-Bulnes [1,2,*]

1 Comparative Physiology Group, SGIT-INIA, 28040 Madrid, Spain; garcia.consolacion@inia.es (C.G.-C.); torres.laura@inia.es (L.T.-R.); astiz.susana@inia.es (S.A.)
2 Faculty of Veterinary Sciences, Universidad Complutense de Madrid, 28040 Madrid, Spain; mvgomez@ucm.es (M.V.-G.); bisabelr@ucm.es (B.I.)
3 Micros Veterinaria, Campus de Vegazana, 24007 Leon, Spain; info@microsvet.com
4 Institute of Biomedical Technology (ITB), Universidad de La Laguna, 38200 Tenerife, Spain; esteban.l.porrini@gmail.com
5 Central Unit of Clinical Research and Clinical Assays (UCICEC), Universitary Hospital of Canary Island, 28010 Tenerife, Spain; magaligch@hotmail.com
* Correspondence: bulnes@inia.es
† These authors contributed equally to this work.

Abstract: Sarcopenia and sarcopenic obesity are currently considered major global threats for health and well-being. However, there is a lack of adequate preclinical models for their study. The present trial evaluated the suitability of aged swine by determining changes in adiposity, fatty acids composition, antioxidant status and lipid peroxidation, development of metabolic disturbances and structural changes in tissues and organs. Iberian sows with clinical evidence of aging-related sarcopenia were fed a standard diet fulfilling their maintenance requirements or an obesogenic diet for 100 days. Aging and sarcopenia were related to increased lipid accumulation and cellular dysfunction at both adipose tissue and non-adipose ectopic tissues (liver and pancreas). Obesity concomitant to sarcopenia aggravates the condition by increasing visceral adiposity and causing dyslipidemia, insulin resistance and lipotoxicity in non-adipose tissues. These results support that the Iberian swine model represents certain features of sarcopenia and sarcopenic obesity in humans, paving the way for future research on physiopathology of these conditions and possible therapeutic targets.

Keywords: animal-model; insulin-resistance; lipotoxicity; obesity; sarcopenia; swine

1. Introduction

Sarcopenia is a syndrome characterized by loss of skeletal muscle mass and function [1], causing negative health outcomes like functional decline and disability [2–4] and increased mortality [5]. This may be further aggravated in case of obesity and increases in fat mass (sarcopenic obesity; [6]) which increases mobility and disability problems [7]. Currently, around 20 and 30% of elderly women and men, respectively, may have sarcopenic obesity [8]. Sarcopenic obesity is also related to metabolic disturbances, like metabolic syndrome and type-2 diabetes [9]; it is, therefore, considered a major global threat to health and well-being [10].

There are currently no drugs for the treatment of sarcopenia [7,11] and the recommended therapeutic interventions are based on lifestyle changes [9], with limited effects and with difficult implementation in elderly individuals with chronic diseases or different disabilities. Hence, there is a strong need for research efforts on pathogenesis and possible treatments. The results will contribute to relevant improvements of individual life-quality and savings in health-care resources.

Almost all the available studies are observational (with their inherent constraints), and interventional research is, therefore, necessary. Such research should be based on adequate translational animal models as elegantly reviewed by Palus in 2017 [12]. Most of the interventional trials on sarcopenia have been performed in rodents and have been based on induced acute muscle atrophy. These models do not represent sarcopenia by ageing [9], which needs long time to be achieved (around 20–24 months [13]). Moreover, the study of metabolic implications of sarcopenic obesity in rodents is constrained by their marked differences in metabolic and endocrine pathways with humans [14]. There is, consequently, a need for complementary preclinical animal models. The use of non-rodent mammals is essential to develop more relevant and predictive models of human disease. In this way, large animals have close similarities to humans in size and in many anatomical, physiological and pathological features. Moreover, large animal models of human diseases can be studied employing the same clinical approach used for human patients. In this sense, the pig has more similar patho-physiological features to humans than rodents [15].

Pigs used for biomedical research can be either random- or purpose-bred. Pigs from random-bred are typically farm animals (e.g., Landrace, Large White, Pietrain), where genetic selection is focused on animal production parameters. Purpose-bred pigs for biomedical research originate from closed colonies selected for a specific phenotype. The most commonly used swine breeds for research on obesity and metabolic diseases are Göttingen, Yucatan and Ossabaw Island pigs. However, all these breeds have a common ancestor: the Iberian pig.

The Iberian pig has an ancient origin, being traced back approximately to year 1000 Before Christ, and has been traditionally reared under extensive free-range conditions, using natural resources like pastures and acorns. Maintenance in semi-feral conditions has induced the pigs to develop an adaptive mechanism to the environment, which is known as *thrifty genotype* and which was firstly described in humans [16]. The *thrifty genotype* facilitates accommodation to seasonal cycles of feasting and famine because the ability to store fat in excess during food abundance enables survival during periods of scarcity. However, these individuals become obese in case of food-excess. Iberian pigs arise therefore as good model for studies on obesity and associated morbidities, since they develop cardiovascular and metabolic disorders in case of obesity, either during juvenile development [17] or adulthood [18].

The Iberian pig may be also useful for studies focused on sarcopenia, since the breed is reared under extensive traditional systems which facilitates the finding of older animals than in the case of breeds used for meat production under intensive management conditions (e.g., Landrace, Large-White, Pietrain). Intensive animal production systems are associated to intense genetic and productive selection and sows identified as having lower performance than the herd average are early culled, as early as age as 3–4 year-old [19]. Conversely, genetic and productive demands are not so strong in extensive traditional systems and culling is more related to either reproductive failures or musculoskeletal and locomotive disorders associated to age (which are similar to those associated with human sarcopenia).

Hence, the present study aimed to characterize a large-animal model for preclinical studies on sarcopenia and sarcopenic obesity, based on the use of old Iberian sows with aging-related sarcopenia and exposed or not to obesogenic diets. The validity of the models was assessed by determining possible links among adiposity, fatty acids composition, antioxidant status and lipid peroxidation, development of metabolic disturbances and structural changes in tissues and organs.

2. Results

2.1. Body-Weight and Adiposity

All the animals fed with the obesogenic diet showed a significant increase in body-weight (123 ± 6.1 to 202.3 ± 4.9 kg, $p < 0.0001$) and adiposity (16.1 ± 2.4 to 45.6 ± 2.9 mm of back-fat depth,

$p < 0.0001$) from Day 0 to 100 (Figure 1). The values in control sows were similar to the initial values in obese sows (127.9 ± 4.0 kg and 19.3 ± 1.3 mm, respectively). The macroscopic findings during necropsy indicated a severe intraabdominal fattening in obese sows, with large amounts of mesenteric fat covering all viscerae and mesenteric tissues. However, intramuscular fat content was similar in obese and non-obese sows (12.9 ± 1.1% vs. 12.8 ± 0.7%).

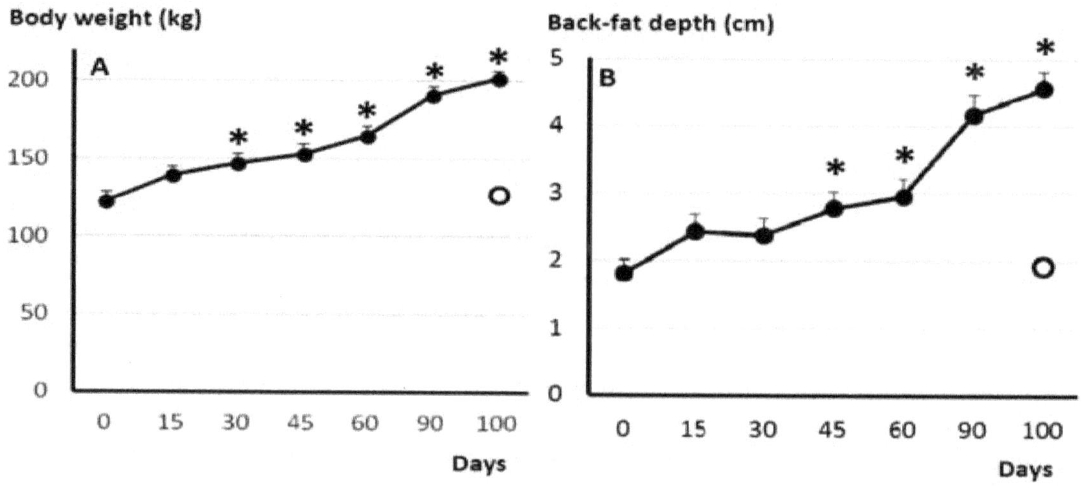

Figure 1. Mean (±S.E.M.) values in body-weight (**A**) and back-fat depth (**B**) in control sows (white dot; $n = 17$) and changes in such values over time after starting differential feeding with a diet enriched with saturated fat in treated sows (black line and dots; $n = 11$). Asterisks (*) denote significant differences between obese and non-obese sows ($p < 0.05$).

2.2. Fatty Acid Composition of Subcutaneous and Visceral Fat and Muscle

The composition of fatty acids (FA) was similar at the outer and inner layers of subcutaneous fat (Supplementary Tables S1 and S2). Overall, when compared to non-obese sows, obese females showed a higher monounsaturated FA (MUFA) content ($p < 0.05$) and lower contents of polyunsaturated FA (PUFA), n-3 and n-6 PUFA ($p < 0.005$ for all). Visceral fat in obese sows also evidenced a higher MUFA content ($p < 0.0001$; Supplementary Table S3) and a lower content of PUFA, n-3 and n-6 PUFA ($p < 0.0001$ for all) than non-obese females. There were no differences at subcutaneous fat, but visceral fat of obese females showed higher ratios of MUFA/saturated FA (SFA) and C18:1/C18:0 ($p < 0.05$ for both).

The analysis of the fatty acid composition in the *longissimus dorsi* showed major effects at the polar lipid fraction (Supplementary Table S4). Obese sows showed a higher MUFA content and a lower content of SFA and PUFA than the controls and, as a consequence, higher MUFA/SFA and C18:1/C18:0 ratios ($p < 0.005$ for all). The content of n-3 and n-6 PUFA were lower, with a higher Σn-6/Σn-3 ratio, in obese than in control sows ($p < 0.005$ for all). The effects from obesity were minor at the neutral fraction (Supplementary Table S5), with MUFA content being lower in obese than in control females ($p < 0.01$).

2.3. Hepatic Architecture, Fatty Acid Composition and Function

The total fat content in the liver was similar in control and obese groups (15.3 ± 0.2% vs. 14.5 ± 0.4%). Histological evaluation of the liver (Figure 2) indicated lipid accumulation in all the obese and in 82.4% of the control sows, with degrees varying from mild (63.6% and 76.5%, respectively) to moderate (36.4% and 23.5%, respectively). Increased presence of lipocytes (also known as perisinusoidal fat-storing cells, stellate cells or Ito cells) was found in all the obese and in 88.2% of the control sows. There were no evidences of inflammation or fibrosis, but hydropic degeneration was observed in 23.5% of the controls and all the obese animals ($p < 0.05$). All the controls had mild degeneration, whilst the obese sows showed mild (27.3%), moderate (63.7%, $p < 0.05$) or even severe degeneration (9.0%, $p < 0.05$).

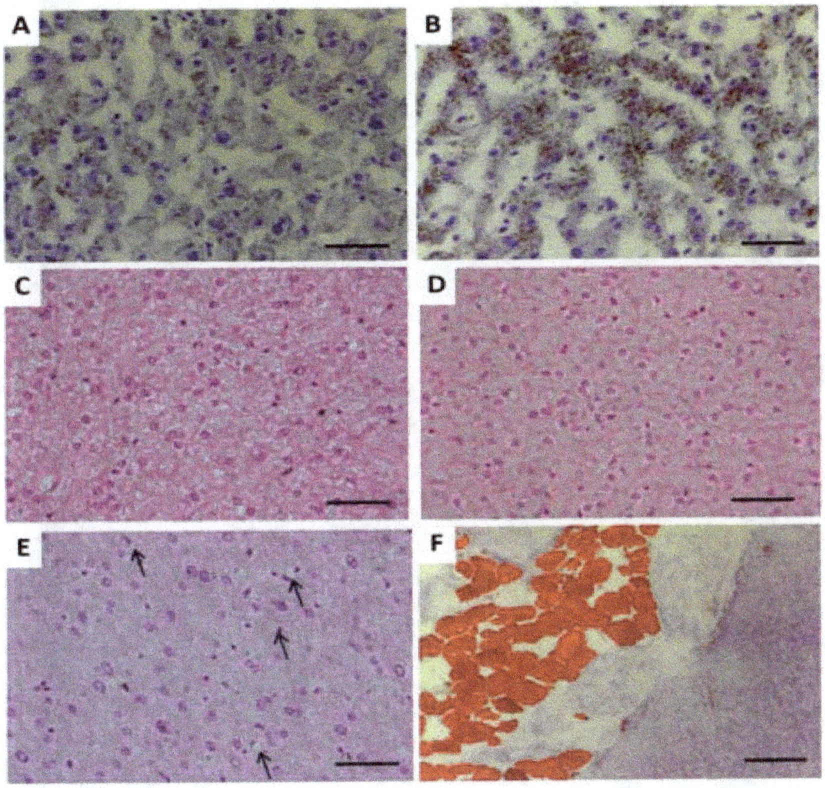

Figure 2. Histological images of liver and pancreas in obese sows. Upper pictures represent mild (**A**) and moderate (**B**) infiltration of lipids, stained in red, in the liver (oil red-O, 400×) Bar 50 µm. Pictures (**C**) and (**D**) of the liver represent mild and severe hydropic degeneration, respectively, whilst picture **E** exemplifies increased presence of lipocytes or Ito cells indicated with arrows (hematoxylin-eosin HE, 400×) Bar 50 µm. Picture **F** represents infiltration of adipocytes with intracytoplasmic accumulation of lipids, stained in red, in the pancreas (oil red-O, 100×) Bar 200 µm.

The major effects of obesity on fatty acids composition of the liver, like in the muscle, were found at the polar fraction (Supplementary Table S6), with higher MUFA/SFA, C18:1/C18:0 and Σn-6/Σn-3 ratios in the obese than in the control females ($p < 0.0001$ for all). The neutral fraction (Supplementary Table S7) was characterized by a higher SFA content ($p < 0.01$) and a higher Σn-6/Σn-3 ratio ($p < 0.0001$) in the obese animals.

The obese sows showed no major changes in the plasma biomarkers of liver function throughout the study, excepting a significant increase in the concentrations of alkaline-phosphatase (56.5 $\pm$ 8.7 to 76.8 $\pm$ 10.1 IU/L, $p < 0.05$) and leucine-aminopeptidase (16.5 $\pm$ 1.9 to 21.4 $\pm$ 0.7 IU/L, $p < 0.01$). Conversely, albumin concentration decreased over time (4.6 $\pm$ 0.1 to 4.1 $\pm$ 0.1 g/dL; $p < 0.05$), from initial values similar to controls (4.7 $\pm$ 0.1 g/dL).

2.4. Plasma Lipid Profile

Plasma concentrations of triglycerides and cholesterol increased with time of treatment in the obese group ($p < 0.05$; Figure 3), starting from values similar to those of control sows at Day 0. The increase in total cholesterol was accompanied by a similar increase in low-density lipoproteins cholesterol (LDL-c) levels ($p < 0.01$) but not in high-density lipoproteins cholesterol (HDL-c). Hence, total cholesterol/HDL-c, LDL-c/HDL-c and atherogenic dyslipidemia ratios increased with time ($p < 0.05$).

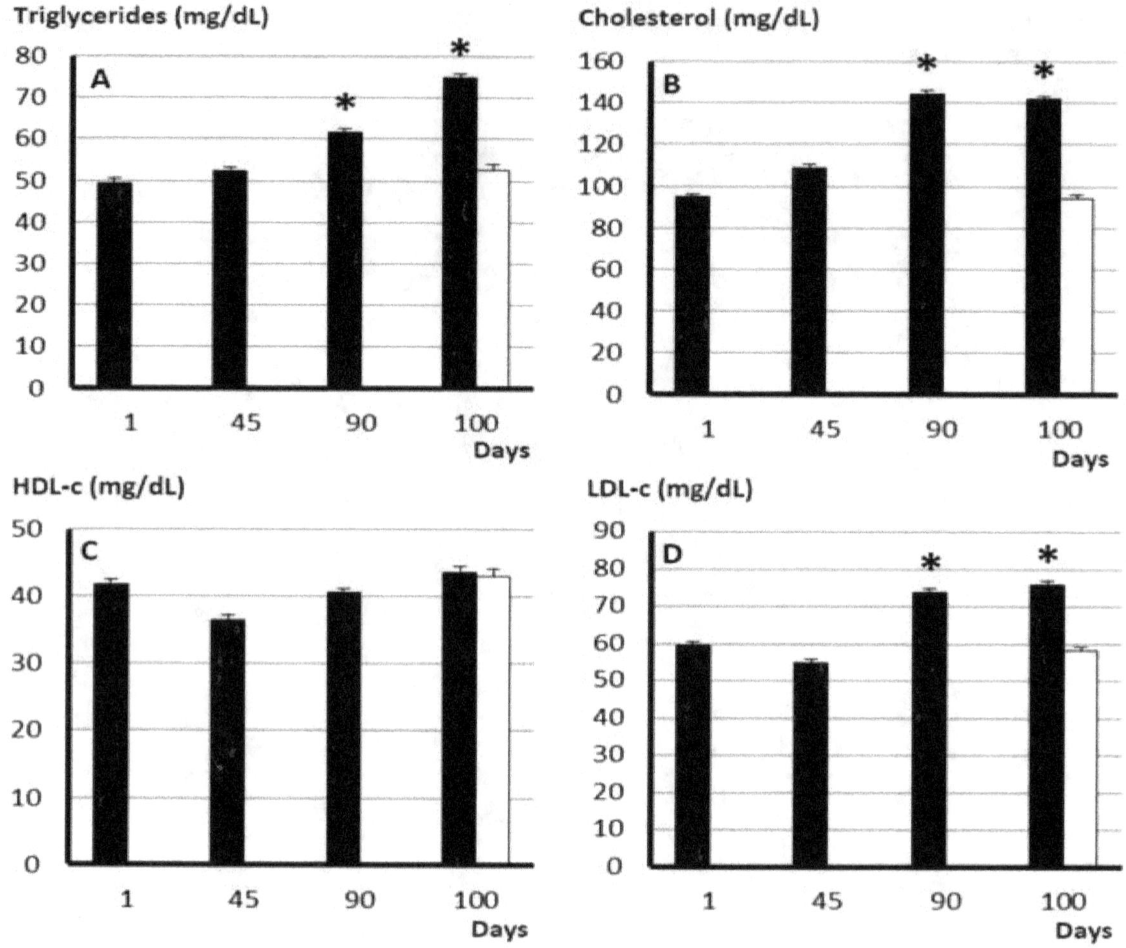

Figure 3. Mean (±S.E.M.) plasma concentrations of triglycerides (**A**), cholesterol (**B**), HDL-c (**C**) and LDL-c (**D**) in control sows (white bar; $n = 17$) and changes in such values over time after starting differential feeding with a diet enriched with saturated fat in treated sows (black bars; $n = 11$). Asterisks (*) denote significant differences between obese and non-obese sows ($p < 0.05$).

2.5. Plasma Antioxidant Capacity and Lipid Oxidation

The plasma antioxidant capacity (measured by FRAP; ferric reducing antioxidant power assay) decreased in the obesogenic-diet group (from 23.6 ± 2.7 at Day 0 to 16.9 ± 2.6 μmol/mL at Day 100, $p < 0.05$), starting from values similar to those of control animals (24.6 ± 4.0 μmol/mL). Concomitantly, the values for total lipid oxidation (assessed as MDA; malondialdehyde) increased with time of treatment in the obese group (from 10.7 ± 0.6 at Day 0 to 12.3 ± 0.3 μmol/mL at Day 100, $p < 0.05$), starting from values similar to those of controls (10.6 ± 0.4 μmol/mL).

2.6. Pancreatic Architecture and Exocrine Function

Microscopic evaluation of the pancreas showed increased lipid accumulation in all the obese sows. Around half of them showed severe infiltration (>66% of the cells; 45.5%), whilst the remaining obese females showed moderate (34–66%; 27.3%) or mild infiltration (5–33%; 27.3%). Conversely, lipid accumulation was found in 12 of the 17 controls (70.6%, $p < 0.05$), with degrees varying from mild (47.1%) to moderate (23.5%), but not severe ($p < 0.01$ with obese sows). On the other hand, no inflammation, fibrosis or cellular injury were observed in any of the animals. Concomitantly, the assessment of plasma biomarkers of exocrine pancreatic function (lipase and amylase) showed no major changes during the period of study.

2.7. Pancreatic Endocrine Function and Insulin Resistance

Mean plasma concentrations of glucose and insulin, and HOMA-IR (Homeostatic Model Assessment for Insulin Resistance) and HOMA-β (Homeostatic Model Assessment for β-cell function) values were similar in controls and obese sows at Day 0. Afterwards, plasma glucose concentrations in obese females were maintained by changes in insulin secretion throughout the period of study (Figure 4). Insulin and HOMA-β index increased at Day 45 ($p < 0.05$ and $p < 0.01$, respectively) and decreased again at Day 90 ($p < 0.05$ and $p < 0.01$, respectively). On the other hand, HOMA-IR increased throughout the study ($p < 0.05$), evidencing insulin resistance (IR). Changes in insulin secretion and glucose elimination were confirmed when analyzing the OGTTs (Oral Glucose Tolerance Tests) performed during the study (Figure 5). In this way, the areas under the curve (AUCs) for glucose and insulin were similar in control and treated sows at Day 0. Afterwards, at 45 and 90 days, AUCs for glucose remained almost stable whilst AUCs for insulin increased 55.7% at Day 45 and 28.3% at Day 90 when compared to Day 0 ($p < 0.01$ and $p < 0.05$, respectively).

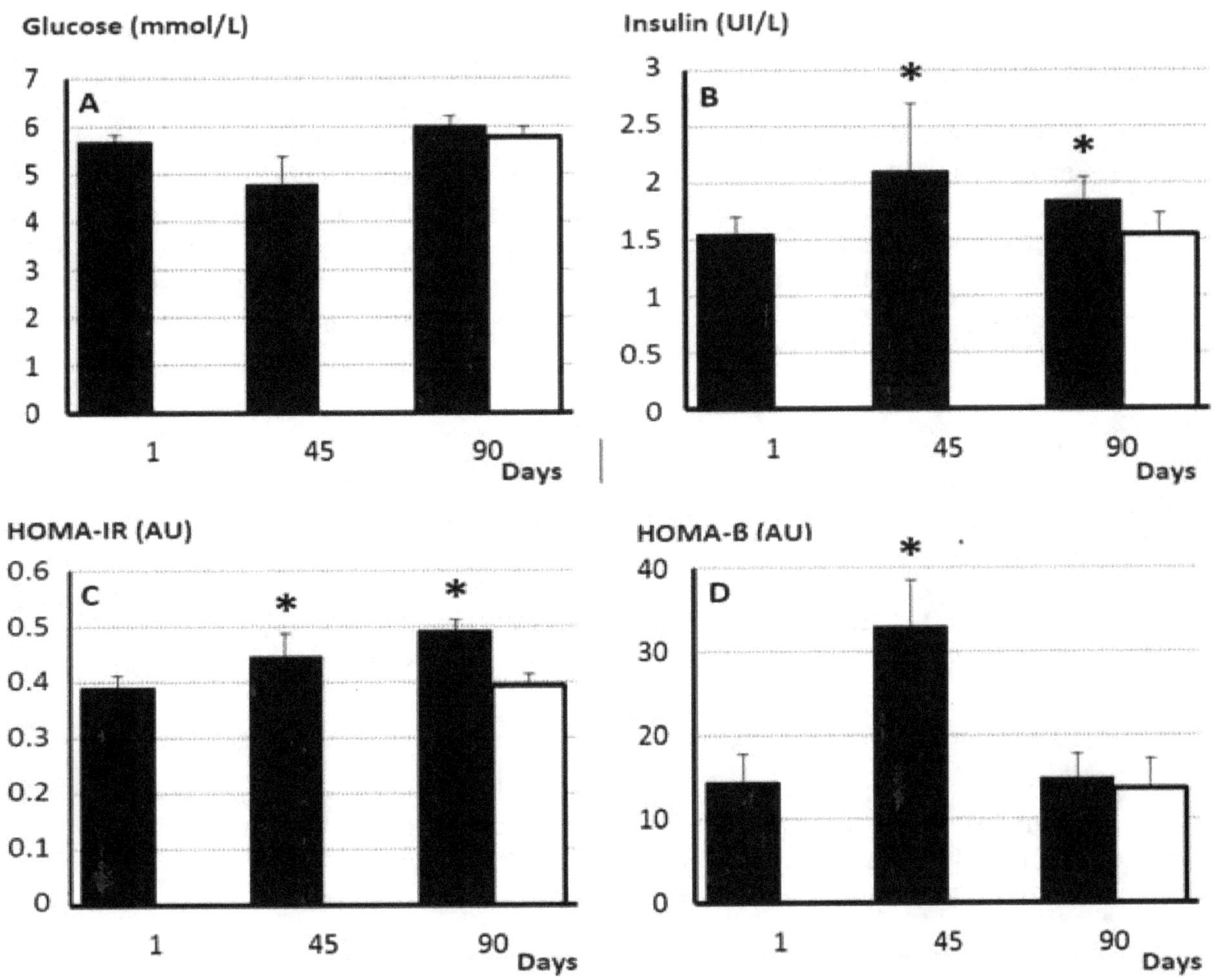

Figure 4. Mean (±S.E.M.) plasma concentrations of glucose (**A**) and insulin (**B**) and values for HOMA-IR and HOMA-β indexes (**C** and **D**, respectively) in control sows (white bar; $n = 17$) and changes in such values over time after starting differential feeding with a diet enriched with saturated fat in treated sows (black bars; $n = 11$). Asterisks (*) denote significant differences between obese and non-obese sows ($p < 0.05$).

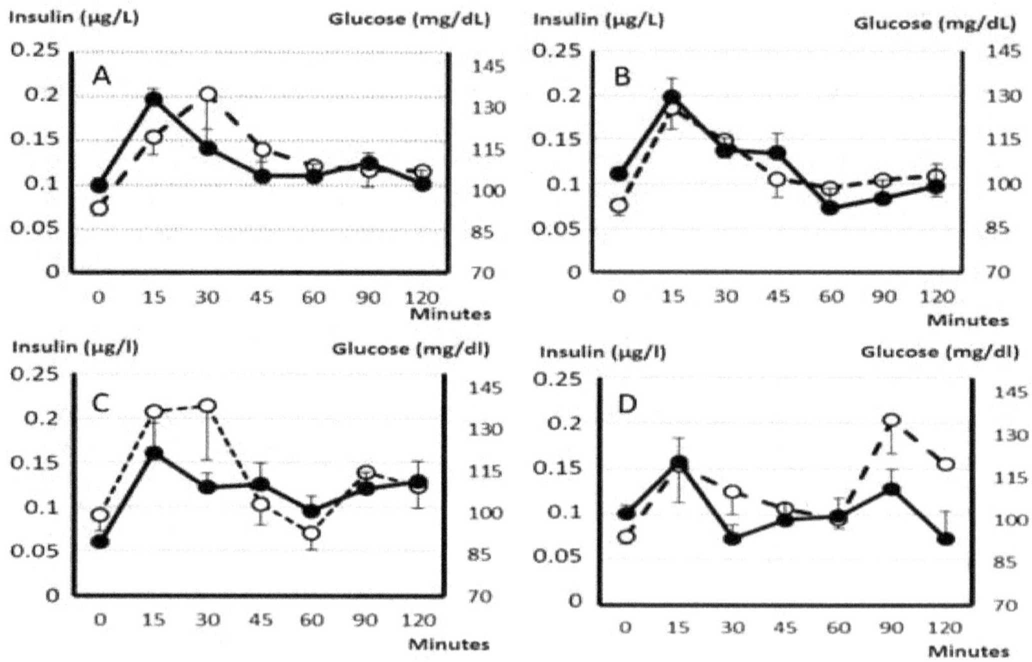

Figure 5. Changes in plasma concentration of glucose (continuous line with black circles) and insulin (discontinuous line with white circles) over time after oral administration of 2 g/kg live weight of D-glucose in control sows (**A**; $n = 17$) and at 0 (**B**), 45 (**C**) and 90 days (**D**) after starting differential feeding with a diet enriched with saturated fat in treated sows ($n = 11$). Areas under the Curve (AUCs) for glucose and insulin were similar in control and treated sows at Day 0. AUCs for glucose remained almost stable at 45 and 90 days but AUCs for insulin increased and were higher at both Day 45 and 90 than at Day 0 ($p < 0.01$ and $p < 0.05$, respectively).

3. Discussion

The present study characterizes aged Iberian pigs as a robust, amenable, and reliable translational model for studies on sarcopenia and sarcopenic obesity. The model represents certain characteristics of the human disease, since aging and sarcopenia were related to increased lipids accumulation and cellular dysfunction, not only at the adipose tissue but also at non-adipose ectopic tissues (liver and pancreas). The food-intake excess leading to sarcopenic obesity worsened the condition by increasing visceral adiposity, dyslipidemia, insulin resistance and lipotoxicity in non-adipose tissues.

3.1. Similarities of the Model with Human Sarcopenia

In the pigs of the current study, aging was characterized, like in humans, by a significant reduction in muscle mass; even 50% when compared to values obtained in younger adults. This sarcopenic state was related to systemic dyslipidemia, insulin resistance (IR) and lipotoxicity in adipose tissue, liver and pancreas (i.e., increased lipids accumulation and cellular dysfunction).

The comparison of lipid profiles in the current trial with data obtained in younger adult pigs in previous studies [18] shows that plasma concentrations of triglycerides and total- and LDL-cholesterol are significantly higher in aged than in young adult sows (around 50 vs. 25 mg/dL for triglycerides, around 95 vs. 55 mg/dL for total cholesterol and around 55 vs. 25 mg/dL for LDL-c). Conversely, increases in HDL-c were smaller (around 35 vs. 25 mg/dL). These data indicate that in our model, ageing and sarcopenia induce a dyslipidemic profile similar to that described in humans [20], resembling the so-called "lipid triad" (elevated triglycerides and LDL-c with normal HDL-c; [21]). In consequence, aged sows have an increased atherogenic dyslipidemia ratio evidencing cardiometabolic risk like human beings [22].

In human medicine, elevated triglycerides in blood and tissues have been largely linked to establishment of glucose intolerance and IR [23,24] and there is a well-known connection between aging, sarcopenia and IR [20]. Concomitantly, in our sows, assessment of the glycemic index showed that HOMA-IR and HOMA-β indexes are higher in aged and sarcopenic individuals than in younger individuals.

The states of dyslipidemia and IR were accompanied by histological evidences of lipotoxicity in the liver, with morphological alterations similar to those found in the early nonalcoholic fatty liver disease (NAFLD) in humans. This finding indicates the main roles of IR and abnormal lipoprotein metabolism in the pathogenesis of NAFLD in swine, like in humans [25]. Around 80–90% of the non-obese sarcopenic sows evidenced lipids infiltration and increased presence of lipocytes (mostly known as Ito cells). This finding supports the relationship between ageing and proliferation of Ito cells previously described in human patients [26]. In 24% of our sows, the presence of ballooning injury, if extrapolated to humans, would be indicative of predisposition to a later development of nonalcoholic steatohepatitis (NASH) [25,27], a condition also known as lipotoxic liver disease [28]. The primary role of Ito cells is the intracytoplasmic storage of fat and vitamin A [29]. However, damage of the liver tissue is associated with proliferation of Ito cells, which plays an important role in the pathogenesis of chronic liver disease [30] since the cells are subsequently transformed in myofibroblasts. Such a process results in fibrogenesis and, in consequence, the normal hepatic tissue is replaced by fibrotic tissue in advanced stages. There was no evidence of hepatic fibrosis in the current study, which indicates early stages of liver disease. This assumption is reinforced by the lack of significant changes in most of the enzymes used as markers of hepatic function that remained within physiological ranges during the whole study [31,32].

Hence, the state of sarcopenia induced by aging in the Iberian sows of the present study represents certain clinical and histological evidences of dyslipidemia, IR, lipotoxicity, NAFLD, and ultimately prodrome of NASH, in human medicine.

3.2. *Similarities of the Model with Human Sarcopenic Obesity*

The obesogenic diet offered to sarcopenic sows affected body weight and adiposity very early after starting the differentiated feeding, like previously described for younger pigs [18].

In the obese sows of the current study, increases in fat accretion were mainly observed at subcutaneous and visceral compartments. In human medicine, it is well-known that aging-related increases in visceral fat favor the development of dyslipidemia and IR [33]. In our model, increases in visceral fat were similarly related to significant changes in the plasma lipids profile, which supports that the lipidomic profile of swine is mainly determined by the visceral fat, as found in humans [33]. The increase in total cholesterol and LDL-c (indicating hyperlipidemia type-2) concurrently with maintained low HDL-c levels found in our obese sarcopenic sows, if extrapolated to human medicine, would be considered as indicative of type 2 of diabetes mellitus (T2DM; [34]. In our pigs, such diagnosis was confirmed by the evidence of impaired glucose regulation throughout the study, with altered β-cell function and IR. However, there were no changes in plasma glucose concentrations, like in the first stages of the human disease [35], and our sows were able to counterbalance the prodrome of T2DM at Day 90. These findings may be related to the short duration of the experiment and/or to the high plasticity of the swine pancreas, in agreement with previous studies [36]. Hence, the data obtained so far pave the way for further studies assessing IR in longer experimental trials.

An elegant revision of Mlinar and Marc [37] analyzes the different factors and steps in the link between adiposity and IR. In brief, a triglyceride overload in non-adipose ectopic tissues occurs when the capacity of the adipose tissue for storing lipids is exceeded. At the same time, the failure of the vasculature to expand together with the adipocyte hypertrophy causes hypoxia of the adipose tissue and, therefore, oxidative stress; in turn, oxidative stress is reinforced by an altered metabolism of the non-adipose tissue. Systemic oxidative stress and steatosis in non-adipose tissues induce low-grade inflammation. Finally, the concurrence of hypertriglyceridemia and ectopic lipid deposition, increased oxidative stress and inflammation trigger IR. All these factors described in humans were also found in the obese sarcopenic sows of the current study.

Moreover, in our study, the assessment of fatty acid composition of subcutaneous and visceral fat, where more than 95% were neutral lipids (triglycerides), offers outstanding information on its changes during sarcopenic obesity. In brief, obesity increases MUFA content and decreases PUFA content (specifically n-3 and n-6 PUFA) at both compartments, but also increases the ratios of MUFA/SFA and C18:1/C18:0 in visceral fat (i.e., increases desaturation index and Stearoyl-CoA desaturase 1 activity; SCD1). In humans, increased desaturation index and SCD1 activity have been related to metabolic disorders, like alterations in lipogenesis and insulin regulation [23,38]. Similar results have been found in the Iberian pig in previous studies [39,40].

In the present study, we observed major effects of obesity on fatty acid composition of the polar fraction of cell membranes at non-adipose ectopic tissues (muscle and liver). Specifically, obese sows showed higher MUFA/SFA, C18:1/C18:0 and Σn-6/Σn-3 ratios than control sows. The implications of the two first ratios have been previously considered, but the changes in the Σn-6/Σn-3ratio also indicate important metabolic impairments. In the skeletal muscle, the n-3 PUFA content of cellular membranes plays a main role favoring the action of insulin; a high Σn-6/Σn-3ratio seems to be deleterious to insulin sensitivity [41] and ultimately results in IR [42]. In the liver, the increase of Σn-6/Σn-3ratio indicates also a pro-inflammatory state related to increased peripheral lipolysis and, therefore, enlarged flux of fatty acids [43].

The histological evidence of lipotoxicity at the liver previously described in a high percentage of the non-obese sarcopenic sows of the current study were also observed in the obese sows. All of them (100%) evidenced lipid infiltration, increased presence of Ito cells and presence of ballooning injury indicating nonalcoholic fatty liver disease (NAFLD) and later development of NASH. These data again mimic results found in aged humans. The increasing prevalence of NAFLD with age was highlighted in the Rotterdam study [44] while its relationship with sarcopenia has been reported, two years ago, in the Korean Sarcopenic Obesity Study [45]. Further analysis of this last database highlighted that this association is independent of obesity [46]. However, these studies are precluded by the inherent limitation in conducting invasive experimentation in humans; hence, animal models for NAFLD are necessary to better understand this pathogenesis. A recent comprehensive review of studies with rodent models of NASH [47] states that the ideal model should encompass all the defining features of the human condition (obesity, IR, steatohepatitis, and ultimately fibrosis). However, no single murine model currently represents all subsets of human NASH. In this scenario, swine models have an outstanding translational value.

In humans, the fatty liver is also closely associated with increased pancreatic fat content (a disorder also known as nonalcoholic fatty pancreas disease, NAFPD) [48]. NAFPD is associated with visceral obesity, dyslipidemia, IR and ultimately T2DM [49,50], which is similar to data from swine models [51]. A similar relationship was found in our current study, where pancreatic steatosis was severe in half of the obese sows and moderate or mild in the remaining animals; conversely, only 70% of the controls showed steatosis and most of them showed it to a mild degree. Moreover, all the obese sows showed pancreatic lipomatosis, defined as fat accumulation around and within the pancreas. This is a condition associated with aging and IR and known to worsen pancreatic dysfunction caused by steatosis [52]. Hence, these results also reinforce the translational value of our model for studies on the effect of aging, obesity and IR on the development of NAFPD.

4. Materials and Methods

4.1. Ethics Statement

The experiment was performed in agreement with the Spanish Policy for Animal Protection RD1201/05, which meets the European Union Directive 86/609. The experiment was specifically assessed and approved by the Committee of Ethics in Animal Research of the National Institute of Agricultural and Food Research and Technology (INIA) (report CEEA 2012/012, 28 January 2012). The sows were housed at the animal facilities of INIA, which meet local, national and European requirements.

4.2. Animals and Management

The experiment involved 28 Iberian sows (8–10 years-old) with established sarcopenia. Presence of sarcopenia was assessed by ultrasonographic evaluation of muscle mass (cross-sectional diameter of the *longissimus dorsi*), with a 5–8 MHz lineal-array probe (SonoSite Inc., Bothell, WA, USA), since ultrasonography is accepted as a reliable method for evaluating muscle mass and sarcopenia [53]. Muscle diameter had a mean value of 21.9 ± 3.2 mm, which is 50% lower than values obtained in adults (2 years-old; around 38–40 mm) and similar to data from young individuals (6 months-old; around 20 mm) of the same breed reared at our facilities.

All the sows were fed, prior to the experimental procedure, with a standard diet (2.8% of polyunsaturated fat and 3.08 Mcal/kg of metabolizable energy) fulfilling their maintenance requirements (2.5 kg/animal/day). For 100 days, seventeen sows (control group) continued being fed with the same diet and amount whilst 11 sows randomly chosen (obese group) were fed with an obesogenic diet (6.8% of saturated fat and 3.36 Mcal/kg of metabolizable energy) for inducing obesity [18]. Meal intake in the obese group was 4 kg/animal/day for the first 45 days and 5 kg/animal/day for the following 55 days.

4.3. Evaluation of Body Weight and Subcutaneous Adiposity

Changes in body-weight and subcutaneous fat-depth in the obese group were measured every 15 days, from Day 0 to 90, and finally at Day 100 together with the control group. Fat depth was evaluated with the ultrasound probe previously described, at the right-side at 4 cm from the midline and the head of the last rib.

4.4. Blood and Tissue Sampling

Plasma samples for assessment of glucose and lipids metabolism were drawn, after fasting, at Days 0, 45, 90 and 100 in the obese group and at Day 100 in the control group and immediately biobanked at −80 °C. Samples obtained at Days 0 and 100 in the obese group and at Day 100 in the control group were also used to determine redox status. In addition, oral glucose tolerance tests (OGTTs) were performed at Days 0, 45 and 90 in the obese and at Day 90 in the control sows by serial blood samplings (0, 15, 30, 60, 90 and 120 min) after giving 2 g/kg live-weight of D-glucose by gavage through a gastric tube.

At the end of the study (Day 100), a systematic necropsy was performed in all the animals, assessing the macroscopic appearance of the organs. Immediately, two portions of subcutaneous and visceral (perirenal) fat, muscle (*longissimus dorsi*), pancreas and left lobe of the liver were collected in 2-mL cryotubes and biobanked at −80 °C for assessment of fatty acids and/or oil red-O staining. A third portion of each tissue was fixed in 10% neutral-buffered-formalin and processed for hematoxylin-eosin (HE).

4.5. Assessment of Plasma Lipid Profiles

Plasma concentrations of triglycerides, total cholesterol and high-density and low-density lipoproteins cholesterol (HDL-c and LDL-c, respectively) were measured with a clinical chemistry analyzer (Saturno 300-plus; Crony Instruments s.r.l., Rome, Italy). Plasma HDL-c ratio and LDL-c ratio were calculated by dividing total cholesterol by HDL-c and LDL-c concentrations, respectively; plasma LDL-c/HDL-c ratio was obtained by dividing LDL-c by HDL-c concentrations. Finally, the atherogenic dyslipidemia ratio was calculated as log(triglycerides)/HDL-c.

4.6. Assessment of Plasma Antioxidant Capacity and Lipid Peroxidation

Values for total antioxidant capacity were determined by FRAP (ferric reducing antioxidant power assay) [54] whilst lipids oxidative damage was assessed by MDA (malondialdehyde) [55].

4.7. Assessment of Hepatic and Exocrine Pancreatic Function

Plasma concentrations of alanine-transaminase, albumin, alkaline-phosphatase, amylase, aspartate-aminotransferase, total and direct bilirubin, creatinine, γ-glutamyl-transpeptidase, leucine-aminopeptidase, lipase and urea were measured with the Saturno 300-plus analyzer (Crony Instruments s.r.l., Rome, Italy).

4.8. Assessment of Glucose Metabolism and Endocrine Pancreatic Function

Plasma concentrations of glucose and insulin were measured, respectively, with the Saturno 300-plus analyzer and with a Porcine Insulin ELISA kit (Mercodia AB, Uppsala, Sweden; 0.26 IU/L of assay sensitivity and 3.5% of intra-assay variation coefficient). Insulin sensitivity/resistance were determined, concomitantly with data from OGTTs, throughout the study of the HOMA-IR index $[(\text{FINS} \times \text{FGLU})/22.5]$, whilst possible changes in β-cell function were assessed by the HOMA-β index $[(20 \times \text{FINS})/(\text{FGLU} - 3.5)]$. FINS accounts for fasting plasma insulin concentration in U/L and FGLU for fasting plasma glucose in mmol/L.

4.9. Histological Assessment of Liver and Pancreas

The stains of liver and pancreas tissue were examined by light microscopy and blindly scored for the presence and severity of histological features indicating fat infiltration, steatosis, inflammation, ballooning injury, fibrosis and vacuolization. Evaluation was based on the scoring developed by Kleiner et al. [56], considering none (<5%), mild (5–33%), moderate (34–66%) and severe degree (>66%).

4.10. Evaluation of Fatty Acids Composition

Fatty acid composition was analysed in subcutaneous (after differentiation of outer and inner layers) and visceral fat, *longissimus dorsi* muscle and liver. Fat was extracted using the *Ball-mill procedure* [57] and gas-chromatography was used for identification and quantification of fatty acids (FA) in total lipid extracts at subcutaneous and visceral fat, and separately for neutral (triacylglycerols or triglycerides) and polar (phospolipids) lipids at muscle and liver [58]. Total saturated FA (SFA), monounsaturated FA (MUFA) and polyunsaturated FA (PUFA) and total content of n-3 and n-6 PUFA and their ratio (Σn-6/Σn-3) were calculated from individual FA percentages. Finally, the desaturation index was obtained from the ratio MUFA/SFA and the activity of the stearoyl-CoA desaturase enzyme 1 (SCD1) was inferred from the proportions of oleic and stearic acids (C18:1n-9 and C18:0; product and precursor of SCD1 activity, respectively).

4.11. Statistical Analysis

Effects of diet on body-weight, adiposity, fatty-acid composition, metabolic and antioxidant/oxidative status were assessed by ANOVA for repeated measures (split-plot ANOVA), whilst changes over time were determined by Pearson correlation procedures. Histological features were assessed by one-way ANOVA or by a Kruskall–Wallis test if a Levene's test showed non-homogeneous variables; Duncan's post-hoc test was performed to contrast the differences among groups. Statistical analysis of results expressed as percentages was performed after arc-sine transformation of the values for each individual percentage, while the response to OGTTs was compared after calculating the Area under the Curve (AUC). All results were expressed as mean ± SEM and statistical significance was accepted from $p < 0.05$.

5. Conclusions

The present study shows that the Iberian swine model represents features of sarcopenia and sarcopenic obesity in humans, paving the way for future research on physiopathology of the condition and possible therapeutic targets. The strength of the model is increased by the availability and low-price of aged individuals of this breed and the short time necessary for inducing obesity. The present study was performed on female individuals, since availability of aged sows is higher than aged boars and because management is easier in females, but sex-related effects may be studied on males in further studies.

Acknowledgments: The authors thank the INIA animal staff for his assistance with animal care and P. Cuesta and I. Cano (Department of Research Support, Universidad Complutense de Madrid) for statistical analyses. Esteban Porrini is aresearcher of the program Ramón y Cajal (RYC-2014-16573). Consolación García-Contreras, Marta Vázquez-Gómez, Laura Torres-Rovira, Susana Astiz and Antonio González-Bulnes are members of the EU COST-Action BM1308 "Sharing Advances on Large Animal Models (SALAAM)".

Author Contributions: Consolacion Garcia-Contreras, Marta Vazquez-Gomez, Esteban Porrini, Magali Gonzalez-Colaço, Susana Astiz and Antonio Gonzalez-Bulnes designed the experiments; Consolacion Garcia-Contreras, Marta Vazquez-Gomez, Laura Torres-Rovira, Jorge Gonzalez, Beatriz Isabel, Susana Astiz and Antonio Gonzalez-Bulnes performed the experiments and analyzed samples; Consolacion Garcia-Contreras, Marta Vazquez-Gomez, Jorge Gonzalez, Susana Astiz, Beatriz Isabel and Antonio Gonzalez-Bulnes analysed the data; Consolacion Garcia-Contreras, Marta Vazquez-Gomez, Esteban Porrini, Magali Gonzalez-Colaço and Antonio Gonzalez-Bulnes wrote the original draft; Susana Astiz, Laura Torres-Rovira, Jorge Gonzalez and Beatriz Isabel revised the manuscript.

References

1. Fielding, R.A.; Vellas, B.; Evans, W.J.; Bhasin, S.; Morley, J.E.; Newman, A.B.; Abellan van Kan, G.; Andrieu, S.; Bauer, J.; Breuille, D.; et al. Sarcopenia: An undiagnosed condition in older adults. Current consensus definition: Prevalence, etiology, and consequences. International working group on sarcopenia. *J. Am. Med. Dir. Assoc.* **2011**, *12*, 249–256. [CrossRef] [PubMed]
2. Delmonico, M.J.; Harris, T.B.; Lee, J.S.; Visser, M.; Nevitt, M.; Kritchevsky, S.B.; Tylavsky, F.A.; Newman, A.B. Alternative definitions of sarcopenia, lower extremity performance, and functional impairment with aging in older men and women. *J. Am. Geriatr. Soc.* **2007**, *55*, 769–774. [CrossRef] [PubMed]
3. Morley, J.E. Anorexia, sarcopenia, and aging. *Nutrition* **2001**, *17*, 660–663. [CrossRef]
4. Castillo, E.M.; Goodman-Gruen, D.; Kritz-Silverstein, D.; Morton, D.J.; Wingard, D.L.; Barrett-Connor, E. Sarcopenia in elderly men and women: The Rancho Bernardo study. *Am. J. Prev. Med.* **2003**, *25*, 226–231. [CrossRef]
5. Metter, E.J.; Talbot, L.A.; Schrager, M.; Conwit, R. Skeletal muscle strength as a predictor of all-cause mortality in healthy men. *J. Gerontol. A Biol. Sci. Med. Sci.* **2002**, *57*, B359–B365. [CrossRef] [PubMed]
6. Malafarina, V.; Úriz-Otano, F.; Iniesta, R.; Gil-Guerrero, L. Sarcopenia in the elderly: Diagnosis, physiopathology and treatment. *Maturitas* **2012**, *71*, 109–114. [CrossRef]
7. Burton, L.A.; Sumukadas, D. Optimal management of sarcopenia. *Clin. Interv. Aging* **2010**, *5*, 217–228. [PubMed]
8. Batsis, J.A.; Mackenzie, T.A.; Lopez-Jimenez, F.; Bartels, S.J. Sarcopenia, sarcopenic obesity, and functional impairments in older adults: National Health and Nutrition Examination Surveys 1999–2004. *Nutr. Res.* **2015**, *35*, 1031–1039. [CrossRef] [PubMed]
9. Cleasby, M.E.; Jamieson, P.M.; Atherton, P.J. Insulin resistance and sarcopenia: Mechanistic links between common co-morbidities. *J. Endocrinol.* **2016**, *229*, R67–R81. [CrossRef] [PubMed]
10. Batsis, J.A.; Mackenzie, T.A.; Barre, L.K.; Lopez-Jimenez, F.; Bartels, S.J. Sarcopenia, sarcopenic obesity and mortality in older adults: Results from the National Health and Nutrition Examination Survey III. *Eur. J. Clin. Nutr.* **2014**, *68*, 1001–1007. [CrossRef] [PubMed]
11. Bouchonville, M.F.; Villareal, D.T. Sarcopenic obesity: How do we treat it? *Curr. Opin. Endocrinol. Diabetes Obes.* **2013**, *20*, 412–419. [CrossRef] [PubMed]

12. Palus, S.; Springer, J.I.; Doehner, W.; von Haehling, S.; Anker, M.; Anker, S.D.; Springer, J. Models of sarcopenia: Short review. *Int. J. Cardiol.* **2017**, *238*, 19–21. [CrossRef] [PubMed]
13. Bollheimer, L.C.; Buettner, R.; Pongratz, G.; Brunner-Ploss, R.; Hechtl, C.; Banas, M.; Singler, K.; Hamer, O.W.; Stroszczynski, C.; Sieber, C.C. Sarcopenia in the aging high-fat fed rat: A pilot study for modeling sarcopenic obesity in rodents. *Biogerontology* **2012**, *13*, 609–620. [CrossRef] [PubMed]
14. Russell, J.C.; Proctor, S.D. Small animal models of cardiovascular disease: Tools for the study of the roles of metabolic syndrome, dyslipidemia, and atherosclerosis. *Cardiovasc. Pathol.* **2006**, *15*, 318–330. [CrossRef] [PubMed]
15. Roura, E.; Koopmans, S.J.; Lalles, J.P.; Le Huerou-Luron, I.; de Jager, N.; Schuurman, T.; Val-Laillet, D. Critical review evaluating the pig as a model for human nutritional physiology. *Nutr. Res. Rev.* **2016**, *29*, 60–90. [CrossRef] [PubMed]
16. Neel, J.V. Diabetes mellitus: A "thrifty" genotype rendered detrimental by "progress"? *Am. J. Hum. Genet.* **1962**, *14*, 353–362. [PubMed]
17. Torres-Rovira, L.; Gonzalez-Anover, P.; Astiz, S.; Caro, A.; Lopez-Bote, C.; Ovilo, C.; Pallares, P.; Perez-Solana, M.L.; Sanchez-Sanchez, R.; Gonzalez-Bulnes, A. Effect of an obesogenic diet during the juvenile period on growth pattern, fatness and metabolic, cardiovascular and reproductive features of Swine with obesity/leptin resistance. *Endocr. Metab. Immune Disord. Drug Targets* **2013**, *13*, 143–151. [CrossRef] [PubMed]
18. Torres-Rovira, L.; Astiz, S.; Caro, A.; Lopez-Bote, C.; Ovilo, C.; Pallares, P.; Perez-Solana, M.L.; Sanchez-Sanchez, R.; Gonzalez-Bulnes, A. Diet-induced swine model with obesity/leptin resistance for the study of metabolic syndrome and type 2 diabetes. *Sci. World J.* **2012**, *2012*, 510149. [CrossRef] [PubMed]
19. Friendship, R.M.; Wilson, M.R.; Almond, G.W.; McMillan, I.; Hacker, R.R.; Pieper, R.; Swaminathan, S.S. Sow wastage: Reasons for and effect on productivity. *Can. J. Vet. Res.* **1986**, *50*, 205–208. [PubMed]
20. Karakelides, H.; Nair, K.S. Sarcopenia of aging and its metabolic impact. *Curr. Top. Dev. Biol.* **2005**, *68*, 123–148. [PubMed]
21. Temelkova-Kurktschiev, T.; Hanefeld, M. The lipid triad in type 2 diabetes—Prevalence and relevance of hypertriglyceridaemia/low high-density lipoprotein syndrome in type 2 diabetes. *Exp. Clin. Endocrinol. Diabetes* **2004**, *112*, 75–79. [CrossRef] [PubMed]
22. Hermans, M.P.; Ahn, S.A.; Rousseau, M.F. The atherogenic dyslipidemia ratio [log(TG)/HDL-C] is associated with residual vascular risk, beta-cell function loss and microangiopathy in type 2 diabetes females. *Lipids Health Dis.* **2012**, *11*, 132. [CrossRef] [PubMed]
23. Roden, M.; Price, T.B.; Perseghin, G.; Petersen, K.F.; Rothman, D.L.; Cline, G.W.; Shulman, G.I. Mechanism of free fatty acid-induced insulin resistance in humans. *J. Clin. Investig.* **1996**, *97*, 2859–2865. [CrossRef] [PubMed]
24. Koyama, K.; Chen, G.; Lee, Y.; Unger, R.H. Tissue triglycerides, insulin resistance, and insulin production: Implications for hyperinsulinemia of obesity. *Am. J. Physiol.* **1997**, *273*, E708–E713. [CrossRef] [PubMed]
25. Angulo, P. Nonalcoholic fatty liver disease. *N. Engl. J. Med.* **2002**, *346*, 1221–1231. [CrossRef] [PubMed]
26. Kim, I.H.; Kisseleva, T.; Brenner, D.A. Aging and liver disease. *Curr. Opin. Gastroenterol.* **2015**, *31*, 184–191. [CrossRef] [PubMed]
27. Chitturi, S.; Farrell, G.C. Etiopathogenesis of nonalcoholic steatohepatitis. *Semin. Liver Dis.* **2001**, *21*, 27–41. [CrossRef] [PubMed]
28. Cusi, K. Role of obesity and lipotoxicity in the development of nonalcoholic steatohepatitis: Pathophysiology and clinical implications. *Gastroenterology* **2012**, *142*, 711–725. [CrossRef] [PubMed]
29. Sankin, A. Discovering Biomarkers within the Genomic Landscape of Renal Cell Carcinoma. *J. Kidney* **2016**, 2. [CrossRef]
30. Flisiak, R. Role of Ito cells in the liver function. *Pol. J. Pathol.* **1997**, *48*, 139–145. [PubMed]
31. Rückert, I.-M.; Heier, M.; Rathmann, W.; Baumeister, S.E.; Döring, A.; Meisinger, C. Association between markers of fatty liver disease and impaired glucose regulation in men and women from the general population: The KORA-F4-study. *PLoS ONE* **2011**, *6*, e22932. [CrossRef] [PubMed]
32. Sanyal, D.; Mukherjee, P.; Raychaudhuri, M.; Ghosh, S.; Mukherjee, S.; Chowdhury, S. Profile of liver enzymes in non-alcoholic fatty liver disease in patients with impaired glucose tolerance and newly detected untreated type 2 diabetes. *Indian J. Endocrinol. Metab.* **2015**, *19*, 597–601. [CrossRef] [PubMed]
33. Despres, J.P. Dyslipidaemia and obesity. *Baillieres Clin. Endocrinol. Metab.* **1994**, *8*, 629–660. [CrossRef]

34. Goldberg, R.B. Lipid disorders in diabetes. *Diabetes Care* **1981**, *4*, 561–572. [CrossRef] [PubMed]
35. Kahn, S.E.; Prigeon, R.L.; McCulloch, D.K.; Boyko, E.J.; Bergman, R.N.; Schwartz, M.W.; Neifing, J.L.; Ward, W.K.; Beard, J.C.; Palmer, J.P.; et al. Quantification of the relationship between insulin sensitivity and beta-cell function in human subjects. Evidence for a hyperbolic function. *Diabetes* **1993**, *42*, 1663–1672. [CrossRef] [PubMed]
36. Koopmans, S.J.; Schuurman, T. Considerations on pig models for appetite, metabolic syndrome and obese type 2 diabetes: From food intake to metabolic disease. *Eur. J. Pharmacol.* **2015**, *759*, 231–239. [CrossRef] [PubMed]
37. Mlinar, B.; Marc, J. New insights into adipose tissue dysfunction in insulin resistance. *Clin. Chem. Lab. Med.* **2011**, *49*, 1925–1935. [CrossRef] [PubMed]
38. Poudyal, H.; Brown, L. Stearoyl-CoA desaturase: A vital checkpoint in the development and progression of obesity. *Endocr. Metab. Immune Disord. Drug Targets* **2011**, *11*, 217–231. [CrossRef] [PubMed]
39. Barbero, A.; Astiz, S.; Lopez-Bote, C.J.; Perez-Solana, M.L.; Ayuso, M.; Garcia-Real, I.; Gonzalez-Bulnes, A. Maternal malnutrition and offspring sex determine juvenile obesity and metabolic disorders in a swine model of leptin resistance. *PLoS ONE* **2013**, *8*, e78424. [CrossRef] [PubMed]
40. Gonzalez-Bulnes, A.; Astiz, S.; Ovilo, C.; Lopez-Bote, C.J.; Sanchez-Sanchez, R.; Perez-Solana, M.L.; Torres-Rovira, L.; Ayuso, M.; Gonzalez, J. Early-postnatal changes in adiposity and lipids profile by transgenerational developmental programming in swine with obesity/leptin resistance. *J. Endocrinol.* **2014**, *223*, M17–M29. [CrossRef] [PubMed]
41. Corcoran, M.P.; Lamon-Fava, S.; Fielding, R.A. Skeletal muscle lipid deposition and insulin resistance: Effect of dietary fatty acids and exercise. *Am. J. Clin. Nutr.* **2007**, *85*, 662–677. [PubMed]
42. Li, Y.; Xu, S.; Zhang, X.; Yi, Z.; Cichello, S. Skeletal intramyocellular lipid metabolism and insulin resistance. *Biophys. Rep.* **2015**, *1*, 90–98. [CrossRef] [PubMed]
43. Valenzuela, R.; Videla, L.A. The importance of the long-chain polyunsaturated fatty acid n-6/n-3 ratio in development of non-alcoholic fatty liver associated with obesity. *Food Funct.* **2011**, *2*, 644–648. [CrossRef] [PubMed]
44. Koehler, E.M.; Schouten, J.N.; Hansen, B.E.; van Rooij, F.J.; Hofman, A.; Stricker, B.H.; Janssen, H.L. Prevalence and risk factors of non-alcoholic fatty liver disease in the elderly: Results from the Rotterdam study. *J. Hepatol.* **2012**, *57*, 1305–1311. [CrossRef] [PubMed]
45. Hong, H.C.; Hwang, S.Y.; Choi, H.Y.; Yoo, H.J.; Seo, J.A.; Kim, S.G.; Kim, N.H.; Baik, S.H.; Choi, D.S.; Choi, K.M. Relationship between sarcopenia and nonalcoholic fatty liver disease: The Korean Sarcopenic Obesity Study. *Hepatology* **2014**, *59*, 1772–1778. [CrossRef] [PubMed]
46. Lee, Y.H.; Jung, K.S.; Kim, S.U.; Yoon, H.J.; Yun, Y.J.; Lee, B.W.; Kang, E.S.; Han, K.H.; Lee, H.C.; Cha, B.S. Sarcopaenia is associated with NAFLD independently of obesity and insulin resistance: Nationwide surveys (KNHANES 2008–2011). *J. Hepatol.* **2015**, *63*, 486–493. [CrossRef] [PubMed]
47. Ibrahim, S.H.; Hirsova, P.; Malhi, H.; Gores, G.J. Animal Models of Nonalcoholic Steatohepatitis: Eat, Delete, and Inflame. *Dig. Dis. Sci.* **2016**, *61*, 1325–1336. [CrossRef] [PubMed]
48. Van Geenen, E.J.; Smits, M.M.; Schreuder, T.C.; van der Peet, D.L.; Bloemena, E.; Mulder, C.J. Nonalcoholic fatty liver disease is related to nonalcoholic fatty pancreas disease. *Pancreas* **2010**, *39*, 1185–1190. [CrossRef] [PubMed]
49. Tushuizen, M.E.; Bunck, M.C.; Pouwels, P.J.; Bontemps, S.; van Waesberghe, J.H.; Schindhelm, R.K.; Mari, A.; Heine, R.J.; Diamant, M. Pancreatic fat content and beta-cell function in men with and without type 2 diabetes. *Diabetes Care* **2007**, *30*, 2916–2921. [CrossRef] [PubMed]
50. Lee, J.S.; Kim, S.H.; Jun, D.W.; Han, J.H.; Jang, E.C.; Park, J.Y.; Son, B.K.; Kim, S.H.; Jo, Y.J.; Park, Y.S.; et al. Clinical implications of fatty pancreas: Correlations between fatty pancreas and metabolic syndrome. *World J. Gastroenterol.* **2009**, *15*, 1869–1875. [CrossRef] [PubMed]
51. Yin, W.; Liao, D.; Kusunoki, M.; Xi, S.; Tsutsumi, K.; Wang, Z.; Lian, X.; Koike, T.; Fan, J.; Yang, Y.; et al. NO-1886 decreases ectopic lipid deposition and protects pancreatic beta cells in diet-induced diabetic swine. *J. Endocrinol.* **2004**, *180*, 399–408. [CrossRef] [PubMed]
52. Noel, P.; Patel, K.; Durgampudi, C.; Trivedi, R.N.; de Oliveira, C.; Crowell, M.D.; Pannala, R.; Lee, K.; Brand, R.; Chennat, J.; et al. Peripancreatic fat necrosis worsens acute pancreatitis independent of pancreatic necrosis via unsaturated fatty acids increased in human pancreatic necrosis collections. *Gut* **2016**, *65*, 100–111. [CrossRef] [PubMed]

53. Minetto, M.A.; Caresio, C.; Menapace, T.; Hajdarevic, A.; Marchini, A.; Molinari, F.; Maffiuletti, N.A. Ultrasound-Based Detection of Low Muscle Mass for Diagnosis of Sarcopenia in Older Adults. *PM R* **2016**, *8*, 453–462. [CrossRef] [PubMed]
54. Benzie, I.F.; Strain, J.J. The ferric reducing ability of plasma (FRAP) as a measure of "antioxidant power": The FRAP assay. *Anal. Biochem.* **1996**, *239*, 70–76. [CrossRef] [PubMed]
55. Larstad, M.; Ljungkvist, G.; Olin, A.C.; Toren, K. Determination of malondialdehyde in breath condensate by high-performance liquid chromatography with fluorescence detection. *J. Chromatogr. B Anal. Technol. Biomed. Life Sci.* **2002**, *766*, 107–114. [CrossRef]
56. Kleiner, D.E.; Brunt, E.M.; Van Natta, M.; Behling, C.; Contos, M.J.; Cummings, O.W.; Ferrell, L.D.; Liu, Y.C.; Torbenson, M.S.; Unalp-Arida, A.; et al. Design and validation of a histological scoring system for nonalcoholic fatty liver disease. *Hepatology* **2005**, *41*, 1313–1321. [CrossRef] [PubMed]
57. Segura, J.; Lopez-Bote, C.J. A laboratory efficient method for intramuscular fat analysis. *Food Chem.* **2014**, *145*, 821–825. [CrossRef] [PubMed]
58. Olivares, A.; Rey, A.I.; Daza, A.; Lopez-Bote, C.J. High dietary vitamin A interferes with tissue alpha-tocopherol concentrations in fattening pigs: A study that examines administration and withdrawal times. *Animal* **2009**, *3*, 1264–1270. [CrossRef] [PubMed]

8

The Newly Normed SKT Reveals Differences in Neuropsychological Profiles of Patients with MCI, Mild Dementia and Depression

Hartmut Lehfeld [1,*] and Mark Stemmler [2]

1 Department of Psychiatry and Psychotherapy, Paracelsus Medical University, 90419 Nuremberg, Germany
2 Institute of Psychology, University of Erlangen-Nuremberg, 91052 Erlangen, Germany; mark.stemmler@fau.de
* Correspondence: Hartmut.Lehfeld@klinikum-nuernberg.de

Abstract: The SKT (Syndrom-Kurztest) is a short cognitive performance test assessing deficits of memory and attention in the sense of speed of information processing. The new standardization of the SKT (2015) aimed at improving its sensitivity for early cognitive decline due to dementia in subjects aged 60 or older. The goal of this article is to demonstrate how the neuropsychological test profile of the SKT can be used to provide valuable information for a differential diagnosis between MCI (mild cognitive impairment), dementia and depression. $n = 549$ patients attending a memory clinic (Nuremberg, Germany) were diagnosed according to ICD-10 and tested with the SKT. The SKT consists of nine subtests, three for the assessment of memory and six for measuring attention in the sense of speed of information processing. The result of the SKT test procedure is a total score, which indicates the severity of overall cognitive impairment. Besides the summary score, two subscores for memory and attention can be interpreted. Using the level of depression as a covariate, statistical comparisons of SKT test profiles between the three patient groups revealed that depressed patients showed more pronounced deficits than MCI patients in all six attention subtests. On the other hand, MCI patients displayed significantly greater mnestic impairment than the depressed group, which was indicated by significant differences in the memory subscore. MCI and dementia patients showed similar deficit patterns dominated by impairment of memory (delayed recall) with MCI patients demonstrating less overall impairment. In sum, the SKT neuropsychological test profiles provided indicators for a differential diagnosis between MCI and beginning dementia vs. depression.

Keywords: differential diagnosis depression vs. MCI/dementia; mild cognitive impairment; dementia; depression in old age; SKT (Syndrom-Kurztest); cognitive assessment

---

1. Introduction

Dementia and depression are the most frequent psychiatric disorders of old age [1]. Both affect quality of life of patients in a more fundamental way and to a much greater extent than many somatic diseases [2]. Depression is also considered a serious risk factor for developing dementia [3,4]. In addition, dementia and depression share a diagnostic deficit. Dementia is often only diagnosed in more advanced stages showing higher degrees of functional impairment [5]. Worldwide, patients suffering from depression frequently are not correctly diagnosed; therefore, in many countries less than 10% of depressed subjects receive adequate treatment [6].

Due to an overlap in symptoms, a valid differential diagnosis between dementia and depression is sometimes difficult to establish: Depressive disorders in old age are associated with cognitive impairment in 40% to 60% of patients [7]. Conversely, about 40% of dementia patients develop depression symptoms [8,9]. Accordingly, among the differential diagnoses of dementia, in the first place the ICD-10 [10] lists depressive disorders, which can show characteristics of incipient dementia with memory impairment, slowed thinking and lack of spontaneity. In the same way, the DSM-5 [11] recommends inspecting the cognitive profiles of patients suggesting memory and executive impairment as typical for Alzheimer's disease, whereas nonspecific and more variable test performance could be expected in major depression. In accordance with this perspective, a number of reviews state a lack of clarity in the neuropsychological profiles of depressive disorders [12,13]. However, other authors consider impairment in speed of information processing, attention or executive functions as cognitive core features of depressed older patients [7,14–16].

Since the cognitive deficits associated with depression are less pronounced than those found in dementia [17–19], making a differential diagnosis much more difficult when it is not a full-blown dementia, but "mild cognitive impairment" (MCI), which has to be differentiated from depression. For almost 30 years, MCI has been conceptualized as a transitional phase between normal aging and dementia; it is discussed as a clinical condition with a high prognostic value for future dementia development, mostly towards Alzheimer's dementia [20–22]. The diagnostic differentiation of MCI and depression is further complicated by the existence of several MCI subtypes (amnestic vs. non-amnestic, single vs. multiple domains) causing a potential variety of neuropsychological performance patterns. Furthermore, nearly one third of MCI patients also will develop depression symptoms [23]. Overall, a wide range of disturbed cognitive functions may be expected in both MCI and depressed subjects. Consequently, attempts to differentiate between MCI and depression by means of psychometric tests often have failed [18,19,24].

Against this background, the present study compared the neuropsychological profiles of patients with MCI, mild dementia and depression tested with the SKT according to Erzigkeit [25]. The SKT (acronym for Syndrom-Kurztest; however, this German term is outdated and not used anymore) is a short cognitive performance test assessing memory and attention, the latter in the sense of speed of information processing. Thus, the SKT addresses exactly those two cognitive domains that are considered to be primarily impaired in patients with mild dementia and depressive disorders, respectively. Furthermore, given the fact that amnestic MCI is the most frequent MCI subtype [24,26], it was expected that patients with MCI or mild dementia would show greater deficits in the memory section of the SKT, while depressed patients would be more impaired in subtests measuring speed of information processing.

2. Methods

2.1. Samples

The present study included all patients referred between 2000 and 2005 to the Memory Clinic of Nuremberg General Hospital fulfilling the following criteria: (1) age 60 years or older, (2) diagnosis of mild cognitive impairment (MCI, in accordance with the consensus criteria according to Winblad et al. 2004 [20]), mild dementia (Alzheimer type, mixed type or vascular dementia; ICD-10 codes F00 or F01) or depressive disorder (ICD-10 codes F32 or F33) and (3) complete assessment with all SKT subtests. As an indicator of the clinical severity of MCI and mild dementia, assignment to stages 3 (MCI) or 4 (mild dementia) of the Global Deterioration Scale (GDS, [27]) was required. Exclusion criteria were (1) age below 60 years, (2) all other diagnoses than the ones required for inclusion, e.g., other forms of dementia (dementia in Parkinson disease and amnesic syndromes due to substance use), other forms of depression (e.g., adjustment disorders or post-traumatic stress disorders) and (3) not being able to complete all SKT subtests (e.g., due to reduced motor abilities, due to not being able to understand the test instructions or being unfamiliar with numbers).

2.2. Measures

The SKT is a cognitive test developed and published in Germany [28] assessing impairment of memory and attention, the latter in the sense of speed of information processing. The SKT comprises nine subtests, three of which refer to visual memory (immediate and delayed recall and recognition memory), the remaining six subtests measure processing speed. An overview of the subtests and the tasks to be completed is given in Table 1, the test materials are shown in Figure 1.

Table 1. Overview of the nine Syndrom-Kurztest (SKT) subtests.

Name of Subtest	Content of Subtest	Domain
I Naming Objects	twelve objects have to be named and memorized at the same time	attention/speed
II Immediate Recall	recall of objects shown in subtest I	memory
III Naming Numerals	two digit numbers written on magnetic blocks placed on a board have to be read out loud	attention/speed
IV Arranging Blocks	the magnetic blocks have to be arranged in ascending order of the numbers	attention/speed
V Replacing Blocks	the blocks have to be replaced in their original positions	attention/speed
VI Counting Symbols	symbols printed on a tableau have to be counted	attention/speed
VII Reversal Naming	two rows composed of two letters in random order are to be read by naming each letter with the name of the other	attention/speed
VIII Delayed Recall	recall of objects shown in subtest I	memory
IX Recognition Memory	identification of objects shown in subtest I from a table containing 48 objects	memory

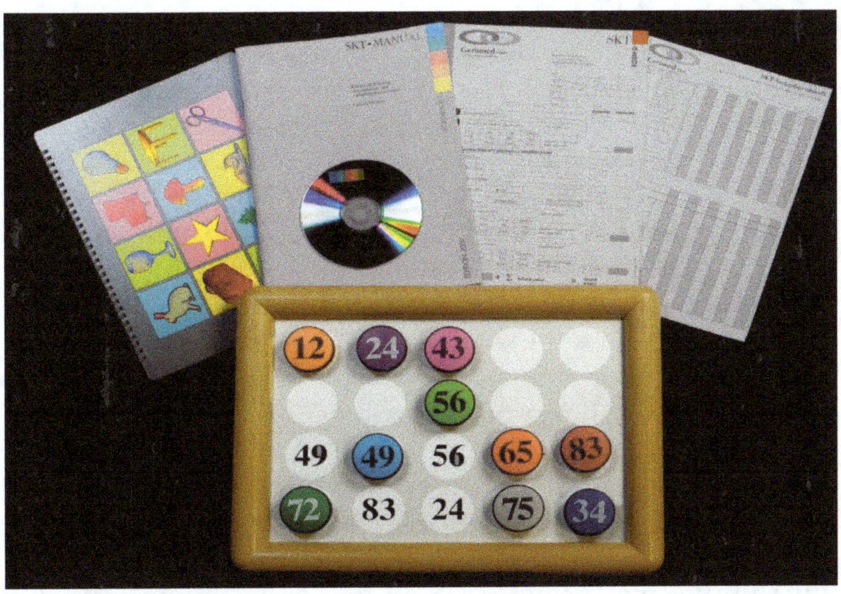

Figure 1. SKT test materials.

The maximum performance time for each subtest is limited to 60 s, so that the total administration time will be approximately 10 to 15 min. In the attention/speed subtests, the patient is instructed to work as fast and accurately as possible. In the memory subtests, all correct answers given within 60 s will be scored. The test was developed in five parallel forms (A to E) for repeated test administration even within short time intervals. In addition to a total summary score, the evaluation also provides subscores for separately interpreting memory and attention performance.

Since its publication in 1977, the SKT has been revised three times. The last revision carried out in 2015 was undertaken to establish new test norms for age groups 60 years and older to improve the sensitivity of the SKT for early cognitive decline due to Alzheimer's disease or other neurocognitive disorders [25]. In a first step, more than 1000 non-demented community dwelling subjects aged between 60 and 91 years were tested with the SKT. On the basis of this data set, conditional expected values were calculated for each of the nine SKT subtests using multiple regressions taking into account age, gender and level of intelligence. Based on the deviations from the predicted performance, in a second step, norm scores of 0, 1 or 2 were defined depending on the size of the deviation of the actual performance from the predicted performance (higher scores indicating greater cognitive impairment). The SKT total summary score ranging between 0 and 18 is obtained by adding the deviation scores (i.e., norm scores) of the nine subtests and is visualized in a traffic light system. Total scores between 0 and 4 indicate "age-appropriate cognitive performance" (green), scores between 5 and 10 points suggest "mild cognitive impairment" (MCI, yellow) and values between 11 and 18 substantiate a "suspicion of beginning dementia" (red). It must be noted that the SKT total summary score can be reliably interpreted in case of a homogeneous test profile, i.e., the memory and attention domain are affected to a similar extent. In case of profile heterogeneity, the summary scores should be interpreted with caution and the severity of impairment should also be assessed separately for the two domains.

Besides the SKT, the standard test battery of the Nuremberg Memory Clinic comprised the CERAD-NP [29] and two different depression scales [30,31]. Furthermore, relatives rated the patient using the Bayer-ADL scale to stage functional capacities [32] and the Neuropsychiatric Interview [33] to assess behavioral disturbances occurring in dementia. The diagnostic classification of a given patient was made taking into account information from different sources (anamnesis, medical examination, neuropsychology, everyday functioning, and neuroimaging or laboratory results).

2.3. Statistics

The raw scores of the nine SKT subtests were converted into norm scores using the EXCEL program "SKT-Analyser-v10.xlsm" [25]. From these, the subscores for memory and attention as well as the SKT total summary score were calculated by adding the corresponding subtest scores (SKT subscores and total summary score are also included in the program printout). Using one-way analyses of variance, differences in the nine subtests, the two subscores and the SKT total summary score were checked for statistical significance between the three study groups. Pairwise group comparisons were based on the Tukey test. A Bonferroni correction for multiple comparisons was not carried out, as the focus of the analyses presented here was on the comparative examination of test profiles and less on the detection of robust group differences. Comparisons of SKT profiles across the nine subtests and the memory and attention subscores were performed using multivariate analyses of variance for repeated measurements. To assess the effect of depression on SKT scores, Pearson correlation coefficients were computed between depression scores [30,31] and the SKT summary score, the SKT memory and attention subscores and the norm scores of the nine SKT subtests. Moreover, we repeated the analyses of variance controlling for depression to establish a "pure" metric of cognitive impairment unbiased by affective disturbances. While we used two different depression scores, we calculated the mean of the transformed z-scores [30,31]. Furthermore, a receiver operator characteristics (ROC) analysis was employed to compute areas under the curve (AUC) for each of the three diagnostic groups using the SKT norming sample comprising 1053 non-demented community dwelling subjects aged between 60 and 91 as a reference group. All analyses were carried out with the statistics program IBM SPSS Statistics (Version 20, Armonk, NY, United States) and were based on a completely anonymized data set. The study was registered in the study centre of the Nuremberg General Hospital as a quality assurance measure according to § 27/4 of the Bavarian Hospital Law.

3. Results

Of the 1362 patients assessed between 2000 and 2005 in the Nuremberg Memory Clinic, a total sample of n = 549 fulfilled the inclusion and exclusion criteria (see Section 2.1). The patients were distributed among the three diagnostic groups as follows: 172 patients were diagnosed with MCI, 166 patients were diagnosed with dementia (F00.0 or F00.1: 89 patients, F00.2: 39 patients and F01: 38 patients), 211 patients suffered from first manifested or recurrent depression (F32: 150 patients and F33:

61 patients). Diagnoses were based on ICD-10 [10]. Sociodemographic data and SKT results (subtests, subscores and SKT total score) of the three study groups were compiled together with the results of the group comparisons in Table 2. The SKT test profiles of the three study samples are depicted in Figure 2.

Table 2. Demographic data, Mini-Mental State Examination (MMSE) and depression scores, SKT norm scores for subtests I to IX, SKT subscores for memory and attention and SKT total score. Frequencies (sample size and gender) or mean values with standard deviations in brackets are given.

	MCI M (SD)	DEM M (SD)	DEP M (SD)	p	Group Comparisons
sample size	172	166	211		
age	73.9 (7.3)	76.6 (7.6)	72.5 (7.5)	0.000	DEP < MCI < DEM
gender (f/m)	90/82	102/64	134/77	0.045	
education *	12,0 (2,8)	11,3 (2,9)	11,4 (2,8)	*n.s.*	
MMSE **	26.5 (2.2)	22.6 (3.1)	26.2 (3.0)	0.000	DEM < MCI = DEP
depression (z-scores) ***	−0.42 (0.77)	−0.27 (0.81)	0.55 (1.04)	0.000	DEM = MCI, MCI < DEP, DEM < DEP
SKT I	0.70 (0.87)	1.17 (0.90)	0.91 (0.93)	0.000	MCI < (tend.) DEP < DEM
SKT II	0.92 (0.93)	1.64 (0,72)	0.78 (0.93)	0.000	MCI = DEP; DEP < DEM; MCI < DEM
SKT III	0.56 (0.83)	0.89 (0.95)	0.69 (0.90)	0.003	MCI = DEP; DEP = DEM; MCI < DEM
SKT IV	1.01 (0.96)	1.49 (0.84)	1.22 (0.94)	0.000	MCI < (tend.) DEP < DEM
SKT V	1.12 (0.95)	1.50 (0.81)	1.28 (0.91)	0.000	MCI = DEP; DEP < (tend.) DEM; MCI < DEM
SKT VI	0.67 (0.87)	0.99 (0.95)	0.91 (0.96)	0.009	MCI < DEP; DEP = DEM; MCI < DEM
SKT VII	1.06 (0.95)	1.39 (0.89)	1.25 (0.93)	0.005	MCI = DEP; DEP = DEM; MCI < DEM
SKT VIII	1.24 (0.92)	1.77 (0.60)	0.86 (0.94)	0.000	DEP < MCI < DEM
SKT IX	0.87 (0.99)	1.46 (0.89)	0.83 (0.99)	0.000	DEP = MCI; DEP < DEM; MCI < DEM
SKT memory	3.03 (1.85)	4.87 (1.44)	2.47 (2.06)	0.000	DEP < MCI < DEM
SKT attention	5.12 (3.58)	7.42 (3.37)	6.27 (3.95)	0.000	MCI < DEP < DEM
SKT sum score	8.15 (3.97)	12.28 (3.55)	8.74 (4.78)	0.000	MCI= DEP; DEP < DEM; MCI < DEM

Abbreviations: MCI: mild cognitive impairment, DEM: dementia, DEP depression; MMSE: Mini-Mental State Examination, f: female, m: male, tend.: statistical tendency ($p < 0.10$);. * 19 missing; ** 1 missing; *** 53 missing.

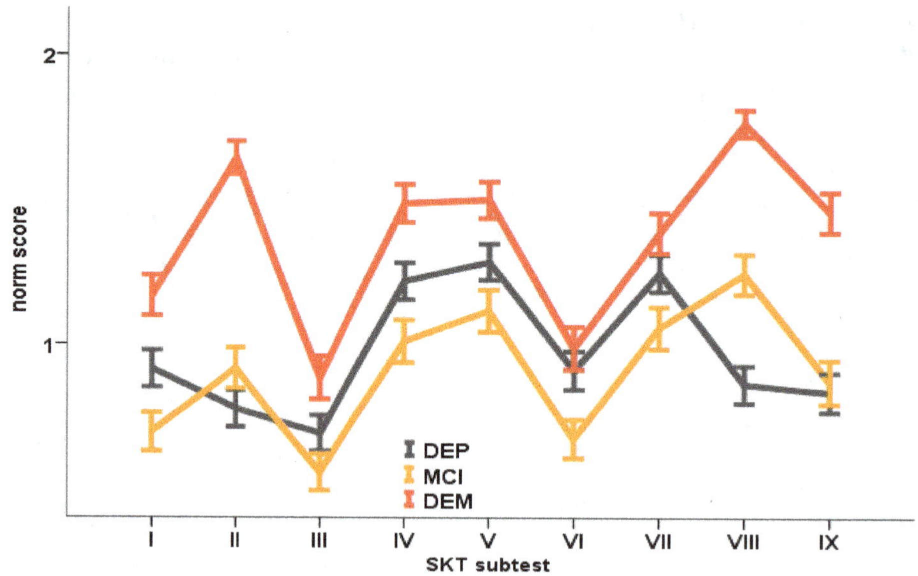

Figure 2. Norm scores (means) of the three study groups for the nine SKT subtests (I: naming objects, II: immediate recall, III: naming numerals, IV: arranging blocks, V: replacing blocks, VI: counting symbols, VII: reversal naming, VIII: delayed recall, IX: recognition memory).

As Figure 2 illustrates, the MCI and dementia group show peaks in their SKT profiles in subtest VIII, which examines the delayed recall of objects. In contrast, depressed patients reveal their most striking performance deficits in the speed subtests IV, V and VII. Furthermore, Figure 2 indicates less overall cognitive impairment in MCI and depressed subjects when compared to dementia patients. SKT total summary scores for the MCI and depressed groups displayed values between 8 and 9 points; they do not differ statistically between both groups (see Table 2). However, striking differences can be detected in their subtest profiles. While mean scores in memory subtests II, VIII and IX of MCI patients are consistently lower than those of subjects with dementia (level significance was reached for subtest VIII), depressed patients show more pronounced deficits than MCI patients in all six speed tests (with only the difference in subtest VI turned out to be significant, statistical tendencies ($p < 0.10$) were found for subtests I and IV). Subsequently, the memory subscore indicated significantly greater cognitive impairment in the MCI group and the attention subscore in the depression group ($p < 0.05$ each).

The comparison of the SKT profiles between the three diagnostic groups included in the study across all nine subtests revealed a highly significant interaction effect 'diagnosis × subtest' (Pillai's Trace = 0.121 with F (16, 1080) = 4.34, $p < 0.000$) in a multivariate analysis of variance with repeated measures (MANOVA), which indicates an overall difference of test profiles. Subsequent pairwise comparisons performed to identify the source of this interaction effect revealed a marginally non-significant interaction (Pillai's Trace = 0.045 with F (8, 329) = 1.59, p = 0.054) for the comparison MCI vs. dementia, indicating a relative similarity of the subtest profiles between these two groups. The two remaining contrasts, MCI vs. depression and dementia vs. depression, were again significant with respect to the interaction term 'diagnosis × subtest' (MCI vs. depression: Pillai's Trace = 0.066; F (8, 329) = 3.31, p < 0.001; depression vs. dementia: Pillai's Trace = 0.0148; F (8, 329) = 8.01, p < 0.000) pointing towards the depression group as the source of the overall difference between profiles.

More clearly than the profile comparisons across subtests, the comparison of the SKT memory and attention subscores revealed the different impairment patterns between diagnostic groups MCI/mild dementia vs. depression. When comparing the three subsamples, the interaction 'diagnosis × subscore' reached significance (Pillai's Trace = 0.034; F (2, 546) = 2.55, p < 0.000). However, when comparing only MCI vs. dementia, the level of significance was missed more clearly for the SKT subscore profile than for the subtest profile (Pillai's Trace = 0.004 with F (1, 336) = 1.18, p = 0.277). This result demonstrates the similarity of the SKT subscore profiles between MCI and mild dementia. The remaining comparisons

(MCI vs. depression and dementia vs. depression) again showed significant interaction effects, which can be interpreted in terms of different subtest compositions in MCI/mild dementia vs. depression (MCI vs. depression: Pillai's Trace = 0.042; F (1, 381) = 16.52, $p < 0.000$; dementia vs. depression: Pillai's Trace = 0.024; F (1, 375) = 9.18, $p < 0.01$).

Pearson correlation coefficients between SKT and depression scores ranged between r = −0.15–0.20 in the total sample and hardly exceeded r = 0.20 in the three subsamples (MCI: range *r* = 0.02–0.20; DEM: range *r* = −0.22–0.15; DEP: range *r* = −0.03–0.17). Accordingly, introducing depression as a covariate into the analyses of variance did not fundamentally change the outcome. Regarding significance, seven out of eight comparisons remained significant, even though less pronounced. Noteworthy, the differences in SKT subtest and subscore profiles between MCI vs. depression outlasted the correction for depression. When comparing these two groups, the interaction terms remained significant (diagnosis × subtest: Pillai's Trace = 0.046; F (8,351) = 2.130, p = 0.033; diagnosis × subscore: Pillai's Trace = 0.017; F (1,358) = 6.29, p = 0.013). Finally, Table 3 displays the results of the ROC analyses examining the ability of the SKT sum score and the subscores to correctly classify MCI, dementia and depression. All SKT scores were based on the SKT norming sample used for developing the regression based norms [25].

Table 3. Results of receiver operating curves (ROC): area under curve (AUC).

	MCI	DEM	DEP
SKT sum score	0.83	0.96	0.81
SKT memory subscore	0.77	0.93	0.68
SKT attention subscore	0.74	0.88	0.79

4. Discussion

In the present analyses, the newly-normed SKT, a short cognitive performance test for assessing deficits of memory and attention, revealed different neuropsychological profiles for patients belonging to the MCI/mild dementia spectrum on the one hand, and patients suffering from depressive disorders on the other. In the MCI and dementia conditions, the deficit patterns displayed their peaks for the delayed memory recall of objects. Since amnestic MCI (isolated or in combination with other cognitive domains) is considered to be the most frequent MCI subtype [24,26] and impaired episodic memory is a prerequisite for a dementia diagnosis according to the ICD-10 criteria, this result is not really surprising. However, it can be taken as an indication of the construct validity of the SKT as a tool to support diagnosis in organic mental disorders. It may be expected that the assessment of patients with other forms of dementia, e.g., Lewy-Body, Frontal Lobe or Parkinson's, might have resulted in different test profiles. In the same vein, an exploratory investigation comparing SKT subtest patterns of patients diagnosed with Alzheimer's and Parkinson's dementia using the old test norms [34] indicated greater impairment of Parkinson patients in subtests assessing speed of information processing with subtest V (replacing blocks) reaching the level of statistical significance. Moreover, the slowing of speed of information processing, especially in tasks with a strong executive component, which could be observed in the depressed sample of the study has been described as a characteristic neuropsychological feature of depression [7,14,15].

To address a common misunderstanding, it must be pointed out that the SKT is not a test exclusively for the area of dementia. Originally, it was developed for usage with patients older than 17 years of age suffering from acute or chronic mental disorders irrespective of their aetiology. Therefore, there is ample experience with the SKT in the cross-sectional and longitudinal assessment of cognitive impairment resulting, e.g., from brain injury, substance abuse or anesthesia [35]. The misclassification of the SKT as a dementia test was surely supported by the fact that the SKT has been used as an outcome measure in more than 50 studies investigating the efficacy of various nootropic compounds, cognition enhancers or antidementia drugs, in the past years with a clear focus on the efficacy of Ginkgo biloba [35].

In line with this shift of test usage towards dementing disorders starting in the 1980s, all three test revisions of the SKT focused on older patients suffering from cognitive impairment. The first modification in 1989 aimed at making test materials more appealing [36]. The second revision suggested a finer classification of age norms beyond the age of 65 and included an option for separate assessment of memory and speed functions allowing for differential diagnostic considerations [37]. Finally, the new norming of 2015 [25] served the purpose of improving the sensitivity of the test for early recognition of dementia in persons aged 60 years or older. First data show the high sensitivity and specificity of the SKT for dementia being 0.83 and 0.84, respectively [38,39]. The results of the ROC analyses reported in the present study support these findings.

Of special interest in the present investigation is the finding that the analysis of the SKT subscores for memory and attention revealed statistically significant differences between MCI and depressed patients. Other working groups, e.g., Barth et al. (2005) [18] using the CERAD-NP test battery did not find significant differences between MCI and depression in any of the CERAD tasks. In the same way, Zihl et al. (2010) [24] analyzing neuropsychological test data of MCI and cognitively impaired depressed patients also applying the CERAD-NP and an additional series of other psychometric instruments did not receive a single significant difference between both diagnostic groups. Nevertheless, they identified a significant reduction in speed of information processing for their depressed patients when comparing the results to cognitively normal older controls. This may be taken as a further indication that processing speed is a core domain affected by depression, which is in full accordance with the present results. Accordingly, our ROC analyses for depression vs. controls revealed a higher discriminative power of the SKT speed subscore in comparison to the memory subscore. Furthermore, the fact that the differences in SKT subscores for memory and speed performance outlasted a correction for (self-rated) depression may cautiously be considered as a hint of reduced speed of information processing as a trait marker for depression. This interpretation is supported by results that speed and executive test performance of depressed patients who were successfully treated was improved, but not normalized [15]. Finally, in a study by Dierckx et al. (2007) [19] a cued recall paradigm discriminated well between Alzheimer patients and depressed subjects, but considerably lost diagnostic accuracy for separating MCI from depression. The authors explain this finding by the heterogeneity among MCI patients and a diagnostic uncertainty induced by misdiagnosing MCI in the presence of affective symptoms as depression.

Differential diagnosis between MCI/dementia and depression is not only complicated by an overlap in cognitive and affective symptoms. Meanwhile, there is evidence that MCI/dementia and depression share common pathophysiological pathways (e.g., [40,41]). On the one hand, depression seems to play a role in the pathogenesis of Alzheimer's disease via stress and a glucocorticoid increase that may cause amyloid-beta production or hippocampal atrophy resulting in an elevated dementia risk in depressed subjects. On the other hand, neurodegenerative and cerebrovascular alterations in the brain are discussed as etiological factors of depression [42,43]. Thus, in the future it is desirable that the clinical and psychometric assessment of patients suffering from cognitive and/or affective symptoms should be supplemented by information available from biomarkers reflecting neuronal or vascular damage. This could allow for defining MCI [21] and depression subgroups bearing a higher risk for cognitive decline towards a dementia syndrome. The next step for our working group will be an analysis of SKT follow-up data that might be available for MCI and depressed patients participating in the present investigation to validate their diagnostic classifications.

A final remark refers to the international validity of the SKT, which up to about 1990 was mainly used in German-speaking countries. However, in the following years an increasing number of international studies were performed, e.g., in the United States, the UK, Greece, Russia, Chile, Mexico, Brazil or South Korea [44–50]. Some of these studies specifically aimed at validating the SKT for the respective target language or culture. To summarize a few findings, the transcultural transfer of the (mostly nonverbal) SKT test materials only required minor adjustments of some objects shown in subtest I (because they were less familiar in the target countries) or the adaptation of letters to be read in subtest VII (especially for countries using non-Latin letters). In many of these studies, the SKT kept the psychometric properties or factor structure comparable to the original German test version. However, the dependency of test results on education becomes critical especially with patients from developing countries with very few years of formal school education [47,49].

In 2019, the German standardization study of 2015, which established the new testing norms was replicated in three testing centers in the USA, Australia and Ireland with a somewhat smaller sample of altogether 285 cognitively unimpaired persons aged between 60 and 96 years [35,51]. As in the German study, the most important predictors of the SKT performance were age, age-squared, gender and intelligence. The explained variance was comparable to that found in the German standardization sample suggesting that the regression-based German SKT norms from 2015 are well matched by those found in 2019 for English speaking subjects. This equivalence may be taken as evidence for the cross-cultural stability of the SKT in German and English speaking countries of the Western world (see also [45]). It indicates that the SKT in its present form may be used without any further adaptations of the testing material in these regions. Taken together, the results of the present study confirm that the SKT can be considered as a neuropsychological test instrument validly assessing impairment in two cognitive domains, i.e., memory and attention (speed of information processing), which should always be addressed for a comprehensive diagnostic work-up within the spectrum of neurodevelopmental (ICD-11) or neurocognitive disorders (DSM-5).

Author Contributions: H.L. and M.S. wrote the manuscript; H.L. did all the statistical analyses.

Acknowledgments: The article is dedicated to the memory of Hellmut Erzigkeit, who passed much too early in 2010. Hellmut Erzigkeit developed and published the SKT in the 1970s. For many years, he directed the Department of Clinical Psychology of the Psychiatric University Hospital Erlangen, Germany. Hartmut Lehfeld worked with him for many years. Hellmut Erzigkeit inspired many scientific projects, he was a visionary of psychometric assessment. We also deeply thank Robert Hoerr (Willmar Schwabe Arzneimittel, Karlsruhe, Germany) for his valuable comments and for proof reading the manuscript and Sophia Schneider (University of Erlangen-Nuremberg, Germany) for completing and correcting the reference list.

References

1. Wernicke, T.F.; Linden, M.; Gilberg, R.; Helmchen, H. Ranges of psychiatric morbidity in the old and the very old–results from the Berlin Aging Study (BASE). *Eur. Arch. Psychiatry Clin. Neurosci.* **2000**, *250*, 111–119. [CrossRef] [PubMed]
2. Murray, C.J.L.; Vos, T.; Lozano, R.; Mohsen, N.; Flaxman, A.D.; Michaud, C.; Ezzati, M.; Shibuya, K.; Salomon, J.A.; Abdalla, S.; et al. Disability-adjusted life years (DALYs) for 291 diseases and injuries in 21 regions, 1990–2010: A systematic analysis for the global burden of disease study 2010. *Lancet* **2012**, *380*, 2197–2223. [CrossRef]
3. Barnes, D.; Yaffe, K.; Byers, A.L.; McCormick, M.; Schaefer, C.; Whitmer, R. Midlife vs Late-Life Depressive Symptoms and Risk of Dementia Differential Effects for Alzheimer Disease and Vascular Dementia. *Arch. Gen. Psychiatry* **2012**, *69*, 493–498. [PubMed]
4. Singh-Manoux, A.; Dugravot, A.; Fournier, A.; Abell, J.; Ebmeier, K.; Kivimäki, M.; Sabia, S. Trajectories of Depressive Symptoms Before Diagnosis of Dementia: A 28-Year Follow-up Study. *JAMA Psychiatry* **2017**. [CrossRef] [PubMed]
5. Amjad, H.; Roth, D.L.; Sheehan, O.C.; Lyketsos, C.G.; Wolff, J.L.; Samus, Q.M. Underdiagnosis of Dementia: An Observational Study of Patterns in Diagnosis and Awareness in US Older Adults. *J. Gen. Intern. Med.* **2018**, *33*, 1131–1138. [CrossRef]
6. Depression: Fact sheet. Available online: https://www.who.int/news-room/fact-sheets/detail/depression (accessed on 7 July 2019).
7. Dybedal, G.S.; Tanum, L.; Sundet, K.; Gaarden, T.L.; Bjølseth, T.M. Neuropsychological functioning in late-life depression. *Front. Psychol.* **2013**, *4*, 381. [CrossRef]

8. Mega, M.S.; Cummings, J.L.; Fiorello, T.; Gornbein, J. The spectrum of behavioral changes in Alzheimer's disease. *Neurology* **1996**, *46*, 130–135. [CrossRef]
9. Zhao, Q.-F.; Tan, L.; Wang, H.-F.; Jiang, T.; Tan, M.-S.; Tan, L.; Xu, W.; Li, J.Q.; Wang, J.; Lai, T.J.; et al. The prevalence of neuropsychiatric symptoms in Alzheimer's disease: Systematic review and meta-analysis. *J. Affect. Disord.* **2016**, *190*, 264–271. [CrossRef]
10. Dilling, H.; Mombour, W.; Schmidt, M.H.; Schulte-Markwort, M. *Weltgesundheitsorganisation: Internationale Klassifikation psychischer Störungen: ICD-10 Kapitel V (F). Diagnostische Kriterien für Forschung und Praxis*, 3rd ed.; Verlag Hans Huber: Toronto, ON, Canada, 1999; pp. 181–183.
11. APA American Psychiatric Association. *Diagnostic and Statistical Manual of Mental Disorders (DSM-5®)*; American Psychiatric Pub: Washington, DC, USA, 2013.
12. Lee, R.S.; Hermens, D.F.; Porter, M.A.; Redoblado-Hodge, M.A. A meta-analysis of cognitive deficits in first-episode major depressive disorder. *J. Affect. Disord.* **2012**, *140*, 113–124. [CrossRef]
13. Beblo, T.; Sinnamon, G.; Baune, B.T. Specifying the neuropsychology of affective disorders: Clinical, demographic and neurobiological factors. *Neuropsychol. Rev.* **2011**, *21*, 337–359. [CrossRef]
14. Butters, M.A.; Whyte, E.M.; Nebes, R.D.; Begley, A.E.; Dew, M.A.; Mulsant, B.H.; Zmuda, M.D.; Bhalla, R.; Meltzer, C.C.; Pollock, B.G.; et al. The nature and determinants of neuropsychological functioning in late-life depression. *Arch. Gen. Psychiatry.* **2004**, *61*, 587–595. [CrossRef] [PubMed]
15. Gualtieri, C.T.; Johnson, L.G.; Benedict, K.B. Neurocognition in depression: Patients on and off medication versus healthy comparison subjects. *J. Neuropsychiatry Clin. Neurosci.* **2016**, *18*, 217–225. [CrossRef] [PubMed]
16. Rock, P.L.; Roiser, J.P.; Riedel, W.J.; Blackwell, A.D. Cognitive impairment in depression: A systematic review and meta-analysis. *Psychol. Med.* **2014**, *44*, 2029–2040. [CrossRef] [PubMed]
17. Künig, G.; Jäger, M.; Stief, V.; Kaldune, A.; Urbaniok, F.; Endrass, J. The impact of the CERAD-NP on diagnosis of cognitive deficiencies in late onset depression and Alzheimer's disease. *Int. J. Geriatr. Psychiatry.* **2006**, *21*, 911–916. [CrossRef]
18. Barth, S.; Schönknecht, P.; Pantel, J.; Schröder, J. Neuropsychologische Profile in der Demenzdiagnostik: Eine Untersuchung mit der CERAD-NP-Testbatterie. [Mild Cognitive Impairment and Alzheimer's Disease: An Investigation of the CERAD–NP Test Battery. *Fortschr. Der. Neurol. Und. Der. Psychiatr* **2005**, *73*, 568–576. [CrossRef]
19. Dierckx, E.; Engelborghs, S.; Raedt, R.D.; Deyn, P.P.D.; Ponjaert-Kristoffersen, I. Differentiation between mild cognitive impairment, Alzheimer's disease and depression by means of cued recall. *Psychol. Med.* **2007**, *37*, 747–755. [CrossRef]
20. Winblad, B.; Palmer, K.; Kivipelto, M.; Jelic, V.; Fratiglioni, L.; Wahlund, L.O.; Nordberg, A.; Bäckman, L.; Albert, M.; Almkvist, O.; et al. Mild cognitive impairment–beyond controversies, towards a consensus: Report of the International Working Group on Mild Cognitive Impairment. *J. Intern. Med.* **2004**, *256*, 240–246. [CrossRef]
21. Albert, M.S.; DeKosky, S.T.; Dickson, D.; Dubois, B.; Feldman, H.H.; Fox, N.C.; Gamst, A.; Holtzman, D.M.; Jagust, W.J.; Petersen, R.C.; et al. The diagnosis of mild cognitive impairment due to Alzheimer's disease: Recommendations from the National Institute on Aging-Alzheimer's Association workgroups on diagnostic guidelines for Alzheimer's disease. *Alzheimer's Dis. Dement.* **2011**, *7*, 270–279. [CrossRef]
22. Petersen, R.C.; Caracciolo, B.; Brayne, C.; Gauthier, S.; Jelic, V.; Fratiglioni, L. Mild cognitive impairment: A concept in evolution. *J. Intern. Med.* **2014**, *275*, 214–228. [CrossRef]
23. Ismail, Z.; Elbayoumi, H.; Fischer, C.E.; Hogan, D.B.; Millikin, C.P.; Schweizer, T.; Mortby, M.E.; Smith, E.E.; Patten, S.B.; Fiest, K.M. Prevalence of depression in patients with mild cognitive impairment: A systematic review and meta-analysis. *JAMA Psychiatry* **2017**, *74*, 58–67. [CrossRef]
24. Zihl, J.; Reppermund, S.; Thum, S.; Unger, K. Neuropsychological profiles in MCI and in depression: Differential cognitive dysfunction patterns or similar final common pathway disorder? *J. Psychiatr. Res.* **2010**, *44*, 647–654. [CrossRef] [PubMed]
25. Stemmler, M.; Lehfeld, H.; Horn, R. *SKT Manual Edition 2015*; Geromed GmbH: Spardorf, Bavaria, Germany, 2015.
26. Roberts, R.O.; Geda, Y.E.; Knopman, D.S.; Cha, R.H.; Pankratz, V.S.; Boeve, B.F.; Tangalos, E.G.; Ivnik, R.J.; Rocca, W.A.; Petersen, R.C. The incidence of MCI differs by subtype and is higher in men: The Mayo Clinic Study of Aging. *Neurology* **2012**, *78*, 342–351. [CrossRef] [PubMed]

27. Reisberg, B.; Ferris, S.H.; de Leon, M.J.; Crook, T. The Global Deterioration Scale for assessment of primary degenerative dementia. *Am. J. Psychiatry* **1982**, *139*, 1136–1139. [PubMed]
28. Erzigkeit, H. *Manual for the Syndrom-Kurztest*; Geromed GmbH: Spardorf, Germany, 1997.
29. Monsch, A. *CERAD—Neuropsychological Test Battery*; Memory Clinic: Basel, Switzerland, 1997.
30. Hautzinger, M.; Bailer, M. *ADS, General Depression Scale*; Hogrefe Publishing GmbH: Göttingen, Germany, 1993.
31. Collegium Internationale Psychiatriae Scalarum (Hrsg.). *International Scales for Psychiatry*, 5th ed; Hogrefe Publishing GmbH: Göttingen, Germany, 2005.
32. Hindmarch, I.; Lehfeld, H.; de Jongh, P.; Erzigkeit, H. The Bayer Activities of Daily Living Scale (B-ADL Scale). *Dement. Geriatr. Cogn. Disord.* **1998**, *9*, 20–26. [CrossRef] [PubMed]
33. Cummings, J.L.; Mega, M.; Gray, K.; Rosenberg-Thompson, S.; Carusi, D.A.; Gornbein, J. The Neuropsychiatric Inventory: Comprehensive assessment of psychopathology in dementia. *Neurology* **1994**, *44*, 2308–2314. [CrossRef] [PubMed]
34. Stroessenreuther, N.; Lehfeld, H.; Niklewski, N. PANDA—A screening tool Parkinson neuropsychometric dementia assessment. In Proceedings of the DGPPN Congress, Berlin, Germany, 24–27 November 2010.
35. Stemmler, M.; Lehfeld, H.; Erzigkeit, A. The English Validation of the SKT according to Erzigkeit. In *SKT Manual Edition 2019*; Geromed GmbH: Spardorf, Bavaria, Germany, 2019.
36. Erzigkeit, H. *Manual for the SKT forms A-E*, 4th ed.; Beltz: Weinheim, Germany, 1989.
37. Lehfeld, H.; Erzigkeit, H. The SKT—A short cognitive performance test for assessing deficits of memory and attention. *Int. Psychogeriatr.* **1997**, *9*, 115–121. [CrossRef]
38. Hessler, J.B.; Stemmler, M.; Bickel, H. Cross-Validation of the newly-normed SKT for the detection of MCI and dementia. *GeroPsych.* **2017**, *30*, 19–25. [CrossRef]
39. Stemmler, M.; Hessler, J.B.; Bickel, H. Predicting cognitive decline and dementia with the newly-normed SKT Short Cognitive Performance Test. *Dement. Geriatr. Cogn. Disord. Extra* **2019**, *9*, 184–193. [CrossRef]
40. Butters, M.A.; Young, J.B.; Lopez, O.; Aizenstein, H.J.; Mulsant, B.H.; Reynolds III, C.F.; DeKosky, S.T.; Becker, J.T. Pathways linking late-life depression to persistent cognitive impairment and dementia. *Dialogues Clin. Neurosci.* **2008**, *10*, 345–357.
41. Wang, L.; Potter, G.G.; Krishnan, R.K.; Dolcos, F.; Smith, G.S.; Steffens, D.C. Neural correlates associated with cognitive decline in late-life depression. *Am. J. Geriatr Psychiatry* **2012**, *20*, 653–663. [CrossRef]
42. Aizenstein, H.J.; Baskys, A.; Boldrini, M.; Butters, M.A.; Diniz, B.S.; Jaiswal, M.K.; Jellinger, K.A.; Kruglov, L.S.; Meshandin, I.A.; Mijajlovic, M.D.; et al. Vascular depression consensus report—A critical update. *Bmc Med.* **2016**, *14*, 161. [CrossRef] [PubMed]
43. Yatawara, C.; Lee, D.; Ng, K.P.; Chander, R.; Ng, D.; Ji, F.; Shim, H.Y.; Hilal, S.; Venketasubramanian, N.; Chen, C.; et al. Mechanisms Linking White Matter Lesions, Tract Integrity and Depression in Alzheimer's Disease. *Am. J. Geriatr. Psychiatry* **2019**. [CrossRef] [PubMed]
44. Kim, Y.S.; Nibbelink, D.W.; Overall, J.E. Factor structure and scoring of the SKT test battery. *J. Clin. Psychol.* **1993**, *49*, 61–71. [CrossRef]
45. Lehfeld, H.; Rudinger, G.; Rietz, C.; Heinrich, C.; Wied, V.; Fornazzari, L.; Pittas, J.; Hindmarch, I.; Erzigkeit, H. Evidence of the cross-cultural stability of the factor structure of the SKT short test for assessing deficits of memory and attention. *Int. Psychogeriatr.* **1997**, *9*, 139–153. [CrossRef] [PubMed]
46. Tsolakis, M.; Pittas, J. The use of SKT for the assessment of dementia in Greece. *Encephalos* **1995**, *32*, 336–345.
47. Flaks, M.K.; Forlenza, O.V.; Pereira, F.S.; Viola, L.F.; Yassuda, M.S. Short cognitive performance test: Diagnostic accuracy and education bias in older Brazilian adults. *Arch. Clin. Neuropsychol.* **2009**, *24*, 301–306. [CrossRef] [PubMed]
48. Fornazzari, L.; Cumsille, F.; Quevedo, F.; Quiroga, P.; Rioseco, P.; Klaasen, G.; Martinez, C.G.; Rhode, G.; Sacks, C.; Rivera, E.; et al. Spanish validation of the Syndrom Kurztest (SKT). *Alzheimer Dis. Assoc. Disord.* **2001**, *15*, 211–215. [CrossRef]
49. Ostrosky-Solís, F.; Davila, G.; Ortiz, X.; Vega, F.; Garcia Ramos, G.; de Celis, M.; Dávila, L.; Gómez, C.; Jiménez, S.; Juárez, S.; et al. Determination of normative criteria and validation of the SKT for use in Spanish-speaking populations. *Int. Psychogeriatr.* **1999**, *11*, 171–180. [CrossRef]

50. Choi, S.H.; Lee, B.H.; Hahm, D.S.; Jeong, J.H.; Ha, C.K.; Han, S.H.; Erzigkeit, H.; Na, D.L. Validation of the Korean version of the Syndrom Kurztest (SKT): A short test for the assessment of memory and attention. *Hum. Psychopharmacol.* **2004**, *19*, 495–501. [CrossRef]
51. Stemmler, M.; Lehfeld, H. Validation of the SKT short cognitive performance test for the detection of early cognitive decline in English-speaking countries. In Proceedings of the CTAD Conference, San Diego CA, USA, 4–7 December 2019.

9

Lower CSF Amyloid-Beta$_{1-42}$ Predicts a Higher Mortality Rate in Frontotemporal Dementia

Daniela Vieira [1,†], João Durães [1,†], Inês Baldeiras [1,2,3], Beatriz Santiago [1], Diana Duro [1], Marisa Lima [1], Maria João Leitão [1,3], Miguel Tábuas-Pereira [1,*,‡] and Isabel Santana [1,2,3,‡]

1 Neurology Department, Centro Hospitalar e Universitário de Coimbra, 3000-045 Coimbra, Portugal; danielacgvieira@gmail.com (D.V.); duraes.jlo@gmail.com (J.D.); ines.baldeiras@sapo.pt (I.B.); hbmcsantiago@hotmail.com (B.S.); diana.duro@gmail.com (D.D.); marisalima5@hotmail.com (M.L.); jajao86@gmail.com (M.J.L.); isabeljsantana@gmail.com (I.S.)
2 Faculty of Medicine, University of Coimbra, 3000-070 Coimbra, Portugal
3 Center for Neuroscience and Cell Biology, University of Coimbra, 3000-070 Coimbra, Portugal
* Correspondence: miguelatcp@gmail.com
† These authors contributed equally to this work.
‡ These authors contributed equally to this work.

Abstract: Frontotemporal lobar degeneration, the neuropathological substrate of frontotemporal dementia (FTD), is characterized by the deposition of protein aggregates, including tau. Evidence has shown concomitant amyloid pathology in some of these patients, which seems to contribute to a more aggressive disease. Our aim was to evaluate cerebrospinal fluid (CSF) amyloid-beta as a predictor of the mortality of FTD patients. We included 99 patients diagnosed with FTD—both behavioral and language variants—with no associated motor neuron disease, from whom a CSF sample was collected. These patients were followed prospectively in our center, and demographic and clinical data were obtained. The survival analysis was carried through a Cox regression model. Patients who died during follow up had a significantly lower CSF amyloid-beta$_{1-42}$ than those who did not. The survival analysis demonstrated that an increased death rate was associated with a lower CSF amyloid-beta$_{1-42}$ (HR = 0.999, 95% CI = [0.997, 1.000], p = 0.049). Neither demographic nor clinical variables, nor CSF total tau or p-tau were significantly associated with this endpoint. These results suggest that amyloid deposition in FTD patients may be associated with a higher mortality.

Keywords: frontotemporal dementia; amyloid; cerebrospinal fluid; mortality

1. Introduction

Frontotemporal dementia (FTD) is a progressive neurodegenerative clinical syndrome, characterized by changes in behavior, executive function, and language. It is generally classified in three clinical variants: behavioral-variant FTD, non-fluent variant primary progressive aphasia, and semantic-variant primary progressive aphasia.

The neuropathological substrate, frontotemporal lobar degeneration, is characterized by neuronal loss, gliosis, and microvacuolar changes of the frontal lobes, anterior temporal lobes, anterior cingulate cortex, and insular cortex. Different subtypes are associated with abnormal deposition of different proteins, namely microtubule-associated protein tau, the TAR DNA-binding protein with molecular weight 43 kDa, or the fused-in-sarcoma protein [1].

On the contrary, amyloid-beta$_{1-42}$ deposition is a hallmark of Alzheimer's disease (AD). However, patients with FTD may have superimposed amyloid pathology [2]. Recently, amyloid-beta plaques have been found to facilitate the aggregation of tau [3] in AD models. Interestingly, in FTD patients with pathogenic mutations, amyloid has also been shown to be associated with a worse performance in several cognitive tests [4]. Additionally, CSF amyloid has been shown to be associated with higher volumetric loss in sporadic FTD patients [5].

We aimed to evaluate the value of cerebrospinal (CSF) amyloid-beta$_{1-42}$ as a predictor of mortality in FTD patients.

2. Materials and Methods

2.1. Patient Selection

Our study included patients that fulfilled the current diagnostic criteria for behavioral variant of FTD [6] or language variants [7] with probable FTD-associated pathology, recruited at the Dementia Outpatient Clinic of the Centro Hospitalar e Universitário de Coimbra (Portugal). Defined inclusion criteria mandated a full neuropsychological evaluation and CSF biomarkers analysis. Patients who presented with motor neuron disorder at any point along the follow-up period were excluded. For the survival analysis, we considered the interval between the time of the lumbar puncture (LP)—baseline—and the time of death.

These patients are part of a prospectively evaluated cohort at our center. For the purpose of this study, we collected demographical data (age of onset, age at LP, gender, family history, and years of formal education), vascular risk factors at the time of the LP (history of diabetes, high blood pressure, dyslipidemia, atrial fibrillation, obesity, heart failure, coronary artery disease, heart valve disease, alcohol abuse, smoking, sleep obstructive apnea, and stroke), Mini-Mental State Examination (MMSE), and Clinical Dementia Rating (CDR) score at the time of LP.

The study was conducted according to the revised Declaration of Helsinki and Good Clinical Practice guidelines. Informed consent was given by all study participants or their legal next of kin. This project was approved by the ethics committee of our center, with the code HUC-43-09, prior to the beginning of the study.

2.2. CSF Biomarkers

CSF samples were collected as part of the routine clinical diagnostic protocol. Pre-analytical and analytical procedures were done in accordance with the Alzheimer's Association guidelines for CSF biomarker determination [8]. CSF samples were collected in sterile polypropylene tubes, immediately centrifuged at 1800 g for 10 min at 4 °C, aliquoted into polypropylene tubes and stored at −80 °C until analysis. CSF Aβ42, T-tau, and P-tau were measured separately by commercially available sandwich ELISA kits (Innotest, Fujirebio, Belgium), as previously described [9,10]. External quality control of the assays was performed under the scope of the Alzheimer's Association Quality Control Program for CSF Biomarkers [8].

2.3. Statistical Analysis

Statistical analysis was performed using the SPSS statistical software (version 20.0; SPSS Inc., Chicago, IL, USA). Categorical data are presented as frequency (percentage) and were compared using χ^2-test. Ordinal or discrete risk factors are represented using median values and compared using the Mann–Whitney U test. Comparison of the measured variables between the different groups was performed using a Student's t-test or γ^2 test.

To assess for independent associations with death, a Cox regression was performed, adjusted for the collected data: age at onset, age at LP, CDR at the time of LP, CSF biomarkers, and behavioral versus language variants. Vascular risk factors with significant differences between patients who died during follow up and those who did not were also included. All the assumptions of these models were verified. Statistical significance was set at $\alpha = 0.05$.

3. Results

We included 116 patients. Eight patients were lost to follow-up. Nine were excluded for having developed a motor neuron disorder. Finally, we included 99 patients, with a mean follow-up duration of 5.0 (±2.8) years. Mean age of onset was 61.4 (±9.3) years old. Male patients composed 46.9% of the cohort. Median education was 4.0 (IQR = 5.0) years. From the whole sample, 32 (33.3%) patients died during the follow-up period (average follow-up period for this subset of 5.0 ± 3.0 years). Table 1 presents the comparison of patients who died and those who did not during the follow-up period in terms of the studied variables. Vascular risk factors prevalence and comparison may be found in Supplementary Table S1.

Table 1. Comparison of the two groups in terms of the studied variables.

Variable	Mean Values for the Whole Sample	Mean Values for Patients Who Died during Follow-Up	Mean Values For Patients Who Did Not Die during Follow-Up	p
Sex (% male)	46.9	50.0	45.3	0.664
Variant (% behavioral variant)	85.4	87.5	84.4	0.683
Family history (% positive)	30.2	28.1	31.3	0.753
Age of onset (years)	61.4 (±9.3)	61.1 (±9.8)	61.5 (±9.2)	0.831
Age at LP (years)	63.5 (±9.6)	62.9 (±10.1)	63.9 (9.6)	0.664
Education (years) (median, IQR)	4.0 (IQR = 5.0)	4.0 (IQR = 5.0)	4.0 (IQR = 5.0)	0.791
MMSE at LP	21.1 (±6.8)	20.0 (±7.1)	21.6 (±6.4)	0.271
CDR at LP (median, IQR)	1.0 (IQR = 1.0)	1.0 (IQR = 1.0)	1.0 (IQR = 0.0)	0.016
Follow-up (years)	5.0 (±2.8)	4.5 (±2.6)	5.0 (±3.0)	0.468
CSF amyloid-beta$_{1-42}$ (pg/mL)	677.5 (±301.8)	532.7 (±306.0)	731.8 (±279.2)	0.002
CSF tau (pg/mL)	338.9 (±371.1)	277.6 (±166.5)	365.2 (±429.4)	0.286
CSF phosphorylated-tau (pg/mL)	41.4 (±38.4)	34.8 (±16.2)	44.7 (±44.4)	0.223

LP: lumbar puncture. MMSE: Mini-Mental State Examination, CDR: Clinical Dementia Rating, CSF: Cerebrospinal Fluid.

In terms of vascular risk factors, patients who died during follow-up had a significant lower prevalence of high blood pressure (28.1% vs. 52.2%, $p = 0.024$), diabetes (6.3% vs. 23.9%, $p = 0.033$), and dyslipidemia (18.8% vs. 49.3%, $p = 0.004$). No significant differences were found in the other vascular risk factors (Supplementary Table S1).

In the univariate analysis, death was associated with CSF amyloid-beta$_{1-42}$ levels and CDR. In Cox regression (Table 2), the risk of death was associated with CSF amyloid-beta$_{1-42}$ levels (HR = 0.999, 95%CI = [0.997, 1.000], $p = 0.049$).

Table 2. Cox regression results of the variables associated with the death rate ($\gamma^2 = 18.799$, df = 10, $p = 0.043$, −2 log likelihood = 225.540).

Variable	HR	95% CI	p
Age of onset	0.951	0.807, 1.120	0.546
Age at lumbar puncture	1.097	0.933, 1.289	0.261
Behavioral variant	0.634	0.147, 2.736	0.542
CDR	1.692	0.983, 2.914	0.058
CSF Amyloid-beta$_{1-42}$	0.999	0.997, 1.000	0.049
CSF total tau	1.001	0.998, 1.004	0.514
CSF phosphorylated tau	0.985	0.956, 1.014	0.305
Diabetes	0.428	0.087, 2.118	0.298
High blood pressure	0.735	0.301. 1.794	0.499
Dyslipidemia	0.403	0.142, 1.147	0.089

HR: Hazard ratio; CI: Confidence interval; CSF: cerebrospinal fluid.

4. Discussion

We report a relatively large size sample of thoroughly studied frontotemporal dementia patients. We found a significant independent association between lower CSF amyloid-beta$_{1-42}$ levels and higher mortality.

There is a lack of good FTD diagnostic and prognostic biomarkers. Neurofilament light chain, total Tau [11], and phosphorylated-Tau/total-Tau ratio have been reported to have some clinical value [5,12–15]. Neurofilament light chain has also been shown to be correlated with disease severity, brain atrophy, annualized brain atrophy, and survival [16]. Additionally, some studies have shown that amyloid-positive patients perform significantly worse in cognitive tests [4]. Also, low baseline amyloid-beta$_{1-42}$ has been associated with faster radiographic change in bvFTD [5].

In our sample, amyloid-beta$_{1-42}$ has shown value as a marker of higher mortality rate (HR = 0.999, 95% CI = [0.997, 1.000], $p = 0.049$). If, on one hand, the clinical value of this association might be low, the biological link it represents may be of great importance in the understanding of the biological processes underlying this (and possibly other) conditions. In fact, it has been recently suggested that amyloid-beta plaques enhance tau-seeded pathologies by facilitating neuritic plaque tau aggregation [3]. This facilitation may happen through different mechanisms, such as the creation of a microenvironment that enhances the recruitment of tau into fibrils, but also by impairment of intracellular protein degradation [17].

This may be one explanation for these findings, but other hypotheses may be put forward, such as the occurrence of co-pathology (19.2% of the patients had reduced CSF amyloid-beta$_{1-42}$). However, the rather young age of these patients makes it less likely that Alzheimer's pathology may cause a great disease burden. On the other hand, it could be that, in the presence of concurring FTD-related pathology, a less advanced Alzheimer's pathology could cause a more severe dysfunction. There is evidence that extracellular tau regulates the production of amyloid-beta, by mediating neuronal hyperactivity [18]. The amyloid-beta$_{1-42}$ values could, therefore, be a reflection of a downstream impact of extracellular tau. In the absence of pathologic confirmation, misdiagnosis in a part of the sample is always a possibility. But these patients have been extensively studied and followed for several years. Moreover, one would expect that AD patients (who would have lower CSF amyloid-beta$_{1-42}$ values) would progress slower than the FTD patients [19], however, this is an inverse relationship of what we found.

One important consideration is concerning vascular risk factors, as there were some differences in their prevalence on univariate analysis. In fact, the patients who did not die during the follow-up have a higher prevalence of some of these risk factors (diabetes, high blood pressure, and dyslipidemia) than those who have died. This is in line with some previous studies [20]. This may mean that the patients with a more rapid course have other strong factors driving the progression (possibly genetic), rather than a more multifactorial disease in the group of patients who did not die. These results could also mean that some of the patients in the group of patients who did not die during follow-up may have vascular dementia rather than frontotemporal dementia, leading to a more slowly progressive disease.

The main limitation of our work is its retrospective nature, although the data were prospectively collected, the hypothesis may be biased. Additionally, we do not have pathological data, and, since frontotemporal dementia may be associated with different pathological patterns and deposition of different proteins, the association with CSF amyloid-beta$_{1-42}$ may be true only for one of these pathologies. However, the hard endpoint that we have measured (progression), and the moderate size of the sample, support the generalizability of these results.

5. Conclusions

Our results suggest that CSF amyloid-beta$_{1-42}$ may modulate mortality in frontotemporal dementia patients.

Author Contributions: Conceptualization—M.T.-P., D.V., J.D. and I.S.; methodology—I.B., B.S., D.D., M.L., M.J.L., I.S. and M.T.-P.; software—M.T.-P.; validation—M.T.-P., I.S.; formal analysis—all authors; investigation, all authors; writing—original draft preparation—D.V., M.T.-P. and J.D.; writing—review and editing—I.S., M.T.-P. and I.B.

References

1. Bang, J.; Spina, S.; Miller, B.L. Frontotemporal dementia. *Lancet* **2015**, *386*, 1672–1682. [CrossRef]
2. Rohrer, J.D.; Lashley, T.; Schott, J.M.; Warren, J.E.; Mead, S.; Isaacs, A.M.; Beck, J.; Hardy, J.; de Silva, R.; Warrington, E.; et al. Clinical and neuroanatomical signatures of tissue pathology in frontotemporal lobar degeneration. *Brain A J. Neurol.* **2011**, *134*, 2565–2581. [CrossRef] [PubMed]
3. He, Z.; Guo, J.L.; McBride, J.D.; Narasimhan, S.; Kim, H.; Changolkar, L.; Zhang, B.; Gathagan, R.J.; Yue, C.; Dengler, C.; et al. Amyloid-beta plaques enhance Alzheimer's brain tau-seeded pathologies by facilitating neuritic plaque tau aggregation. *Nat. Med.* **2018**, *24*, 29–38. [CrossRef] [PubMed]
4. Naasan, G.; Rabinovici, G.D.; Ghosh, P.; Elofson, J.D.; Miller, B.L.; Coppola, G.; Karydas, A.; Fong, J.; Perry, D.; Lee, S.E.; et al. Amyloid in dementia associated with familial FTLD: Not an innocent bystander. *Neurocase* **2016**, *22*, 76–83. [CrossRef]
5. Ljubenkov, P.A.; Staffaroni, A.M.; Rojas, J.C.; Allen, I.E.; Wang, P.; Heuer, H.; Karydas, A.; Kornak, J.; Cobigo, Y.; Seeley, W.W.; et al. Cerebrospinal fluid biomarkers predict frontotemporal dementia trajectory. *Ann. Clin. Transl. Neurol.* **2018**, *5*, 1250–1263. [CrossRef]
6. Rascovsky, K.; Hodges, J.R.; Knopman, D.; Mendez, M.F.; Kramer, J.H.; Neuhaus, J.; van Swieten, J.C.; Seelaar, H.; Dopper, E.G.; Onyike, C.U.; et al. Sensitivity of revised diagnostic criteria for the behavioural variant of frontotemporal dementia. *Brain* **2011**, *134*, 2456–2477. [CrossRef] [PubMed]
7. Gorno-Tempini, M.L.; Hillis, A.E.; Weintraub, S.; Kertesz, A.; Mendez, M.; Cappa, S.F.; Ogar, J.M.; Rohrer, J.D.; Black, S.; Boeve, B.F.; et al. Classification of primary progressive aphasia and its variants. *Neurology* **2011**, *76*, 1006–1014. [CrossRef] [PubMed]
8. Mattsson, N.; Andreasson, U.; Persson, S.; Arai, H.; Batish, S.D.; Bernardini, S.; Bocchio-Chiavetto, L.; Blankenstein, M.A.; Carrillo, M.C.; Chalbot, S.; et al. The Alzheimer's Association external quality control program for cerebrospinal fluid biomarkers. *Alzheimer's Dement.* **2011**, *7*, 386–395. [CrossRef] [PubMed]
9. Baldeiras, I.E.; Ribeiro, M.H.; Pacheco, P.; Machado, A.; Santana, I.; Cunha, L.; Oliveira, C.R. Diagnostic value of CSF protein profile in a Portuguese population of sCJD patients. *J. Neurol.* **2009**, *256*, 1540–1550. [CrossRef] [PubMed]

10. Kapaki, E.; Kilidireas, K.; Paraskevas, G.P.; Michalopoulou, M.; Patsouris, E. Highly increased CSF tau protein and decreased beta-amyloid (1-42) in sporadic CJD: A discrimination from Alzheimer's disease? *J. Neurol. Neurosurg. Psychiatry* **2001**, *71*, 401–403. [CrossRef] [PubMed]
11. Borroni, B.; Benussi, A.; Cosseddu, M.; Archetti, S.; Padovani, A. Cerebrospinal fluid tau levels predict prognosis in non-inherited frontotemporal dementia. *Neuro.-Degener. Dis.* **2014**, *13*, 224–229. [CrossRef] [PubMed]
12. Meeter, L.H.H.; Vijverberg, E.G.; Del Campo, M.; Rozemuller, A.J.M.; Donker Kaat, L.; de Jong, F.J.; van der Flier, W.M.; Teunissen, C.E.; van Swieten, J.C.; Pijnenburg, Y.A.L. Clinical value of neurofilament and phospho-tau/tau ratio in the frontotemporal dementia spectrum. *Neurology* **2018**, *90*, e1231–e1239. [CrossRef] [PubMed]
13. Borroni, B.; Benussi, A.; Archetti, S.; Galimberti, D.; Parnetti, L.; Nacmias, B.; Sorbi, S.; Scarpini, E.; Padovani, A. Csf p-tau181/tau ratio as biomarker for TDP pathology in frontotemporal dementia. *Amyotroph. Lateral Scler. Front. Degener.* **2015**, *16*, 86–91. [CrossRef] [PubMed]
14. Hu, W.T.; Watts, K.; Grossman, M.; Glass, J.; Lah, J.J.; Hales, C.; Shelnutt, M.; Van Deerlin, V.; Trojanowski, J.Q.; Levey, A.I. Reduced CSF p-Tau181 to Tau ratio is a biomarker for FTLD-TDP. *Neurology* **2013**, *81*, 1945–1952. [CrossRef] [PubMed]
15. Pijnenburg, Y.A.; Verwey, N.A.; van der Flier, W.M.; Scheltens, P.; Teunissen, C.E. Discriminative and prognostic potential of cerebrospinal fluid phosphoTau/tau ratio and neurofilaments for frontotemporal dementia subtypes. *Alzheimer's Dement.* **2015**, *1*, 505–512. [CrossRef] [PubMed]
16. Meeter, L.H.; Dopper, E.G.; Jiskoot, L.C.; Sanchez-Valle, R.; Graff, C.; Benussi, L.; Ghidoni, R.; Pijnenburg, Y.A.; Borroni, B.; Galimberti, D.; et al. Neurofilament light chain: A biomarker for genetic frontotemporal dementia. *Ann. Clin. Transl. Neurol.* **2016**, *3*, 623–636. [CrossRef] [PubMed]
17. Almeida, C.G.; Takahashi, R.H.; Gouras, G.K. Beta-amyloid accumulation impairs multivesicular body sorting by inhibiting the ubiquitin-proteasome system. *J. Neurosci.* **2006**, *26*, 4277–4288. [CrossRef] [PubMed]
18. Bright, J.; Hussain, S.; Dang, V.; Wright, S.; Cooper, B.; Byun, T.; Ramos, C.; Singh, A.; Parry, G.; Stagliano, N.; et al. Human secreted tau increases amyloid-beta production. *Neurobiol. Aging* **2015**, *36*, 693–709. [CrossRef] [PubMed]
19. Kertesz, A. Rate of progression differs in frontotemporal dementia and Alzheimer disease. *Neurology* **2006**, *66*, 1607. [CrossRef] [PubMed]
20. Irimata, K.E.; Dugger, B.N.; Wilson, J.R. Impact of the Presence of Select Cardiovascular Risk Factors on Cognitive Changes among Dementia Subtypes. *Curr. Alzheimer Res.* **2018**, *15*, 1032–1044. [CrossRef] [PubMed]

10

Articular Cartilage Aging-Potential Regenerative Capacities of Cell Manipulation and Stem Cell Therapy

Magdalena Krajewska-Włodarczyk [1,2,3,*], Agnieszka Owczarczyk-Saczonek [4], Waldemar Placek [4], Adam Osowski [3] and Joanna Wojtkiewicz [3,5]

1 Department of Rheumatology, Municipal Hospital in Olsztyn, 10-900 Olsztyn, Poland
2 Department of Internal Medicine, School of Medicine, Collegium Medicum, University of Warmia and Mazury, 10-900 Olsztyn, Poland
3 Department of Pathophysiology, School of Medicine, Collegium Medicum, University of Warmia and Mazury, 10-900 Olsztyn, Poland; adam.osowski@uwm.edu.pl (A.O.); joanna.wojtkiewicz@uwm.edu.pl (J.W.)
4 Department of Dermatology, Sexually Transmitted Diseases and Clinical Immunology, School of Medicine, Collegium Medicum, University of Warmia and Mazury, 10-900 Olsztyn, Poland; aganek@wp.pl (A.O.-S); w.placek@wp.pl (W.P.)
5 Laboratory for Regenerative Medicine, School of Medicine, Collegium Medicum, University of Warmia and Mazury, 10-900 Olsztyn, Poland
* Correspondence: magdalenakw@op.pl

Abstract: Changes in articular cartilage during the aging process are a stage of natural changes in the human body. Old age is the major risk factor for osteoarthritis but the disease does not have to be an inevitable consequence of aging. Chondrocytes are particularly prone to developing age-related changes. Changes in articular cartilage that take place in the course of aging include the acquisition of the senescence-associated secretory phenotype by chondrocytes, a decrease in the sensitivity of chondrocytes to growth factors, a destructive effect of chronic production of reactive oxygen species and the accumulation of the glycation end products. All of these factors affect the mechanical properties of articular cartilage. A better understanding of the underlying mechanisms in the process of articular cartilage aging may help to create new therapies aimed at slowing or inhibiting age-related modifications of articular cartilage. This paper presents the causes and consequences of cellular aging of chondrocytes and the biological therapeutic outlook for the regeneration of age-related changes of articular cartilage.

Keywords: aging; articular cartilage; cell manipulation; stem cells

---

1. Introduction

The motor system is the basis for the motion of the human body and the processes that take place in it during aging result not only in limiting the self-sufficiency in performing everyday activities, changes in attitude and gait and increased risk of falling but they also affect the function of internal organs and the quality of life [1].

Attempts to elucidate the causes of age-related changes in articular cartilage and the development of osteoarthritis (OA) include several theories, including the wear and tear theory [2]. Causes of OA development are also sought in processes related to cellular aging, such as the acquisition of the so-called senescence-associated secretory phenotype (SASP), which derives from a change of gene expression in old cells [3], the weakening of the chondrocyte response to growth factors, including the insulin-like growth factor-1 (IGF-1) and transforming growth factor-β (TGF-β) [4], mitochondria function disorders and the effect of oxidative stress [5] as well as the accumulation of advanced glycation end products (AGEs) [6]. Therefore, the destruction of articular cartilage which progresses with age is not only a result of mechanical overload caused by obesity, posture, gait disorders or trauma. Depletion of cartilage that penetrates into the sub-cartilage bone is a gate to non-differentiated mesenchymal cells which—depending on numerous local factors—can differentiate towards osteoblasts which produce bone tissue, towards fibroblasts which contribute to the formation of fibrous connective tissue or towards chondroblasts, which can produce fibrous or hyaline-like cartilage [7]. Unfortunately, physiological regenerative capability of articular cartilage is highly limited and, in cases of significant damage, only external therapeutic intervention can improve the local condition.

2. Cellular Senescence

Cellular senescence affects all cells. After the number of divisions (ca. 30–60) determined by the replication limit (Hayflick's limit) in an in vitro culture, cells lose their replication potential and stop dividing while continuing to age but they do not die at once and can remain metabolically active for a long time [8]. The aging of cells and organs is probably caused by the accumulation of old cells, which—because of changed metabolism and secreted proteins—create their own microenvironment, affecting their own activity and adjacent cells. The low-grade inflammation which develops as a result of these processes accompanies a majority of old-age diseases [9]. Cellular senescence not only reflects the aging of the body but it also plays a significant role in tissue regeneration in young individuals and probably reduces the risk of neoplasm formation by inhibiting mitotic divisions of cells with damaged genetic material [10]. Unlike in apoptotic cells, the activity of senescence associated β-galactosidase (SA-β-gal) increases in the aging process [11]. As a result of DNA damage, aging cells acquire a specific secretory phenotype which leads to their elimination by immune system phages, while at the same time contributing to the development of age-related diseases. The essence of SASP lies in secretion to the environment of a range of cytokines (interleukin: IL-1, -6, -7, -13, -15), inflammatory chemokines (CCL2/MCP-1, CCL8/MCP-2, CCL26, CXCL8/IL-8, CXCL12/SDF-1), growth factors (amphiregulins, EGF, hFGF, HGF, heregulins, KGF, NGF, VEGF), metalloproteinases (MMP) -1, -3, -10, -12, -13, -14, other proteases and their modulators (TIMP-2, PAI-1,PAI-2, t-PA, u-PA) [12].

Two types of cellular senescence are distinguished: replicative and accelerated [13]. Replicative senescence is associated with exhaustion of the division limit. This is caused by shortening of telomeres, whose function is to protect the ends of chromosomes from joining and preserving the genome integrity. Human telomeres consist of thousands of repetitions of motifs made up of six pairs of bases TTAGGG and they constitute a specific counter of cell divisions. The telomere structure is supported by shelterins—proteins that ensure maintenance of their specific structure. Telomeres are multiplied with a specific reverse transcriptase (RT)—telomerase in a complex process, coordinated by genomic replication. Human telomerase is made up of two main subunits—the telomerase RNA template (hTERC) and the catalytic enzyme telomerase reverse transcriptase (hTERT), which are responsible for replication of base pairs in a specific sequence and for the length of telomeres, respectively [14]. Activity of telomerases in regular human tissues is not sufficient to keep the telomere length constant, which results in telomeres becoming shorter with each cellular division [15]. When telomeres are shortened down to half of their original length on five chromosomes, phenotypic cell senescence occurs [16]. Stress-induced premature senescence (SIPS), associated with DNA damage, is another type of cellular senescence that takes place regardless of physiological telomere shortening. Accelerated senescence can be triggered by oxidative stress, oncogenes, UV radiation or a chronic inflammation [17]. This process is faster than replicative senescence and it does not result directly from exhausting the division potential. The causes of each of these types of senescence is different but they are associated with activation of the same path of response to DNA damage. Such a signal in replicative senescence is generated by shortened telomeres or ones without shelterins. A similar response in accelerated senescence is triggered by a rupture of a double strand of DNA in telomere sections which are inaccessible to the repair systems due to their specific structure and protective proteins [17]. A response to DNA damage is controlled, inter alia, with protein p53, which is an inhibitor of cyclin-dependent kinases, which is responsible for inhibiting cellular divisions and hypophosphorylated Rb (retinoblastoma protein), which is responsible for recruiting enzymes associated with epigenetic chromatin modification [18].

3. Senescence-Related Changes of Articular Cartilage

Homeostasis of cartilage depends on the regularity of function of mature chondrocytes and progenitor cells. With age, the matrix of articular cartilage also undergoes molecular, structural and mechanical changes, there are some changes in the composition and structure of proteoglycans, collagen cross-linking increases and the elongation strength of cartilage decreases. The balance between anabolic activity of chondrocytes and destructive processes is disturbed. Articular cartilage thins slowly as the matrix reduces, cartilage hydration decreases and the chondrocyte count decreases (Figure 1). An age-related decrease in the number of chondrocytes in articular cartilage has been observed in people without clinical symptoms of arthritis, although more pronounced chondrocyte loss is present in patients with OA [19]. The number of chondrocytes in the hip joint cartilage in people aged 30–70 years was reduced by ca. 40% [20]; similar differences have been observed in animal studies [21]. However, in a study of human knee joint cartilage, no significant changes in the number of chondrocytes were observed [22]. The frequency of chondrocyte divisions observed in articular cartilage in adults is low, which—with a very small number of local progenitor cells—may suggest that chondrocytes in elderly people are the same cells as many years earlier but are considerably changed. It also appears that the number of apoptotic cells in human articular cartilage does not increase significantly with progressing age [22].

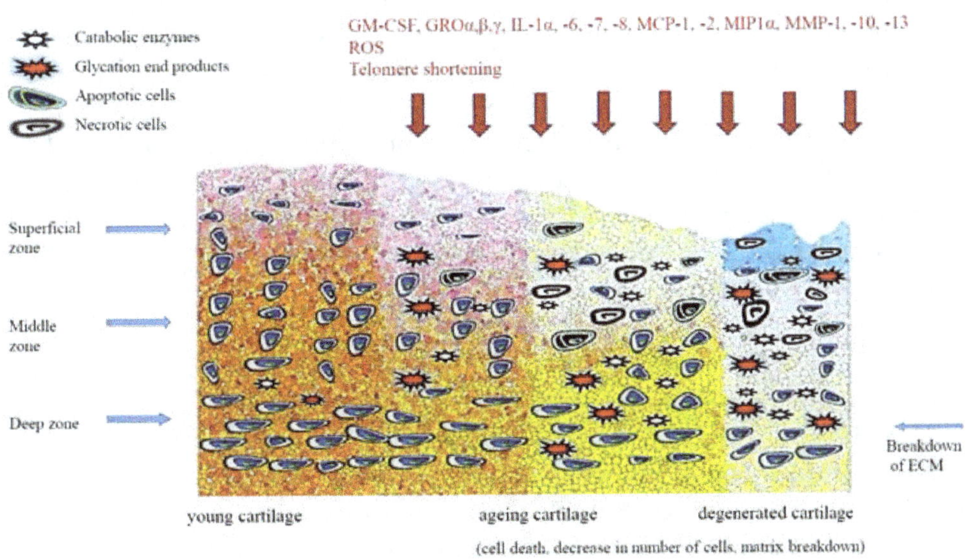

Figure 1. The age-related changes in cartilage.

Senescence of chondrocytes is accompanied by aging-related changes in extracellular cartilage matrix (ECM). The unique properties of extracellular matrix of cartilage have their source in collagenic and non-collagenic glycoproteins, proteoglycans and hyaluronic acid. ECM in articular cartilage plays a crucial role in regulating chondrocyte functions via cell-matrix interaction, organized cytoskeleton and integrin-mediated signalling [23]. A reduction in cartilage volume can be caused by a reduction of water content dependent largely on the content of aggrecan, which is the principal proteoglycan in an articular cartilage matrix. Sulphated, negatively-charged glycosaminoglycans (GAG), which make up aggrecan, are characterised by high hydrophilicity and are responsible for cartilage elasticity.

There have been reports describing age-related changes of size, structure and degree of sulphation of aggrecan which resulted in a decrease in hydration and elasticity of cartilage [24].

3.1. Telomere Shortening

Like in cells of other tissues, telomeres have been found to be significantly shortened in chondrocytes of articular cartilage which have passed through a larger number of cellular divisions [25]; larger numbers of shortened telomeres have also been reported in chromosomes of chondrocytes in elderly people [25]. Age-dependent shortening of telomeres has been observed recently in a study conducted with people with no symptoms of arthritis and in a group of OA patients [26]. The activity of telomerase is higher in chondrocytes in young individuals, which enables repair procedures in young chondrocytes; this activity is reduced considerably after puberty [27]. Attempts have been made to explain the importance of telomeres shortening for senescence of chondrocytes and their precursors—mesenchymal stem cells (MSCs). The length of telomeres varies depending on the donor's age. Embryonic or foetal cells have longer telomeres, telomerase activity in them is higher and they senesce later than cells collected from adult individuals [28]. The length of telomeres in chondrocytes has been reported as 9 to 11 kbp in donors over 55 years old and below 12 kbp in donors under 22 years old [3]. Guillot et al. report that telomeres in foetal stem cells were significantly longer (10 to 11 kbp) than in MSCs obtained from the bone marrow of adult individuals (under 7 kbp) [28], whereas Mareschi et al. found the length of telomeres in MSCs of young donors to be approx. 10 kbp [29]. In these in vitro studies, the telomere length in bone marrow MSCs decreased by 1.5–2 kbp per passage. Telomere length in bone marrow MSCs decreased by 17 bp a year, as found in an in vivo study [30]. Interesting findings were presented in a paper by Parsch et al. where telomeres in bone marrow MSC remained shorter than in chondrocytes even after they were chondrogenically differentiated and their shortening was inhibited at a length of approx. 10 kbp [31]. Apart from the length reduction caused by replicative senescence, telomeres shortening is caused by oxidative stress and destruction of DNA strands [32]. Telomeres in chondrocytes and in MSCs have been found to shorten considerably in cell culture subjected both to sublethal oxidative stress and to prolonged low-level stress [33,34]. A relationship has been described between a considerable shortening of telomeres in chondrocytes and intensified senescence of chondrocytes and the severity of OA [35], although no differences have been observed in another study in the length of telomeres in regular chondrocytes and in those collected from OA lesions [36]. The reason for the large differences between these studies may be the use of different telomere length estimation methods.

3.2. Oxidative Stress

Chondrocytes and MSCs are known to be exposed naturally to under-physiological oxygen concentrations. Reactive oxygen species (ROS) induce telomere shortening stimulated by DNA damage [37,38]. The amount of ROS in chondrocytes increases with age, excessive mechanical load and activity of inflammatory cytokines [39]. The addition of ROS to a chondrocyte culture resulted in developing aging-related phenotypic traits in chondrocytes [39]. The amount of proteins (which are shelterins) associated with telomerase TRF1, TRF2 (telomeric repeat binding factor 1, 2) increases considerably in chondrocytes under oxidative stress during early cell division. These proteins are responsible for the formation and maintaining the structure of telomeres, protein XRCC5 (X-ray repair complementing defective repair in Chinese hamster cells 5) participating in the repair of two-strand DNA and sirtulin 1 (SIRT1), which suppresses protein p53 and prevents inhibition of cell divisions. Secretion of these shelterins is much weaker in later divisions [37]. This study suggests a protective effect of proteins TRF1, TRF2, XRCC5 and SIRT1 on young chondrocytes against shortening of telomeres associated with damage to DNA strands under oxidative stress, whereas in chondrocytes which divide later, a decrease in the activity of these regulatory proteins results in decreased tolerance to ROS and in the accumulation of damaged DNA, which may induce aging-related processes. ROS appear to induce acceleration of chondrocyte senescence by intensifying expression of p53 and p21 and by activation of p38 MAPK (mitogen-activated protein kinase) and phosphatidylinositol 3-kinase/Akt (PI3K/Akt) signalling pathways [40]. Chondrocytes in areas of cartilage affected by OA have been found to contain an increased amount of nitrotyrosine—an oxidative damage marker—which was proportionate to intensification of histological changes [41]. Oxidative stress affecting chondrocytes participates in inducing apoptosis, decreases the cells sensitivity to growth factors, leads to mitochondria dysfunction, telomere-related genomic instability and loss of cartilage matrix [42–45]. ROS also contribute to senescence of MSCs, which are precursors of chondrocytes. The presence of antioxidants (such as *N*-acetylcysteine (NAC) and ascorbic acid) in cell cultures, increased the proliferative activity of MSCs [44,46] and the proliferative and differentiating capability of MSCs in low oxygen concentration (3–5%) was higher than in physiological concentrations (20%) [47,48].

With age, excessive formation of ROS takes place and the oxidative-antioxidative equilibrium is disturbed in cartilage matrix. In reaction with the core protein of proteoglycans, reactive oxygen species modify amino acid residues and cause ruptures of the polypeptide chain of the core protein and formation of proteoglycan fragmentation products in the form of glycosaminoglycan chains bound to core protein residues and free glycosaminoglycans [49].

3.3. Inflammatory Cytokines

Epidemiological studies indicate a relationship between a low-level systemic inflammation and an increase in a concentration of inflammatory cytokines, including C-reactive protein (CRP), IL-6 and TNF-α and the development of OA [50,51]. Inflammatory cytokines can be generated locally in chondrocytes, synovial membrane cells and infrapatellar fat pad-derived cells [50]. Articular cartilage aging may result from the acquisition of a specific secretory phenotype by chondrocytes, whose characteristic features include an increase in the production and secretion of interleukins, matrix metalloproteinases and growth factors, including epidermal growth factor (EGF) [38,52]. SASP-inducing factors include granulocyte macrophage colony stimulating factor (GM-CSF), growth regulated oncogene-α, -β, -γ (GRO-α, -β, -γ), IL-1α, IL-6, IL-7, IL-8, monocyte chemoatractant protein (MCP)-1, -2, IGF-1, macrophage inflammatory protein-1α (MIP-1α) as well as MMP-1, MMP-10 and MMP-13 [50]. Literature reports have described increased expression of metalloproteinases MMP-1 and MMP-13 in aging cartilage [53] and the accumulation of neoepitopes of collagens formed as a result of denaturation and fragmentation of collagen [54]. Other studies have found the capability for production and secretion of IL-1 [55] and IL-7 [56] by isolated chondrocytes to significantly increase with the donor's age and an increase in IL-7 secretion to be associated with increased production of MMP-13 [56]. Moreover, the inflammation process induced by the administration of IL-1β was associated with an increase in the expression of $p16^{INK4a}$, resulting in increased production of MMP-1 and MMP-13 [52].

The total amount of all proteoglycans in cartilage decreases with age. Age-related modifications of proteoglycans in cartilage matrix are related to synthesis disorders and enzymatic and non-enzymatic degradation. Degradation of proteoglycan macromolecules which intensifies with age is accompanied by overexpression of MMP, including MMP-1, MMP-8, MMP-13 with a concomitant decrease in their tissue inhibitors (TIMP) [57]. The activity of disintegrin and metalloproteinase with thrombospondin motifs (ADAMTS), including aggrecanases ADAMTS-4 and ADAMTS-5, which participate in the digestion of core proteins of aggrecans, increases with age [58]. Apart from a direct effect degrading the extracellular matrix of cartilage, these enzymes stimulate the secretion of inflammatory cytokines, e.g.,: IL-1, IL-6 and the tumour necrosis factor-α (TNF-α) [38]. IL-1, IL-6 and TNF-α induce chondrocytes to synthesise increased amounts of matrix metalloproteinases, at the same time inhibiting the production of natural inhibitors of these endopeptidases [58]. Additionally, IL-1 and TNF-α stimulate the production of insulin-like growth factor-binding protein-1 (IGFBP-1). IGFBP-1 binds IGF-1, thereby decreasing its binding capability with an appropriate receptor on chondrocytes, which leads to a decreased response of mature chondrocytes to IGF-1 [59]. An effect of IL-1 and TNF-α results in an increase in the activity of inducible nitric oxide synthase (iNOS), and—secondarily—in an increase in secretion to the matrix of catabolic metalloproteinases and prostaglandins [58].

3.4. Altered Responsiveness to Growth Factors

With time, the anabolic activity of chondrocytes in cartilage decreases and the chondrocyte metabolic equilibrium shifts towards catabolic mechanisms.

Chondrocyte response to IGF-1 decreases with age [4]. Similar disturbances also occur in isolated chondrocytes from cartilage with symptoms of OA [60]. IGF-1 stimulates the proliferation of cartilage cells, supports the synthesis of cartilage matrix cells and inhibits chondrocytes apoptosis through phosphoinositide 3-kinase (PI3K) and extracellular signal-regulated kinase (ERK) [61]. IGF-1 increases the synthesis of proteoglycans of cartilage matrix under in vitro conditions by activating the kinases PI3K/Akt/mTOR/p70S6 pathway [62]. Through PI3K, IGF-1 stimulates MSCs to chondrogenic differentiation [62].

Expression and amount in cartilage of osteogenic protein OP-1 (BMP-7), which is a member of the bone morphogenetic proteins superfamily, decreases with age. The addition of anabolic protein OP-1 to a culture of chondrocytes collected from mature individuals does not affect the activity of telomerase, whereas an addition of inflammatory cytokine IL-1α inhibits its activity [27].

The concentration of TGF-β2 and TGF-β3 (but not TGF-β1) in cartilage also decreases in an age-related manner, like the number of TGF-β receptors [21]. TGF-β is secreted by cells as a latent form (latent TGF-β, L-TGF-β). An active form is generated after dissociation of the non-covalently bonded latency-associated peptide (LAP). LAP dissociation is effected by the plasminogen/plasmin proteolytic system [63], thrombospondin-1 (TSP-1) [64], metalloproteases [65] as well as by mechanical stress [66]. After TGF-β binds to the II type receptor, an activin receptor-like kinase 5 (ALK5) recruiting complex is formed, which is a TGF-β type I receptor. Such a compound induces phosphorylation of serine and threonine residues of type I receptor by type II receptor. The primed receptor transmits the signal directly to cytoplasm, where R–SMAD proteins are phosphorylated and translocated to the cell nucleus [67]. TGF-β signal transmission can be mediated by an alternative ALK1 type I receptor, resulting in the final cellular differentiation and hypertrophy [68]. Binding of TGF-β to the ALK5 receptor leads to phosphorylation of proteins: SMAD2 and SMAD3, whereas binding of TGF-β to the ALK1 results in phosphorylation of SMAD1, SMAD5 and SMAD8. Activation of SMAD2/3 and SMAD1/5/8 pathways differs by the response. Signal transduction by SMAD2/3 is associated with a protective effect and by SMAD1/5/8—with terminal differentiation and hypertrophy [69]. Activation of signal pathways is necessary for in vitro development of MSCs population. Inhibition of TGF-β pathways in rat and human cultures prevented their differentiation [70]. TGF-β in MSCs cultures can be a factor used in the induction of chondrogenesis [71]; on the other hand, TGF-β can accelerate processes of cellular senescence by increasing the activity of senescence-associated-galactosidase (SA-Gal) and the production of mitochondrial reactive oxygen species (mROS) [72]. Philipot et al. found that—during chondrogenic differentiation of BM-MSCs caused by TGF-β3—expression of $p16^{INK4a}$ accompanying the production of type IIB collagen and MMP13 took place, which was a sign of terminal cell differentiation [52].

3.5. Advanced Glycation End-Products

Modifications of proteoglycans of articular cartilage taking place with time are caused by the catabolic effect of enzymes and oxidative stress but also by accumulation of products of late glycation in cartilage (advanced glycation end-products, AGEs). The production of AGEs takes place as a result of spontaneous, non-enzymatic glycation of proteins which, in turn, is a result of reaction of reducing sugars, including sucrose, fructose and ribose with lysine and arginine residues. Due to its relatively slow metabolism, cartilage is particularly predisposed to form AGEs. The half-life of type II collagen, which is the most widespread protein of extracellular cartilage matrix, has been estimated to exceed 100 years [73]. Although products of late glycation decrease the sensitivity of proteoglycans to proteolytic effect of metalloproteinases, the total pool of proteoglycans in cartilage is decreased proportionally to the amount of AGEs [74]. The effect of AGEs on processes that take place in aging cartilage has not been fully elucidated. The appropriate receptors (receptor for advanced glycation end products, RAGE) on the chondrocyte cell membrane are probably responsible for inhibition of synthesis and secretion of proteoglycans to cartilage extracellular matrix and for inducing the synthesis of matrix metalloproteinases (MMP-1, MMP-3, MMP-13) and prostaglandine E2 [57].

3.6. Autophagy

Autophagy has gained interest in the past decade due to its role in regulation of the aging process. Autophagy is a naturally occurring catabolic process that removes unnecessary of dysfunctional cellular components in cytoplasm as aggregated proteins and redundant or damaged organelles [75]. Little is known about the role of autophagy in articular cartilage. In articular cartilage, which has a very low rate of cell turnover, autophagy appears to be protective process for maintaining cartilage homeostasis. Autophagy regulates maturation and promotes survival of terminally differentiated chondrocytes under stress and hypoxia conditions [76]. Transiently increased autophagy is a compensatory response to cellular stress. During the early degenerative phase, autophagy is increased in cartilage, with increased accumulation of autophagic proteins, such as ULK-1, LC3 and Beclin-1 messenger RNA in chondrocytes [77]. Reduced expression of ULK1, Beclin-1 and LC3 protein was observed in aging joints in humans and mice [78]. The reduction in these major autophagy regulators was accompanied by increased chondrocyte apoptosis [77,78]. Many studies identified correlations between autophagy and the mTOR signalling pathway. The cartilage-specific deletion of mTOR upregulates autophagy and results in increased autophagy signalling and a significant protection from the articular cartilage degradation, apoptosis and synovial fibrosis [79]. The intra-articular injection of rapamycin- an mTOR inhibitor [80], or intra-articular administration of gelatin hydrogels incorporating rapamycin-micelles [81], inhibited mTOR expression suppressed the development of the articular cartilage degeneration. Additionally, REDD1- an endogenous inhibitor of mTOR that regulates cellular stress responses is highly expressed in normal human articular cartilage and reduced with age [82]. Chondrocytes are adapted to hypoxic conditions. Two main HIF hypoxia-inducible factors isoforms (HIF-1α and HIF-2α) mediate the response of chondrocytes to hypoxia. HIF-1α supports metabolic adaptation to a hypoxic environment and by suppression of mTOR causes increased autophagy [83]. In contrast, HIF-2α has been shown to be a suppressor of autophagy under hypoxic conditions in vitro [84].

4. Possible Anti-Aging Strategies

Old age and, obviously, the aging of tissues and organs pose a challenge to contemporary medicine. Neither the treatment of pain as the main symptom of changes related to aging of the motor system, nor burdensome surgeries are fully satisfying to patients; hence, the need for alternative methods for slowing down the aging process and supporting regeneration of articular cartilage.

4.1. Cell Manipulation

4.1.1. Telomerase Activators

Several studies have been conducted to assess the effect of an increase in the hTERT activity on the lifespan of MSCs. Increased expression of hTERT by transduction in MSCs resulted in extended in vitro cell replication capability and in maintaining the potential for in vitro adipo-, chondro- and in vivo osteogenic differentiation [85,86]. Neither a tendency for neoplasm formation nor changes in the MSCs caryotype were observed in these studies. Recently, several telomerase-inducing factors have been discovered and described [87–89]. Astragaloside (AST) and its active metabolite cysloastragenole (CAG) activated telomerase and slowed down the aging process in human embryonic kidney HEK293 fibroblasts [90]. Cynomorium songaricum polysaccharide increased telomerase activity and led to elongation of telomeres in murine cells [91]. Tichon et al. found chemical telomerase activators: AGS-499 and AGS-500 to induce expression of TERT in MSCs, to increase the length of telomeres and to stimulate cell resistance to apoptosis induced by oxidative stress. No chromosomal aberrations or MSCs differentiation disorders were observed [92]. Telomerase differentiation in vitro was increased by curcuminoid derivatives with the core and at least one *n*-pentylpyridine side chain [93]. An extract of Astragalus membranaceus root (TA-65) used in another study extended the proliferative activity of T cells [94] and it significantly decreased the amount of extremely short telomeres in a study of mice [95].

4.1.2. Antioxidants and Hypoxia

Several antioxidants have been described with a protective effect on chondrocytes and MSC against cellular senescence and oxidative stress-induced apoptosis. NAC inhibited apoptosis in chondrocytes [40] and MSCs [44] subjected to oxidative stress. In the study by Liu et al., stimulation of chondrocytes with IL-1β caused a significant up-regulation of TLR4 and its downstream targets MyD88 and TRAF6 resulting in NF-κB activation associated with the synthesis of IL-1β and TNFα. These IL-1β-induced inflammatory responses were all effectively reversed by resveratrol- a polyphenol of plant origin. Furthermore, activation of NF-κB in chondrocytes treated with TLR4 siRNA was significantly attenuated but not abolished and exposure to resveratrol further reduced NF-κB translocation [96]. In another study, following resveratrol injection, the expression of collagen type II was retained but the expression of inducible nitric oxide synthase and matrix metalloproteinase-13 was reduced in OA cartilage. Moreover, the administration of resveratrol significantly induced the activation of SIRT1 expression in mouse OA cartilage and in IL-1β-treated human chondrocytes [97]. The effectiveness of antioxidants in preventing damage to chondrocytes seems to increase when biomaterial scaffolds are used [98]. A cell-free collagen/resveratrol (Col/Res) complex in the form of hydrogel significantly reduced the activity of IL-1β, MMP-13 and COX-2 in an animal OA model; additionally, it improved the condition of articular cartilage after only 12 weeks [99]. The physiological oxygen concentration was found to weaken the growth of human chondrocytes and MSCs in a culture and an increase in antioxidant production as a response to these oxygen concentrations resulted in cell destruction [100,101]. Hypoxia in culturing regular human chondrocytes enabled maintaining the chondrogenic cell potential [102] but this was not observed in a study with osteoarthritic human chondrocytes [103]. In the study by Choi et al. chondrogenic differentiation of ASCs was found to be increased under hypoxia as evidenced by the greater amount of proteoglycan formation and increased chondrogenic genes expression, ACAN, COL2 and SOX9 [104]. It appears that human MSCs acquire aging-related traits in cultures under hypoxic conditions later than under normoxic ones. Additionally, the frequency of MSC divisions increases at low oxygen concentrations with the intact genotype maintained [105]. An increase in the chondrogenic potential of MSCs caused by hypoxia has been reported [104,106], although—as with chondrocytes—the direction of MSCs differentiation depends on the oxygen concentration but also on other factors, such as the substrate used [107,108].

4.1.3. Mechanical Load

Mechanical load stimulates the metabolic activity of chondrocytes, which is responsible for keeping the metabolic balance of matrix proteins [109] and participates in processes which regulate MSCs differentiation towards chondrogenesis [110]. Dynamic compressive loading is the most common system of mechanical stimulation of MSC-dependent cartilage regeneration used in mechanobiological studies. The process of mechano-transduction is, at least partly, mediated by the TGF-β signalling pathway [111–113]. Synthesis of matrix proteins by MSCs stimulated by multiaxial pressure is more effective than with monoaxial stimulation [114]. Multidirectional forces support the production of type II collagen, aggrecan and GAG, with or without the participation of external growth factors, including TGF-β [113]; intensification of the production and activity of endogenous TGF-β caused by mechanical load has been reported [111]. In a human MSCs culture, dynamic compressive loading significantly inhibited the expression of hypertrophy markers, such as type X collagen X, MMP-13 and alkaline phosphatase (ALP) [114]. In another study, mechanical inhibition of chondrocyte hypertrophy was mediated by TGF-β/SMAD and integrin β1/focal adhesion kinase (FAK)/extracellular-signal-regulated kinase (ERK) pathways [115]. These findings suggest that applying a mechanical load to a joint following the implantation of cartilage obtained by bioengineering or applying a load to cellular structures before intra-articular implantation can support cartilage maturation and inhibit its hypertrophy, giving better results than immobilisation of the joint, which can have significant application in clinical practice.

4.2. Cell-Based Therapy

Attempts have been made for a long time to surgically stimulate local regeneration of weakened articular cartilage in such procedures as abrasion arthroplasty, drilling and microfracture. Alternatively, there are therapies based on autologous chondrocyte implantation (ACI), autologous matrix-induced chondrogenesis (AMIC) and intra-articular injection of mesenchymal stem cells [116–119].

4.2.1. Autologous Chondrocyte Implantation

ACI is an example of the application of tissue engineering in the treatment of small- and medium-size cartilage loss. This technique includes a surgical biopsy of cartilage from an affected joint, isolation of chondrocytes with collagenase and creation of a monolayer culture, which requires a series of cellular passages to achieve sufficient propagation of chondrocytes. At the next stage, cells acquired in vitro are implanted at the site of a loss and immobilised with a periosteal patch, which has a protective role but which also has chondrogenic capability, or they are protected with a collagenic layer [120]. The results of the ACI procedure observed in population studies have been encouraging—pain within the joint decreased and the formation of high-strength tissue was observed [121]. However, there are some limitations to the application of ACI. However, it seems that the proliferative capability and the chondrocytes' ability to propagate in a one-layer culture decrease with the age of a donor [122]. The study by Barbero et al. did not show any difference in the proliferative activity of chondrocytes collected from donors under 40 years of age, whereas proliferation of chondrocytes from donors over 40 years of age slowed down considerably [123]. A decrease in the proliferative capability of chondrocytes collected from older donors can obviously limit the use of ACI in treating age-related changes. Changes in the phenotype are also an issue in monolayer chondrocyte cultures. The culture conditions do not reflect fully the in vivo conditions. When cultured in vitro, cells can change shape from polygonal or round to flat after as few as four passages; at the time, they start synthesising type X collagen, which is a sign of a loss of the chondrocytal phenotype. With a growing number of passages, aging and dedifferentiation of chondrocytes in a monolayer culture is taking place, which is associated with a decrease in the production of type II collagen, proteoglycans and glycoproteins [40]. Transplantation of old and dedifferentiated cells results in an unwanted growth of fibrous cartilage at the site under treatment [124]. Apart from a conventional monolayer chondrocyte culture, there are methods currently in use using growth factors [62], pellet culture [125] and bioreactors [126]. De-differentiation can be inhibited and chondrogenicity can be regained successfully by functionalization of the dynamic culture surfaces with ECM [127], culture on a continuously expanding surface [128], surface coating with Col I [129] and by applying a mechanical load [130]. Although the methods are effective in maintaining the chondrocytal phenotype, they may not be able to achieve sufficient cell expansion [131]. Much attention has been recently devoted to supplying genes associated with cellular growth factors, including TGF-β1, BMP, IGF-1, fibroblast growth factor (FGF) and transcription factors, i.e., SRY (sex-determining region Y)-box 9 (SOX9), RUNX2 and SMAD; microRNAs and Col II promoter-binding proteins [132].

4.2.2. Mesenchymal Stem Cells

Mesenchymal stem cells are able to differentiate in multiple directions and to self-regenerate [133]. Since MSCs are present in many embryonic tissues (embryonic stem cells, ESC) and in adult individuals (adult stem cells, ASC), there are many methods of acquiring them. Embryonic stem cells can be collected from umbilical cord blood after delivery, from Wharton's jelly, from the placenta and amniotic fluid and as well as from the subamniotic membrane and perivascular area of the umbilical cord. MSCs have been identified in the following tissues in adult individuals: marrow, adipose tissue, skin, lungs, dental pulp, periosteum, skeletal muscles, tendons and synovial membrane [134] but clinical application of "adult" MSCs is limited mainly to bone marrow-derived mesenchymal stromal cells (BM-MSCs) and adipose-derived stem cells (ADSC, ASC) [135]. According to criteria issued by The International Society for Cellular Therapy (ISCT), characteristic features of mesenchymal cells include the ability to adhere to a plastic base, the presence of three surface antigens: CD105 (endoglin), CD90 (Thy-1), CD73 (ecto-5′-nucleotidase) and concomitant absence of antigens CD45, CD34, CD14 or CD11a, CD79a, or CD19 and class II HLA and the capability of in vitro differentiation towards three cellular lines: osteoblasts, adipocytes and chondroblasts (Figure 2) [133]. Additionally, a detailed description of stem cells includes information, such as the cell origin (tissue, organ, systemic), culture conditions, medium composition, the presence of other antigens of positive identification and absence of negative markers, potential for differentiation, cloning, proteomes, secretomes and transcriptone data [136]. MSCs have a clinically promising immunomodulatory and regenerative potential but it must be noted that MSC also age and die in cultures after several passages [137].

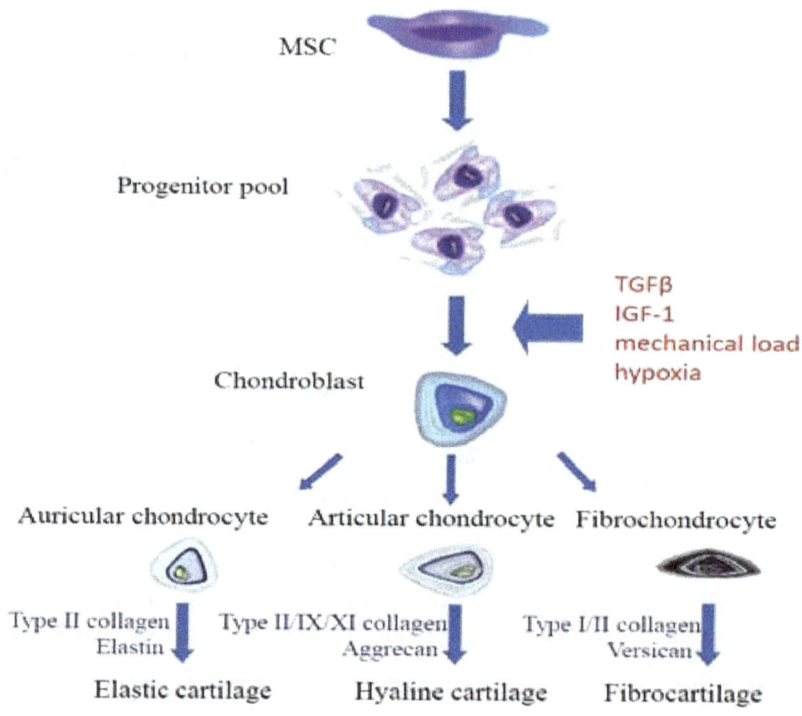

Figure 2. Chondrogenic differentiation of mesenchymal stem cells.

The results of the application of MSCs in regeneration of articular cartilage are promising. In a study by Davatchi et al., intra-articular administration of MSCs to the knee joint ($8–9 \times 10^6$ cells/patient) resulted in a significant, long term reduction of pain as assessed with the visual analogue scale (VAS), as well as in a reduction of flexion contracture in the joint, of cracking during movements and in an extension of the walking distance [138]. In a randomised, multi-centre clinical trial, a considerable reduction of pain assessed in the VAS and an improvement of the function assessed in the WOMAC (Western Ontario and McMaster Universities OA Index) scale and by measurement of the joint movement range was observed in patients following intra-articular administration of autologous BM-MSCs at 100 $\times$ 10^6 cells/patient in combination with hyaluronic acid. Conversely, an improvement was observed only initially in patients who received BM-MSCs in smaller amounts (10 $\times$ 10^6 cells/patient) but when measured after six months, the change in the parameters under assessment was not significant [139]. An improvement after the administration of even small doses of autologous BM-MSCs into the knee joint (2 $\times$ 10^6 cells/patient) was reported recently by Pers et al. [140]. In the study by Emadedin et al. BM-MSCs at 5 $\times$ 10^5 cells/kg/bw (body weight) were administered to patients with OA of knee joints but also to patients with OA of the ankle and of the hip joint. An improvement of the clinical parameters was observed in these patients for a year but it gradually decreased over the next 18 months [141]. A clinical improvement in all the studies corresponded to that observed in imaging examinations (MRI). Reports published later also confirmed the efficacy and safety of the use of autologous MSCs (Table 1) [138,140,142–156]. Use of allogeneic cells could be an alternative to therapy with autologous MSCs (Table 2) [157–160]. Administration to the knee joint of allogeneic BM-MSCs at 40 $\times$ 10^6 cells/patient [158], 50 $\times$ 10^6 cells/patient, 150 $\times$ 10^6 cells/patient [157] was safe and resulted in a clinical improvement, observed in MRI examinations. Similar results were reported in a recent study by de Windt et al. in which a mixture of allogeneic BM-MSCs and autologous chondrones (chondrocytes with their native pericellular matrix) was used [159,160]. However, a growing body of evidence has been emerging of the time of survival of MSCs at the implantation site being much shorter than expected [161]. Therefore, it cannot be ruled out that MSCs have a regenerative effect on articular cartilage, not only as a source of cells which differentiate towards chondrocytes but also through the secretome that they secrete, which covers a broad spectrum of paracrine factors [162]. After intra-articular administration, MSCs use cytokines to stimulate secretion of extracellular matrix proteases and growth factors, including TGF-β, IGF-1 and FGF [163]. After in vitro addition of articular fluid collected from patients in an early and late stage of OA, larger amounts of factors secreted by MSCs were observed, such as: chemokine (C–X–C motif) ligands, chemokine (C–C motif) ligands and IL-6 in the fluid taken from patients in the initial phase of OA [164]. These findings are indicative of different reactions of MSCs following an intra-articular administration, depending on the degree of local cartilage damage, which can determine the therapeutic indications.

However, there are a number of unknowns associated with the use of MSCs. When administered intra-articularly, MSCs after long culturing may lose their chondrogenic phenotype and die quickly [165]. There have been many attempts at maintaining or restoring the chondrogenic differentiation capability of MSCs, which includes the addition of growth factors, modification of culture conditions and specifying the sources of MSCs; however, there are currently no recommendations in this regard [166–168]. Most of the studies conducted to date have been based on MSCs obtained from a patient's own bone marrow or adipose tissue, which was supposed to limit the immune response; allogeneic MSCs were used only in a few studies. The follow-up period in the published studies conducted to assess the efficacy and safety of intra-articular administration of cultured MSCs (except in studies by Davatchi et al. [138] and Wakitani et al. [145]) was short: from six months to two years. A clinical issue is the tendency of implanted MSCs to differentiate towards fibro-like tissue instead of towards hyaline cartilage [169], which considerably affects the properties of the newly-formed tissue. New sources of MSCs from tissues are sought with a high potential of differentiation towards chondrocytes. Synovial membrane was thought to be such a place. Intra-articular administration of autologous synovium stem cells (SSC) in studies with animal models [170] and in human studies [154,171] proved to cause improvement in imaging and histological parameters of articular cartilage. There are some ongoing studies into maintaining the chondroidal phenotype with advanced methods of genetic modifications and epigenetic regulations.

Table 1. List of publications of autologous mesenchymal stem cells application for cartilage repair.

Author Year Study Type	Number of Patients	Stem Cell Origin	Number of Cells	Control Group	Follow-up Time	Co-Treatment	Delivery System	Assessments
Wakitani et al. Case and control study [142]	12	Autologous BM-MSCs from iliac crest	1.3×10^7	12 cell free	28–95 weeks	High tibial osteotomy; gel-cell composite; autologous periosteum	Implantation of collagen cell sheets	Arthroscopic photography; Histological samples; Clinical evaluation
Niejadnik et al. Cohort study [143]	36	Autologous BM-MSCs from iliac crest	$1.0–1.5 \times 10^7$	36 autologous chondrocyte implantation	24 months	Fibrin glue	Implantation upon autologous periosteal patch	ICRS; Lysholm score; Tegner activity scale X-ray; Clinical evaluation
Buda et al. Case series study [144]	20	Autologous BM-MSCs from iliac crest	N/A (2 mL of bone marrow concentrate)	None	24 months	Arthroscopic debridement; Hyaluronic acid membrane scaffold	Transplantation of Arthroscopic Bone-Marrow-Derived Mesenchymal Stem Cells	Clinical evaluation (IKDC, KOOS); MRI; Histochemical analysis
Wakitani et al. Case series [145]	41	Autologous BM-MSCs from iliac crest	5.0×10^6/mL	None	5–137 months	Gel-cell composite	Implantation cell sheets	X-ray; Clinical evaluation
Saw et al. Case series study [146]	5	Autologous peripheral blood progenitor cells	N/A (7–8 mL of peripheral blood progenitor cells	None	10–26 months	Microfracture; Hyaluronic acid intra-articular injections	Intra-articular injection	Second-look arthroscopy; Histological samples;
Davatchi et al. Case series study [147]	4	Autologous BM-MSCs from iliac crest	$8.0–9.0 \times 10^6$	None	12 months	Saline with 2% human serum albumine	Intra-articular injection	X-ray; Clinical evaluation; VAS
Koh et al. Case and control study [148]	25	Autologous A-MSCs from infrapatellar fat pad	$1.2–2.3 \times 10^6$	25 cell free	12–18 months	Arthroscopic debridement; Synovectomy	Intra-articular injection	Lysholm score; Tegner activity scale; VAS
Koh et al. Case series study [149]	18	Autologous A-MSCs from infrapatellar fat pad	$0.3–2.7 \times 10^6$	None	24–26 months	Arthroscopic debridement; Synovectomy; Platelet-rich plasma	Intra-articular injection	Lysholm score; Tegner activity scale; VAS; MRI
Saw et al. Randomised control trial [150]	49	Autologous peripheral blood progenitor cells	N/A (7–8 mL of PBPC)	25 cell free	24 months	Microfracture; Hyaluronic acid intra-articular injections	Intra-articular injection	IKDC; MRI; Second-look arthroscopy; Histological samples
Orozko et al. Case series study [151]	12	Autologous BM-MSCs from iliac crest	40×10^6	None	12 months	Ringer lactate, human albumin, glucose	Intra-articular injection	VAS; Clinical evaluation: WOMAC; MRI

Table 1. *Cont.*

Author Year Study Type	Number of Patients	Stem Cell Origin	Number of Cells	Control Group	Follow-up Time	Co-Treatment	Delivery System	Assessments
Wong et al. Randomized control trial [152]	28	Autologous BM-MSCs from iliac crest	1.46×10^6	28 cell free	24 months	Microfracture and high tibial osteotomy; Hyaluronic acid;	Intra-articular injection	IKDC; Lysholm score; Tegner activity scale; MOCART
Jo et al. Cohort study [153]	18	Autologous A-MSCs from abdominal subcutaneous fats	1.0×10^7, 5.0×10^7, 1.0×10^8	None	6 months	None	Intra-articular injection	WOMAC; VAS, KSS; X-ray, MRI; Second-look arthroscopy; Histological samples
Akgun et al. Prospective, single-site, randomized, single-blind pilot study. [154]	7	Autologous synovium-derived MSCs	4.0×10^6	7 matrix-induced autologous chondrocyte implantation	24 months	Type I/III collagen membrane (2 cm × 2 cm)	Implantation of MSC preloaded collagen membrane	Clinical evaluation: VAS, KOOS; MRI
Davatchi et al. Case series study [138]	4	Autologous BM-MSCs	$8.0–9.0 \times 10^6$	None	60 months	Glucosamine was permitted	Intra-articular injection	X-ray; Clinical evaluation: VAS, walking time to pain
Fodor et al. Case series study [155]	6	Adipose-derived stromal vascular cells (the stromal vascular fraction of adipose tissue)	14.0×10^6	None	12 months	None	Intra-articular injection	Clinical evaluation: WOMAC, VAS, ROM, TUG; MRI.
Koh et al. Randomized control trial [156]	40	Autologous A-MSCs	5.0×10^6	40 Microfracture treatment	24 months	Debridement; Microfracture, Fibrin glue	Arthroscopic implantation of MSC loaded in fibrin glue	Second-look arthroscopy; the Lysholm score, KOOS, VAS; MRI; Histological samples
Pers et al. Cohort study [140]	18	Autologous A-MSCs	2.0×10^6, 10.0×10^6, 50.0×10^6	None	6 months	None	Intra-articular injection	WOMAC, VAS, PGA, SAS, KOOS; Histological samples

A-MSCs: adipose-derived mesenchymal stem cells; BM-MSCs: bone marrow-derived mesenchymal stem cells; ICRS: International Cartilage Repair Society score; IKDC: International Knee Documentation Committee; KOOS: the Knee Injury and Osteoarthritis Outcome; KSS: Knee Society Clinical Rating System score; MOCART: Magnetic Resonance Observation of Cartilage Repair Tissue score; MRI: magnetic resonance imaging; MSCs: mesenchymal stem cells; N/A: not available; PGA: Patient Global Assessment; ROM: range of motion; SAS: Short Arthritis Assessment Scale; TUG: timed up-and-go; VAS: visual analogue pain scale; WOMAC: the Western Ontario and McMaster Universities Arthritis Index.

Table 2. List of publications of allogenic mesenchymal stem cells application for cartilage repair.

Author Year Study Type	Number of Patients	Stem Cell Origin	Number of Cells	Control Group	Follow-up Time	Co-Treatment	Delivery System	Assessments
Vangsness et al. Randomized, double-blind, controlled study [157]	36	Allogenic BM-MSCs from 18–30-year old donors	5.0×10^7, 1.5×10^8	20 cell free vehicle control	24 months	Partial medial meniscectomy	Intra-articular injection	Measurement of immune cell markers; MRI; VAS; Lysholm score
Vega et al. Randomized control trial [158]	15	Allogenic BM-MSCs	40×10^6	15 Hyaluronic acid (60 mg, single dose)	12 months	None	Intra-articular injection	VAS, WOMAC, SF-12; MRI
De Windt et al. Case series study [159]	10	Allogenic BM-MSCs from the iliac crest of 2 healthy donors (age 2 and 5)	N/A. Mixed cells in the fibrinogen component of fibrin glue at 1.5–2 $\times 10^6$ cells/mL	10% or 20% autologous chondrons (a standard or a high yield mixture)	12 months	None	Defect site-specific implantation	KOOS, VAS; Second-look arthroscopy; Histological analysis;
De Windt et al. Case series study [160]	35	Allogenic cryopreserved BM-MSCs	N/A. Mixed cells in the fibrinogen component of fibrin glue at 1.5–2 $\times 10^6$ cells/mL. Approximately 0.9 mL cell product/cm^2 defect	10% or 20% autologous chondrons (a standard or a high yield mixture)	18 months	None	Defect site-specific implantation	KOOS, VAS; Second-look arthroscopy; Histological analysis;

BM-MSCs: bone marrow-derived mesenchymal stem cells; KOOS: the Knee Injury and Osteoarthritis Outcome; MRI: magnetic resonance imaging; N/A: not available; SF-12: short form-12 life quality questionnaire; VAS: visual analogue pain scale; WOMAC: the Western Ontario and McMaster Universities Arthritis Index.

4.3. Cell-Free Procedures

Currently numerous, single-phase scaffold-based cartilage repair techniques exist. Chondral scaffolds used in cartilage repair can be based on components of cartilaginous matrix, such as collagen or hyaluronate [172,173], proteins and natural polymers (such as fibrin, agarose, alginate and chitosan) [174] or synthetic polyesters (such as polylactic acid, polyglycolic acid, polylactide glycolide, polyethylene oxide and polypropylene oxide) [175]. Chondral scaffolds consist of a monolayer material (monophasic scaffold) or they are multi-layer structures, which copy the architecture of cartilage more effectively. Currently, matrices consisting of collagen are used more commonly in regeneration of damaged articular cartilage [118].

As an alternative to cell seeded scaffolds, another treatment approach involves the implantation of acellular biomaterials for cartilage regeneration by stimulating bone marrow stem-cell recruitment and differentiation induced by the scaffold. One of these cell-free procedures is autologous matrix-induced chondrogenesis (AMIC). The method of autologous matrix-induced chondrogenesis is often used in treatment of small, mainly post-traumatic, loss of articular cartilage. AMIC combines stimulation of bone marrow through microfractures with the use of a no-cell membrane made up of type I/III collagen. A collagen membrane stabilises the clot, creates a biological chamber, protects progenitor cells and stimulates the cells to differentiate towards chondrocytes. Collagen membranes are fixed with partial autologous fibrin glue or surgical sutures [176]. Gille et al. showed a significant improvement in all clinical parameters in up to 87% of patients. An analysis of MRI examinations revealed in most cases the total or moderate filling of the cartilage loss with a normal-to-incidentally hyperintense signal. However, an improvement in joint mobility seems to depend on the age of the patients [118]. Moreover, the application of the AMIC technique is recommended in the treatment of local, small cartilage loss and it is contraindicated in cases of multiple cartilage loss, rheumatic diseases and a considerable restriction of joint mobility [176], which considerably limits AMIC applicability in the treatment of aging-related changes.

5. Summary

Aging-related changes in articular cartilage lower the possibility of maintaining the properties and regeneration of cartilage. Obviously, time-related factors, such as chondrocytes secretory phenotype, weakening of chondrocytes' response to growth factors, oxidative stress and accumulation of final glycation products in cartilage can also lead to osteoarthritis, which is frequent in the population of the elderly. Aging of cartilage with time is inevitable and the changes it causes are irreversible. Because of the aging of the global population, age-related diseases of the motor system are a significant social issue. Studies aimed at elucidating the mechanisms of intensified aging of articular cartilage may help to introduce a therapy to slow down the aging-related changes or to support local processes of regeneration of articular cartilage. Due to a growing number of reports published in recent years, increasing attention has been attracted by cell therapies, including the possibility of using MSCs in the regeneration of cartilage. Therapies which employ MSCs offer great potential. However, use of MSCs in the regeneration of aging cartilage raises a lot of doubt. There are no detailed recommendations regarding the culture conditions, the tissue origin and the dosage of stem cells. The degree of changes and the presence of inflammation are the issues which occur in elderly people. Additionally, autologous MSCs in elderly people exhibit lower proliferative activity and there is some difficulty regarding the production of cells with a chondrogenic phenotype and a specific biological activity. However, due to the importance of the issue, further studies are needed of the methods for improving the quality of aging cartilage.

Acknowledgments: The study was supported by the School of Medicine, University of Warmia and Mazury in Olsztyn, Poland.

References

1. Bijlsma, J.W.; Berenbaum, F.; Lafeber, F.P. Osteoarthritis: An update with relevance for clinical practice. *Lancet* **2011**, *377*, 2115–2126. [CrossRef]
2. Aigner, T.; Rose, J.; Martin, J.; Buckwalter, J. Aging theories of primary osteoarthritis: From epidemiology to molecular biology. *Rejuvenation Res.* **2004**, *7*, 134–145. [CrossRef] [PubMed]
3. Martin, J.A.; Buckwalter, J.A. The role of chondrocyte senescence in the pathogenesis of osteoarthritis and in limiting cartilage repair. *J. Bone Jt. Surg. Am.* **2003**, *85*, 106–110. [CrossRef]
4. Messai, H.; Duchossoy, Y.; Khatib, A.M.; Mitrovic, D.R. Articular chondrocytes from aging rats respond poorly to insulin-like growth factor-1: An altered signalling pathway. *Mech. Ageing Dev.* **2000**, *115*, 21–37. [CrossRef]
5. Blanco, F.J.; Rego, I.; Ruiz-Romero, C. The role of mitochondria in osteoarthritis. *Nat. Rev. Rheumatol.* **2011**, *7*, 161–169. [CrossRef] [PubMed]
6. Huang, C.Y.; Lai, K.Y.; Hung, L.F.; Wu, W.L.; Liu, F.C.; Ho, L.J. Advanced glycation end products cause collagen II reduction by activating Janus kinase/signal transducer and activator of transcription 3 pathway in porcine chondrocytes. *Rheumatology (Oxford)* **2011**, *50*, 1379–1389. [CrossRef] [PubMed]
7. Galle, J.; Bader, A.; Hepp, P.; Grill, W.; Fuchs, B.; Käs, J.A.; Krinner, A.; Marquass, B.; Müller, K.; Schiller, J.; et al. Mesenchymal Stem Cells in Cartilage Repair: State of the Art and Methods to monitor Cell Growth, Differentiation and Cartilage Regeneration. *Curr. Med. Chem.* **2010**, *17*, 2274–2291. [CrossRef] [PubMed]
8. Hayflick, L. Intracellular determinants of cell aging. *Mech. Ageing Dev.* **1984**, *28*, 177–185. [CrossRef]
9. Sikora, E.; Arendt, T.; Bennett, M.; Narita, M. Impact of cellular senescence signature on ageing research. *Ageing Res. Rev.* **2011**, *10*, 146–152. [CrossRef] [PubMed]
10. López-Otín, C.; Blasco, M.A.; Partridge, L.; Serrano, M.; Kroemer, G. The hallmarks of aging. *Cell* **2013**, *153*, 1194–1217. [CrossRef] [PubMed]
11. Hunt, A.; Betts, D.; King, W.A.; Madan, P. Senescence or apoptosis? The choice bovine fibroblasts make in the presence of increasing concentrations of extracellular H_2O_2. *SURG J.* **2010**, *3*, 64–68.
12. Coppe, J.P.; Desprez, P.Y.; Krtolica, A.; Campisi, J. The senescence-associated secretory phenotype: The dark side of tumor suppression. *Annu. Rev. Pathol.* **2010**, *5*, 99–118. [CrossRef] [PubMed]
13. Von Zglinicki, T.; Petrie, J.; Kirkwood, T.B. Telomere-driven replicative senescence is a stress response. *Nat. Biotechnol.* **2003**, *21*, 229–230. [CrossRef] [PubMed]
14. Lu, W.; Zhang, Y.; Liu, D.; Songyang, Z.; Wan, M. Telomeres-structure, function and regulation. *Exp. Cell Res.* **2013**, *319*, 133–141. [CrossRef] [PubMed]
15. Gilley, D.; Herbert, B.S.; Huda, N.; Tanaka, H.; Reed, T. Factors impacting human telomere homeostasis and age-related disease. *Mech. Ageing Dev.* **2008**, *129*, 27–34. [CrossRef] [PubMed]
16. Kaul, Z.; Cesare, A.J.; Huschtscha, L.I.; Neumann, A.A.; Reddel, R.R. Five dysfunctional telomeres predict onset of senescence in human cells. *EMBO Rep.* **2011**, *13*, 52–59. [CrossRef] [PubMed]
17. Bielak-Zmijewska, A.; Wnuk, M.; Przybylska, D.; Grabowska, W.; Lewinska, A.; Alster, O.; Korwek, Z.; Cmoch, A.; Myszka, A.; Pikula, S.; et al. A comparison of replicative senescence and doxorubicin-induced premature senescence of vascular smooth muscle cells isolated from human aorta. *Biogerontology* **2014**, *15*, 47–64. [CrossRef] [PubMed]
18. D'Adda di Fagagna, F. Living on a break: Cellular senescence as a DNA-damage response. *Nat. Rev. Cancer* **2008**, *8*, 512–522. [CrossRef] [PubMed]
19. Kühn, K.; D'Lima, D.D.; Hashimoto, S.; Lotz, M. Cell death in cartilage. *Osteoarthr. Cartil.* **2004**, *12*, 1–16. [CrossRef] [PubMed]
20. Vignon, E.; Arlot, M.; Patricot, L.M.; Vignon, G. The cell density of human femoral head cartilage. *Clin. Orthop. Relat. Res.* **1976**, *121*, 303–308. [CrossRef]
21. Blaney Davidson, E.N.; Scharstuhl, A.; Vitters, E.L.; van der Kraan, P.M.; van den Berg, W.B. Reduced transforming growth factor-beta signalling in cartilage of old mice: Role in impaired repair capacity. *Arthritis Res. Ther.* **2005**, *7*, 1338–1347. [CrossRef] [PubMed]
22. Aigner, T.; Hemmel, M.; Neureiter, D.; Gebhard, P.M.; Zeiler, G.; Kirchner, T.; McKenna, L. Apoptotic Cell Death Is Not a Widespread Phenomenon in Normal Aging and Osteoarthritis Human Articular Knee Cartilage: A Study of Proliferation, Programmed Cell Death (Apoptosis) and Viability of Chondrocytes in Normal and Osteoarthritic Human Knee Cartilage. *Arthritis Rheum.* **2001**, *44*, 1304–1312. [PubMed]

23. Ding, C.; Cicuttini, F.; Blizzard, L.; Scott, F.; Jones, G. A longitudinal study of the effect of sex and age on rate of change in knee cartilage volume in adults. *Rheumatology (Oxford)* **2007**, *46*, 273–279. [CrossRef] [PubMed]
24. Wells, T.; Davidson, C.; Morgelin, M.; Bird, J.L.E.; Bayliss, M.T.; Dudhia, J. Age-related changes in the composition, the molecular stoichiometry and the stability of proteoglycan aggregates extracted from human articular cartilage. *Biochem. J.* **2003**, *370*, 69–79. [CrossRef] [PubMed]
25. Parsch, D.; Brümmendorf, T.H.; Richter, W.; Fellenberg, J. Replicative aging of human articular chondrocytes during ex vivo expansion. *Arthritis Rheum.* **2002**, *46*, 2911–2916. [CrossRef] [PubMed]
26. Harbo, M.; Delaisse, J.M.; Kjaersgaard-Andersen, P.; Soerensen, F.B.; Koelvraa, S.; Bendix, L. The relationship between ultra-short telomeres, aging of articular cartilage and the development of human hip osteoarthritis. *Mech. Ageing Dev.* **2013**, *134*, 367–372. [CrossRef] [PubMed]
27. Wilson, B.; Novakofski, K.D.; Donocoff, R.S.; Liang, Y.X.; Fortier, L.A. Telomerase Activity in Articular Chondrocytes Is Lost after Puberty. *Cartilage* **2014**, *5*, 215–220. [CrossRef] [PubMed]
28. Guillot, P.V.; Gotherstrom, C.; Chan, J.; Kurata, H.; Fisk, N.M. Human first-trimester fetal MSC express pluripotency markers and grow faster and have longer telomeres than adult MSC. *Stem Cells* **2007**, *25*, 646–654. [CrossRef] [PubMed]
29. Mareschi, K.; Ferrero, I.; Rustichelli, D.; Aschero, S.; Gammaitoni, L.; Aglietta, M.; Madon, E.; Fagioli, F. Expansion of mesenchymal stem cells isolated from pediatric and adult donor bone marrow. *J. Cell. Biochem.* **2006**, *97*, 744–754. [CrossRef] [PubMed]
30. Baxter, M.A.; Wynn, R.F.; Jowitt, S.N.; Wraith, J.E.; Fairbairn, L.J.; Bellantuono, I. Study of telomere length reveals rapid aging of human marrow stromal cells following in vitro expansion. *Stem Cells* **2004**, *22*, 675–682. [CrossRef] [PubMed]
31. Parsch, D.; Fellenberg, J.; Brümmendorf, T.; Eschlbeck, A.M.; Richter, W. Telomere length and telomerase activity during expansion and differentiation of human mesenchymal stem cells and chondrocytes. *J. Mol. Med.* **2004**, *82*, 49–55. [PubMed]
32. Dai, S.M.; Shan, Z.Z.; Nakamura, H.; Masuko-Hongo, K.; Kato, T.; Nishioka, K.; Yudoh, K. Catabolic stress induces features of chondrocyte senescence through overexpression of caveolin 1: Possible involvement of caveolin 1-induced down-regulation of articular chondrocytes in the pathogenesis of osteoarthritis. *Arthritis Rheum.* **2006**, *54*, 818–831. [CrossRef] [PubMed]
33. Jallali, N.; Ridha, H.; Thrasivoulou, C.; Butler, P.; Cowen, T. Modulation of intracellular reactive oxygen species level in chondrocytes by IGF-1, FGF and TGF-beta1. *Connect. Tissue Res.* **2007**, *48*, 149–158. [CrossRef] [PubMed]
34. Brandl, A.; Meyer, M.; Bechmann, V.; Nerlich, M.; Angele, P. Oxidative stress induces senescence in human mesenchymal stem cells. *Exp. Cell Res.* **2011**, *317*, 1541–1547. [CrossRef] [PubMed]
35. Harbo, M.; Bendix, L.; Bay-Jensen, A.C.; Graakjaer, J.; Soe, K.; Andersen, T.L.; Kjaersgaard-Andersen, P.; Koelvraa, S.; Delaisse, J.M. The distribution pattern of critically short telomeres in human osteoarthritic knees. *Arthritis Res. Ther.* **2012**, *14*, R12. [CrossRef] [PubMed]
36. Rose, J.; Söder, S.; Skhirtladze, C.; Schmitz, N.; Gebhard, P.M.; Sesselmann, S.; Aigner, T. DNA damage, discoordinated gene expression and cellular senescence in osteoarthritic chondrocytes. *Osteoarthr. Cartil.* **2012**, *20*, 1020–1028. [CrossRef] [PubMed]
37. Brandl, A.; Hartmann, A.; Bechmann, V.; Graf, B.; Nerlich, M.; Angele, P. Oxidative stress induces senescence in chondrocytes. *J. Orthop. Res.* **2011**, *29*, 1114–1120. [CrossRef] [PubMed]
38. Loeser, R.F. Aging and osteoarthritis. *Curr. Opin. Rheumatol.* **2011**, *23*, 492–496. [CrossRef] [PubMed]
39. Jallali, N.; Ridha, H.; Thrasivoulou, C.; Underwood, C.; Butler, P.E.; Cowen, T. Vulnerability to ROS-induced cell death in ageing articular cartilage: The role of antioxidant enzyme activity. *Osteoarthr. Cartil.* **2005**, *13*, 614–622. [CrossRef] [PubMed]
40. Yu, S.M.; Kim, S.J. Thymoquinone-induced reactive oxygen species causes apoptosis of chondrocytes via PI3K/Akt and p38kinase pathway. *Exp. Biol. Med.* **2013**, *238*, 811–820. [CrossRef] [PubMed]
41. Yudoh, K.; van Trieu, N.; Nakamura, H.; Hongo-Masuko, K.; Kato, T.; Nishioka, K. Potential involvement of oxidative stress in cartilage senescence and development of osteoarthritis: Oxidative stress induces chondrocyte telomere instability and downregulation of chondrocyte function. *Arthritis Res. Ther.* **2005**, *7*, R380–R391. [CrossRef] [PubMed]

42. Ashraf, S.; Cha, B.H.; Kim, J.S.; Ahn, J.; Han, I.; Park, H.; Lee, S.H. Regulation of senescence associated signalling mechanisms in chondrocytes for cartilage tissue regeneration. *Osteoarthr. Cartil.* **2016**, *24*, 196–205. [CrossRef] [PubMed]
43. Loeser, R.F.; Gandhi, U.; Long, D.L.; Yin, W.; Chubinskaya, S. Aging and oxidative stress reduce the response of human articular chondrocytes to insulin-like growth factor 1 and osteogenic protein 1. *Arthritis Rheumatol.* **2014**, *66*, 2201–2209. [CrossRef] [PubMed]
44. Li, C.J.; Sun, L.Y.; Pang, C.Y. Synergistic Protection of N-acetylcysteine and ascorbic acid 2-phosphate on human mesenchymal stem cells against mitoptosis, necroptosis and apoptosis. *Sci. Rep.* **2015**, *5*, 9819. [CrossRef] [PubMed]
45. Sakata, S.; Hayashi, S.; Fujishiro, T.; Kawakita, K.; Kanzaki, N.; Hashimoto, S.; Iwasa, K.; Chinzei, N.; Kihara, S.; Haneda, M.; et al. Oxidative stress-induced apoptosis and matrix loss of chondrocytes is inhibited by eicosapentaenoic acid. *J. Orthop. Res.* **2015**, *33*, 359–365. [CrossRef] [PubMed]
46. Lin, T.M.; Tsai, J.L.; Lin, S.D.; Lai, C.S.; Chang, C.C. Accelerated growth and prolonged lifespan of adipose tissue-derived human mesenchymal stem cells in a medium using reduced calcium and antioxidants. *Stem Cells Dev.* **2005**, *14*, 92–102. [CrossRef] [PubMed]
47. Estrada, J.C.; Torres, Y.; Benguria, A.; Dopazo, A.; Roche, E.; Carrera-Quintanar, L.; Pérez, R.A.; Enríquez, J.A.; Torres, R.; Ramírez, J.C.; et al. Human mesenchymal stem cell-replicative senescence and oxidative stress are closely linked to aneuploidy. *Cell Death Dis.* **2013**, *4*, e691. [CrossRef] [PubMed]
48. Munir, S.; Foldager, C.; Lind, M.; Zachar, V.; Søballe, K.; Koch, T. Hypoxia enhances chondrogenic differentiation of human adipose tissue-derived stromal cells in scaffold-free and scaffold systems. *Cell. Tissue Res.* **2014**, *355*, 89–102. [CrossRef] [PubMed]
49. Lomri, A. Role of reactive oxygen species and superoxide dismutase in cartilage aging and pathology. *Future Reumatol.* **2008**, *3*, 381–392. [CrossRef]
50. Greene, M.A.; Loeser, R.F. Aging-related inflammation in osteoarthritis. *Osteoarthr. Cartil.* **2015**, *23*, 1966–1971. [CrossRef] [PubMed]
51. Livshits, G.; Zhai, G.; Hart, D.J.; Kato, B.S.; Wang, H.; Williams, F.M.; Spector, T.D. Interleukin-6 is a significant predictor of radiographic knee osteoarthritis: The Chingford study. *Arthritis Rheum.* **2009**, *60*, 2037–2045. [CrossRef] [PubMed]
52. Philipot, D.; Guerit, D.; Platano, D.; Chuchana, P.; Olivotto, E.; Espinoza, F.; Dorandeu, A.; Pers, Y.M.; Piette, J.; Borziet, R.M.; et al. p16INK4a and its regulator miR-24 link senescence and chondrocyte terminal differentiation-associated matrix remodeling in osteoarthritis. *Arthritis Res. Ther.* **2014**, *16*, R58. [CrossRef] [PubMed]
53. Wu, W.; Billinghurst, R.C.; Pidoux, I.; Antoniou, J.; Zukor, D.; Tanzer, M.; Poole, A.R. Sites of collagenase cleavage and denaturation of type II collagen in aging and osteoarthritic articular cartilage and their relationship to the distribution of matrix metalloproteinase 1 and matrix metalloproteinase 13. *Arthritis Rheum.* **2002**, *46*, 2087–2094. [CrossRef] [PubMed]
54. Aurich, M.; Poole, A.R.; Reiner, A.; Mollenhauer, C.; Margulis, A.; Kuettner, K.E.; Cole, A.A. Matrix homeostasis in aging normal human ankle cartilage. *Arthritis Rheum.* **2002**, *46*, 2903–2910. [CrossRef] [PubMed]
55. Forsyth, C.B.; Cole, A.; Murphy, G.; Bienias, J.L.; Im, H.J.; Loeser, R.F. Increased matrix metalloproteinase-13 production with aging by human articular chondrocytes in response to catabolic stimuli. *J. Gerontol. A Biol. Sci. Med. Sci.* **2005**, *60*, 1118–1124. [CrossRef] [PubMed]
56. Long, D.; Blake, S.; Song, X.Y.; Lark, M.; Loeser, R.F. Human articular chondrocytes produce IL-7 and respond to IL-7 with increased production of matrix metalloproteinase-13. *Arthritis Res. Ther.* **2008**, *10*, R23. [CrossRef] [PubMed]
57. Loeser, R.F. Aging and osteoarthritis: The role of chondrocyte senescence and aging changes in the cartilage matrix. *Osteoarthr. Cartil.* **2009**, *17*, 971–979. [CrossRef] [PubMed]
58. Hashimoto, M.; Nakasa, T.; Hikata, T.; Asahara, H. Molecular network of cartilage homeostasis and osteoarthritis. *Med. Res. Rev.* **2008**, *28*, 464–481. [CrossRef] [PubMed]
59. Goldberg, A. Effects of growth factors on articular cartilage. *Ortop. Traumatol. Rehab.* **2001**, *3*, 190–193.
60. De Ceuninck, F.; Caliez, A.; Dassencourt, L.; Anract, P.; Renard, P. Pharmacological disruption of insulin-like growth factor 1 binding to IGF-binding proteins restores anabolic responses in human osteoarthritic chondrocytes. *Arthritis Res. Ther.* **2004**, *6*, 393–403. [CrossRef] [PubMed]

61. Yin, W.; Park, J.I.; Loeser, R.F. Oxidative stress inhibits insulin-like growth factor-I induction of chondrocyte proteoglycan synthesis through differential regulation of phosphatidylinositol 3-Kinase-Akt and MEK-ERK MAPK signaling pathways. *J. Biol. Chem.* **2009**, *284*, 31972–31981. [CrossRef] [PubMed]
62. Starkman, B.G.; Cravero, J.D.; Delcarlo, M.; Loeser, R.F. IGF-I stimulation of proteoglycan synthesis by chondrocytes requires activation of the PI 3-kinase pathway but not ERK MAPK. *Biochem. J.* **2005**, *389*, 723–729. [CrossRef] [PubMed]
63. Allan, E.H.; Martin, T.J. The plasminogen activator inhibitor system in bone cell function. *Clin. Orthop. Relat. Res.* **1995**, *313*, 54–63.
64. Murphy-Ullrich, J.E.; Poczatek, M. Activation of latent TGF-beta by thrombospondin-1: Mechanisms and physiology. *Cytokine Growth Factor Rev.* **2000**, *11*, 59–69. [CrossRef]
65. Dangelo, M.; Sarment, D.P.; Billings, P.C.; Pacifici, M. Activation of transforming growth factor beta in chondrocytes undergoing endochondral ossification. *J. Bone Miner. Res.* **2001**, *16*, 2339–2347. [CrossRef] [PubMed]
66. Albro, M.B.; Cigan, A.D.; Nims, R.J.; Yeroushalmi, K.J.; Oungoulian, S.R.; Hung, C.T.; Ateshian, G.A. Shearing of synovial fluid activates latent TGF-β. *Osteoarthr. Cartil.* **2012**, *20*, 1374–1382. [CrossRef] [PubMed]
67. Gordon, K.J.; Blobe, G.C. Role of transforming growth factor-beta superfamily signaling pathways in human disease. *Biochim. Biophys. Acta* **2008**, *1782*, 197–228. [CrossRef] [PubMed]
68. Blaney Davidson, E.N.; Remst, D.F.; Vitters, E.L.; van Beuningen, H.M.; Blom, A.B.; Goumans, M.J.; van den Berg, W.B.; van der Kraan, P.M. Increase in ALK1/ALK5 ratio as a cause for elevated MMP-13 expression in osteoarthritis in humans and mice. *J. Immunol.* **2009**, *182*, 7937–7945. [CrossRef] [PubMed]
69. Finnson, K.W.; Parker, W.L.; ten Dijke, P.; Thorikay, M.; Philip, A. ALK1 opposes ALK5/Smad3 signaling and expression of extracellular matrix components in human chondrocytes. *J. Bone Miner. Res.* **2008**, *23*, 896–906. [CrossRef] [PubMed]
70. Li, W.; Ding, S. Generation of novel rat and human pluripotent stem cells by reprogramming and chemical approaches. *Methods Mol. Biol.* **2010**, *636*, 293–300. [CrossRef] [PubMed]
71. Johnstone, B.; Hering, T.M.; Caplan, A.I.; Goldberg, V.M.; Yoo, J.U. In vitro chondrogenesis of bone marrow-derived mesenchymal progenitor cells. *Exp. Cell Res.* **1998**, *238*, 265–272. [CrossRef] [PubMed]
72. Wu, J.; Niu, J.; Li, X.; Wang, X.; Guo, Z.; Zhang, F. TGF-β1 induces senescence of bone marrow mesenchymal stem cells via increase of mitochondrial ROS production. *BMC Dev. Biol.* **2014**, *14*, 21. [CrossRef] [PubMed]
73. Ahmed, U.; Anwar, A.; Savage, R.S.; Thornalley, P.J.; Rabbani, N. Protein oxidation, nitration and glycation biomarkers for early-stage diagnosis of osteoarthritis of the knee and typing and progression of arthritic disease. *Arthritis Res. Ther.* **2016**, *18*, 250. [CrossRef] [PubMed]
74. Saudek, D.M.; Kay, J. Advanced glycation endproducts and osteoarthritis. *Curr. Reumatol. Rep.* **2003**, *5*, 33–40. [CrossRef]
75. Mizumura, K.; Choi, A.M.; Ryster, S.W. Emerging role of selective autophagy in human diseases. *Front. Pharmacol.* **2014**, *5*, 244. [CrossRef] [PubMed]
76. Srinivas, V.; Bohensky, J.; Shapiro, I.M. Autophagy: A new phase in the maturation of growth plate chondrocytes is regulated by HIF, mTOR and AMP kinase. *Cells Tissues Organs* **2009**, *189*, 88–92. [CrossRef] [PubMed]
77. Shapiro, I.M.; Layfield, R.; Lotz, M.; Settembre, C.; Whitehouse, C. Boning up on autophagy: The role of autophagy in skeletal biology. *Autophagy* **2014**, *10*, 7–19. [CrossRef] [PubMed]
78. Carames, B.; Taniguchi, N.; Otsuki, S.; Blanco, F.J.; Lotz, M. Autophagy is a protective mechanism in normal cartilage and its aging-related loss is linked with cell death and osteoarthritis. *Arthritis Rheum.* **2010**, *62*, 791–801. [CrossRef] [PubMed]
79. Zhang, Y.; Vasheghani, F.; Li, Y.H.; Blati, M.; Simeone, K.; Fahmi, H.; Lussier, B.; Roughley, P.; Lagares, D.; Pelletier, J.P.; et al. Cartilage-specific deletion of mTOR upregulates autophagy and protects mice from osteoarthritis. *Ann. Rheum. Dis.* **2015**, *74*, 1432–1440. [CrossRef] [PubMed]
80. Takayama, K.; Kawakami, Y.; Kobayashi, M.; Greco, N.; Cummins, J.H.; Matsushita, T.; Kuroda, R.; Kurosaka, M.; Fu, F.H.; Huard, J. Local intra-articular injection of rapamycin delays articular cartilage degeneration in a murine model of osteoarthritis. *Arthritis Res. Ther.* **2014**, *16*, 482–485. [CrossRef] [PubMed]

81. Matsuzaki, T.; Matsushita, T.; Tabata, Y.; Saito, T.; Matsumoto, T.; Nagai, K.; Kuroda, R.; Kurosaka, M. Intra-articular administration of gelatin hydrogels incorporating rapamycin-micelles reduces the development of experimental osteoarthritis in a murine model. *Biomaterials* **2014**, *35*, 9904–9911. [CrossRef] [PubMed]
82. Alvarez-Garcia, O.; Olmer, M.; Akagi, R.; Akasaki, Y.; Fisch, K.M.; Shen, T.; Su, A.I.; Lotz, M.K. Suppression of REDD1 in osteoarthritis cartilage, a novel mechanism for dysregulated mTOR signaling and defective autophagy. *Osteoarthr. Cartil.* **2016**, *24*, 1639–1647. [CrossRef] [PubMed]
83. Zhang, F.J.; Luo, W.; Lei, G.H. Role of HIF-1alpha and HIF-2alpha in osteoarthritis. *Jt. Bone Spine* **2015**, *82*, 144–147. [CrossRef] [PubMed]
84. Bohensky, J.; Terkhorn, S.P.; Freeman, T.A.; Adams, C.S.; Garcia, J.; Shapiro, I.M.; Srinivas, V. Regulation of autophagy in humanand murine cartilage: Hypoxia-inducible factor 2 suppresses chondrocyteautophagy. *Arthritis Rheum.* **2009**, *60*, 1406–1415. [CrossRef] [PubMed]
85. Simonsen, J.L.; Rosada, C.; Serakinci, N.; Justesen, J.; Stenderup, K.; Rattan, S.I.; Jensen, T.G.; Kassem, M. Telomerase expression extends the proliferative life-span and maintains the osteogenic potential of human bone marrow stromal cells. *Nat. Biotechnol.* **2002**, *20*, 592–596. [CrossRef] [PubMed]
86. Shi, S.; Gronthos, S.; Chen, S.; Reddi, A.; Counter, C.M.; Robey, P.G.; Wang, C.Y. Bone formation by human postnatal bone marrow stromal stem cells is enhanced by telomerase expression. *Nat. Biotechnol.* **2002**, *20*, 587–591. [CrossRef] [PubMed]
87. Pearce, V.P.; Sherrell, J.; Lou, Z.; Kopelovich, L.; Wright, W.E.; Shay, J.W. Immortalization of epithelial progenitor cells mediated by resveratrol. *Oncogene* **2008**, *27*, 2365–2374. [CrossRef] [PubMed]
88. Sprouse, A.A.; Steding, C.E.; Herbert, B.S. Pharmaceutical regulation of telomerase and its clinical potential. *J. Cell. Mol. Med.* **2012**, *16*, 1–7. [CrossRef] [PubMed]
89. Shen, C.Y.; Jiang, J.G.; Yang, L.; Wang, D.W.; Zhu, W. Anti-aging active ingredients from herbs and nutraceuticals used in TCM: Pharmacological mechanisms and implications for drug discovery. *Br. J. Pharmacol.* **2017**, *174*, 1395–1425. [CrossRef] [PubMed]
90. Yung, L.Y.; Lam, W.S.; Ho, M.K.; Hu, Y.; Ip, F.C.; Pang, H.; Chin, A.C.; Harley, C.B.; Ip, N.Y.; Wong, Y.H. Astragaloside IV and cycloastragenol stimulate the phosphorylation of extracellular signal-regulated protein kinase in multiple cell types. *Planta Med.* **2012**, *78*, 115–121. [CrossRef] [PubMed]
91. Meng, H.C.; Wang, S.; Li, Y.; Kuang, Y.Y.; Ma, C.M. Chemical constituents and pharmacologic actions of Cynomorium plants. *Chin. J. Nat. Med.* **2013**, *11*, 321–329. [CrossRef] [PubMed]
92. Tichon, A.; Eitan, E.; Kurkalli, B.G.; Braiman, A.; Gazit, A.; Slavin, S.; Beith-Yannai, E.; Priel, E. Oxidative stress protection by novel telomerase activators in mesenchymal stem cells derived from healthy and diseased individuals. *Curr. Mol. Med.* **2013**, *13*, 1010–1022. [CrossRef] [PubMed]
93. Taka, T.; Changtam, C.; Thaichana, P.; Kaewtunjai, N.; Suksamrarn, A.; Lee, T.R.; Tuntiwechapikul, W. Curcuminoid derivatives enhance telomerase activity in an in vitro TRAP assay. *Bioorg. Med. Chem. Lett.* **2014**, *24*, 5242–5246. [CrossRef] [PubMed]
94. Molgora, B.; Bateman, R.; Sweeney, G.; Finger, D.; Dimler, T.; Effros, R.B.; Valenzuela, H.F. Functional assessment of pharmacological telomerase activators in human T cells. *Cells* **2013**, *2*, 57–66. [CrossRef] [PubMed]
95. De Jesus, B.B.; Schneeberger, K.; Vera, E.; Tejera, A.; Harley, C.B.; Blasco, M.A. The telomerase activator TA-65 elongates short telomeres and increases health span of adult/old mice without increasing cancer incidence. *Aging Cell.* **2011**, *10*, 604–621. [CrossRef] [PubMed]
96. Liu, L.; Gu, H.; Liu, H.; Jiao, Y.; Li, K.; Zhao, Y.; An, L.; Yang, J. Protective effect of resveratrol against IL-1β-induced inflammatory response on human osteoarthritic chondrocytes partly via the TLR4/MyD88/NF-κB signaling pathway: An "in vitro study". *Int. J. Mol. Sci.* **2014**, *15*, 6925–6940. [CrossRef] [PubMed]
97. Li, W.; Cai, L.; Zhang, Y.; Cui, L.; Shen, G. Intra-articular resveratrol injection prevents osteoarthritis progression in a mouse model by activating SIRT1 and thereby silencing HIF-2α. *J. Orthop. Res.* **2015**, *33*, 1061–1070. [CrossRef] [PubMed]
98. Toh, W.S.; Loh, X.J. Advances in hydrogel delivery systems for tissue regeneration. *Mater. Sci. Eng. C. Mater. Biol. Appl.* **2014**, *45*, 690–697. [CrossRef] [PubMed]
99. Wang, W.; Sun, L.; Zhang, P.; Song, J.; Liu, W. An anti-inflammatory cell-free collagen/resveratrol scaffold for repairing osteochondral defects in rabbits. *Acta Biomater.* **2014**, *10*, 4983–4995. [CrossRef] [PubMed]

100. Moussavi-Harami, F.; Duwayri, Y.; Martin, J.A.; Moussavi-Harami, F.; Buckwalter, J.A. Oxygen effects on senescence in chondrocytes and mesenchymal stem cells: Consequences for tissue engineering. *Iowa Orthop. J.* **2004**, *24*, 15–20. [PubMed]
101. Martin, J.A.; Klingelhutz, A.J.; Moussavi-Harami, F.; Buckwalter, J.A. Effects of oxidative damage and telomerase activity on human articular cartilage chondrocyte senescence. *J. Gerontol. A. Biol. Sci. Med. Sci.* **2004**, *59*, B324–B336. [CrossRef]
102. Egli, R.J.; Bastian, J.D.; Ganz, R.; Hofstetter, W.; Leunig, M. Hypoxic expansion promotes the chondrogenic potential of articular chondrocytes. *J. Orthop. Res.* **2008**, *26*, 977–985. [CrossRef] [PubMed]
103. Schrobback, K.; Klein, T.J.; Crawford, R.; Upton, Z.; Malda, J.; Leavesley, D.I. Effects of oxygen and culture system on in vitro propagation and redifferentiation of osteoarthritic human articular chondrocytes. *Cell Tissue Res.* **2012**, *347*, 649–663. [CrossRef] [PubMed]
104. Choi, J.R.; Pingguan-Murphy, B.; Wan Abas, W.A.B.; Noor Azmi, M.A.; Omar, S.Z.; Chua, K.H.; Wan Safwani, W.K. Impact of low oxygen tension on stemness, proliferation and differentiation potential of human adipose-derived stem cells. *Biochem. Biophys. Res. Commun.* **2014**, *448*, 218–224. [CrossRef] [PubMed]
105. Tsai, C.C.; Chen, Y.J.; Yew, T.L.; Chen, L.L.; Wang, J.Y.; Chiu, C.H.; Hung, S.C. Hypoxia inhibits senescence and maintains mesenchymal stem cell properties through down-regulation of E2A-p21 by HIF-TWIST. *Blood* **2011**, *117*, 459–469. [CrossRef] [PubMed]
106. Wan Safwani, W.K.Z.; Choi, J.R.; Yong, K.W.; Ting, I.; Mat Adenan, N.A.; Pingguan-Murphy, B. Hypoxia enhances the viability, growth and chondrogenic potential of cryopreserved human adipose-derived stem cells. *Cryobiology* **2017**, *75*, 91–99. [CrossRef] [PubMed]
107. Wan Safwani, W.K.Z.; Wong, C.W.; Yong, K.W.; Choi, J.R.; Mat Adenan, N.A.; Omar, S.Z.; Wan Abas, W.A.B.; Pingguan-Murphy, B. The effects of hypoxia and serum-free conditions on the stemness properties of human adipose-derived stem cells. *Cytotechnology* **2013**, *68*, 1859–1872. [CrossRef] [PubMed]
108. Öztürk, E.; Hobiger, S.; Despot-Slade, E.; Pichler, M.; Zenobi-Wong, M. Hypoxia regulates RhoA and Wnt/β-catenin signaling in a context-dependent way to control re-differentiation of chondrocytes. *Sci. Rep.* **2017**, *7*, 9032. [CrossRef] [PubMed]
109. Grodzinsky, A.J.; Levenston, M.E.; Jin, M.; Frank, E.H. Cartilage tissue remodeling in response to mechanical forces. *Annu. Rev. Biomed Eng.* **2000**, *2*, 691–713. [CrossRef] [PubMed]
110. Schätti, O.; Grad, S.; Goldhahn, J.; Salzmann, G.; Li, Z.; Alini, M.; Stoddart, M.J. A combination of shear and dynamic compression leads to mechanically induced chondrogenesis of human mesenchymal stem cells. *Eur. Cell Mater.* **2011**, *22*, 214–225. [CrossRef] [PubMed]
111. Gardner, O.F.; Fahy, N.; Alini, M.; Stoddart, M.J. Differences in human mesenchymal stell cell secretomes during chondrogenic induction. *Eur. Cell Mater.* **2016**, *31*, 221–235. [CrossRef] [PubMed]
112. Li, Z.; Kupcsik, L.; Yao, S.J.; Alini, M.; Stoddart, M.J. Mechanical Load Modulates Chondrogenesis of Human Mesenchymal Stem Cells through the TGFβ Pathway. *J. Cell Mol. Med.* **2010**, *14*, 1338–1346. [CrossRef] [PubMed]
113. Guo, T.; Yu, L.; Lim, C.G.; Goodley, A.S.; Xiao, X.; Placone, J.K.; Ferlin, K.M.; Nguyen, B.N.; Hsieh, A.H.; Fisher, J.P. Effect of Dynamic Culture and Periodic Compression on Human Mesenchymal Stem Cell Proliferation and Chondrogenesis. *Ann. Biomed. Eng.* **2016**, *44*, 2103–2113. [CrossRef] [PubMed]
114. Bian, L.; Zhai, D.Y.; Zhang, E.C.; Mauck, R.L.; Burdick, J.A. Dynamic compressive loading enhances cartilage matrix synthesis and distribution and suppresses hypertrophy in hMSC-laden hyaluronic acid hydrogels. *Tissue Eng. Part A* **2012**, *18*, 715–724. [CrossRef] [PubMed]
115. Zhang, T.; Wen, F.; Wu, Y.; Goh, G.S.; Ge, Z.; Tan, L.P.; Hui, J.H.; Yang, Z. Cross-talk between TGF-beta/SMAD and integrin signaling pathways in regulating hypertrophy of mesenchymal stem cell chondrogenesis under deferral dynamic compression. *Biomaterials* **2015**, *38*, 72–85. [CrossRef] [PubMed]
116. Simon, T.M.; Jackson, D.W. Articular Cartilage: Injury Pathways and Treatment Options. *Sports Med. Arthrosc. Rev.* **2018**, *26*, 31–39. [CrossRef] [PubMed]
117. Al-Najar, M.; Khalil, H.; Al-Ajlouni, J.; Al-Antary, E.; Hamdan, M.; Rahmeh, R.; Alhattab, D.; Samara, O.; Yasin, M.; Abdullah, A.A.; et al. Intra-articular injection of expanded autologous bone marrow mesenchymal cells in moderate and severe knee osteoarthritis is safe: A phase I/II study. *J. Orthop. Surg. Res.* **2017**, *12*, 190. [CrossRef] [PubMed]

118. Gille, J.; Behrens, P.; Volpi, P.; de Girolamo, L.; Reiss, E.; Zoch, W.; Anders, S. Outcome of Autologous Matrix Induced Chondrogenesis (AMIC) in cartilage knee surgery: Data of the AMIC Registry. *Arch. Orthop. Trauma Surg.* **2013**, *133*, 87–93. [CrossRef] [PubMed]
119. Jo, C.H.; Chai, J.W.; Jeong, E.C.; Oh, S.; Shin, J.S.; Shim, H.; Yoon, K.S. Intra-articular Injection of Mesenchymal Stem Cells for the Treatment of Osteoarthritis of the Knee: A 2-Year Follow-up Study. *Am. J. Sports Med.* **2017**, *45*, 2774–2783. [CrossRef] [PubMed]
120. Brittberg, M.; Lindahl, A.; Nilsson, A.; Ohlsson, C.; Isaksson, O.; Peterson, L. Treatment of deep cartilage defects in the knee with autologous chondrocyte transplantation. *N. Engl. J. Med.* **1994**, *331*, 889–895. [CrossRef] [PubMed]
121. Peterson, L.; Brittberg, M.; Kiviranta, I.; Akerlund, E.L.; Lindahl, A. Autologous chon-drocyte transplantation. Biomechanics and long-term durability. *Am. J. Sports Med.* **2002**, *30*, 2–12. [CrossRef] [PubMed]
122. Li, Y.; Wei, X.; Zhou, J.; Wei, L. The age-related changes in cartilage and osteoarthritis. *BioMed Res. Int.* **2013**, *2013*, 916530. [CrossRef] [PubMed]
123. Barbero, A.; Grogan, S.; Schafer, D.; Heberer, M.; Mainil-Varlet, P.; Martin, I. Age related changes in human articular chondrocyte yield, proliferation and post-expansion chondrogenic capacity. *Osteoarthr. Cartil.* **2004**, *12*, 476–484. [CrossRef] [PubMed]
124. Schulze-Tanzil, G. Activation and dedifferentiation of chondrocytes: Implications in cartilage injury and repair. *Ann. Anat.* **2009**, *191*, 325–338. [CrossRef] [PubMed]
125. Caron, M.M.; Emans, P.J.; Coolsen, M.M.; Voss, L.; Surtel, D.A.; Cremers, A.; van Rhijn, L.W.; Welting, T.J. Redifferentiation of dedifferentiated human articular chondrocytes: Comparison of 2D and 3D cultures. *Osteoarthr. Cartil.* **2012**, *20*, 1170–1178. [CrossRef] [PubMed]
126. Meinert, C.; Schrobback, K.; Hutmacher, D.W.; Klein, T.J. A novel bioreactor system for biaxial mechanical loading enhances the properties of tissue-engineered human cartilage. *Sci. Rep.* **2017**, *7*, 16997. [CrossRef] [PubMed]
127. Rosenzweig, D.H.; Solar-Cafaggi, S.; Quinn, T.M. Functionalization of dynamic culture surfaces with a cartilage extracellular matrix extract enhances chondrocyte phenotype against dedifferentiation. *Acta Biomater.* **2012**, *8*, 3333–3341. [CrossRef] [PubMed]
128. Rosenzweig, D.H.; Matmati, M.; Khayat, G.; Chaudhry, S.; Hinz, B.; Quinn, T.M. Culture of primary bovine chondrocytes on a continuously expanding surface inhibits dedifferentiation. *Tissue Eng. Part A* **2012**, *18*, 2466–2476. [CrossRef] [PubMed]
129. Kino-Oka, M.; Yashiki, S.; Ota, Y.; Mushiaki, Y.; Sugawara, K.; Yamamoto, T.; Takezawa, T.; Taya, M. Subculture of chondrocytes on a collagen type I-coated substrate with suppressed cellular dedifferentiation. *Tissue Eng.* **2005**, *11*, 597–608. [CrossRef] [PubMed]
130. Das, R.H.; Jahr, H.; Verhaar, J.A.; van der Linden, J.C.; van Osch, G.J.; Weinans, H. In vitro expansion affects the response of chondrocytes to mechanical stimulation. *Osteoarthr. Cartil.* **2008**, *16*, 385–391. [CrossRef] [PubMed]
131. Barbero, A.; Martin, I. Human articular chondrocytes culture. *Methods Mol. Med.* **2007**, *140*, 237–247. [PubMed]
132. Gurusinghe, S.; Strappe, P. Gene modification of mesenchymal stem cells and articular chondrocytes to enhance chondrogenesis. *BioMed Res. Int.* **2014**, *2014*, 369528. [CrossRef] [PubMed]
133. Dominici, M.; Le Blanc, K.; Mueller, I.; Slaper-Cortenbach, I.; Marini, F.; Krause, D.; Deans, R.; Keating, A.; Prockop, D.J.; Horwitz, E. Minimal criteria for defining multipotent mesenchymal stromal cells. The International Society for Cellular Therapy position statement. *Cytotherapy* **2006**, *8*, 315–317. [CrossRef] [PubMed]
134. Girlovanu, M.; Susman, S.; Soritau, O.; Rus-Ciuca, D.; Melincovici, C.; Constantin, A.M.; Mihu, C.M. Stem cells—Biological update and cell therapy progress. *Clujul. Med.* **2015**, *88*, 265–271. [CrossRef] [PubMed]
135. Im, G.I. Bone marrow-derived stem/stromal cells and adipose tissue-derived stem/stromal cells: Their comparative efficacies and synergistic effects. *J. Biomed. Mater. Res. A* **2017**, *105*, 2640–2648. [CrossRef] [PubMed]
136. Keating, A. Mesenchymal stromal cells: New directions. *Cell Stem Cell* **2012**, *10*, 709–716. [CrossRef] [PubMed]

137. Ho, A.D.; Wagner, W.; Franke, W. Heterogeneity of mesenchymal stromal cell preparations. *Cytotherapy* **2008**, *10*, 320–330. [CrossRef] [PubMed]
138. Davatchi, F.; Sadeghi Abdollahi, B.; Mohyeddin, M.; Nikbin, B. Mesenchymal stem cell therapy for knee osteoarthritis: 5 years follow-up of three patients. *Int. J. Rheum. Dis.* **2016**, *19*, 219–225. [CrossRef] [PubMed]
139. Lamo-Espinosa, J.M.; Mora, G.; Blanco, J.F.; Granero-Moltó, F.; Nuñez-Córdoba, J.M.; Sánchez-Echenique, C.; Bondía, J.M.; Aquerreta, J.D.; Andreu, E.J.; Ornilla, E.; et al. Intra-articular injection of two different doses of autologous bone marrow mesenchymal stem cells versus hyaluronic acid in the treatment of knee osteoarthritis: Multicenter randomized controlled clinical trial (phase I/II). *J. Transl. Med.* **2016**, *14*, 246. [CrossRef] [PubMed]
140. Pers, Y.M.; Rackwitz, L.; Ferreira, R.; Pullig, O.; Delfour, C.; Barry, F.; Sensebe, L.; Casteilla, L.; Fleury, S.; Bourin, P.; et al. Adipose Mesenchymal Stromal Cell-Based Therapy for Severe Osteoarthritis of the Knee: A Phase I Dose-Escalation Trial. *Stem Cells Transl. Med.* **2016**, *5*, 847–856. [CrossRef] [PubMed]
141. Emadedin, M.; Ghorbani Liastani, M.; Fazeli, R.; Mohseni, F.; Moghadasali, R.; Mardpour, S.; Hosseini, S.E.; Niknejadi, M.; Moeininia, F.; Aghahossein Fanni, A.; et al. Long-Term Follow-up of Intra-articular Injection of Autologous Mesenchymal Stem Cells in Patients with Knee, Ankle, or Hip Osteoarthritis. *Arch. Iran. Med.* **2015**, *18*, 336–344. [PubMed]
142. Wakitani, S.; Imoto, K.; Yamamoto, T.; Saito, M.; Murata, N.; Yoneda, M. Human autologous culture expanded bone marrow mesenchymal cell transplantation for repair of cartilage defects in osteoarthritic knees. *Osteoarthr. Cartil.* **2002**, *10*, 199–206. [CrossRef] [PubMed]
143. Nejadnik, H.; Hui, J.H.; Feng Choong, E.P.; Tai, B.C.; Lee, E.H. Autologous bone marrow-derived mesenchymal stem cells versus autologous chondrocyte implantation: An observational cohort study. *Am. J. Sports Med.* **2010**, *38*, 1110–1116. [CrossRef] [PubMed]
144. Buda, R.; Vannini, F.; Cavallo, M.; Grigolo, B.; Cenacchi, A.; Giannini, S. Osteochondral lesions of the knee: A new one-step repair technique with bone-marrow-derived cells. *J. Bone Jt. Surg. Am.* **2010**, *92*, 2–11. [CrossRef] [PubMed]
145. Wakitani, S.; Okabe, T.; Horibe, S.; Mitsuoka, T.; Saito, M.; Koyama, T.; Nawata, M.; Tensho, K.; Kato, H.; Uematsu, K.; et al. Safety of autologous bone marrow-derived mesenchymal stem cell transplantation for cartilage repair in 41 patients with 45 joints followed for up to 11 years and 5 months. *J. Tissue Eng. Regen. Med.* **2011**, *5*, 146–150. [CrossRef] [PubMed]
146. Saw, K.Y.; Anz, A.; Merican, S.; Tay, Y.G.; Ragavanaidu, K.; Jee, C.S.; McGuire, D.A. Articular cartilage regeneration with autologous peripheral blood progenitor cells and hyaluronic acid after arthroscopic subchondral drilling: A report of 5 cases with histology. *Arthroscopy* **2011**, *27*, 493–506. [CrossRef] [PubMed]
147. Davatchi, F.; Abdollahi, B.S.; Mohyeddin, M.; Shahram, F.; Nikbin, B. Mesenchymal stem cell therapy for knee osteoarthritis. Preliminary report of four patients. *Int. J. Rheum. Dis.* **2011**, *14*, 211–215. [CrossRef] [PubMed]
148. Koh, Y.G.; Choi, Y.J. Infrapatellar fat pad-derived mesenchymal stem cell therapy for knee osteoarthritis. *Knee* **2012**, *19*, 902–907. [CrossRef] [PubMed]
149. Koh, Y.G.; Jo, S.B.; Kwon, O.R.; Suh, D.S.; Lee, S.W.; Park, S.H.; Choi, Y.J. Mesenchymal stem cell injections improve symptoms of knee osteoarthritis. *Arthroscopy* **2013**, *29*, 748–755. [CrossRef] [PubMed]
150. Saw, K.Y.; Anz, A.; Siew-Yoke Jee, C.; Merican, S.; Ching-Soong Ng, R.; Roohi, S.A.; Ragavanaidu, K. Articular cartilage regeneration with autologous peripheral blood stem cells versus hyaluronic acid: A randomized controlled trial. *Arthroscopy* **2013**, *29*, 684–694. [CrossRef] [PubMed]
151. Orozco, L.; Munar, A.; Soler, R.; Alberca, M.; Soler, F.; Huguet, M.; Sentís, J.; Sánchez, A.; García-Sancho, J. Treatment of knee osteoarthritis with autologous mesenchymal stem cells: A pilot study. *Transplantation* **2013**, *95*, 1535–1541. [CrossRef] [PubMed]
152. Wong, K.L.; Lee, K.B.; Tai, B.C.; Law, P.; Lee, E.H.; Hui, J.H. Injectable cultured bone marrow-derived mesenchymal stem cells in varus knees with cartilage defects undergoing high tibial osteotomy: A prospective, randomized controlled clinical trial with 2 years' follow-up. *Arthroscopy* **2013**, *29*, 2020–2028. [CrossRef] [PubMed]
153. Jo, C.H.; Lee, Y.G.; Shin, W.H.; Kim, H.; Chai, J.W.; Jeong, E.C.; Kim, J.E.; Shim, H.; Shin, J.S.; Shin, I.S.; et al. Intra-articular injection of mesenchymal stem cells for the treatment of osteoarthritis of the knee: A proof-of-concept clinical trial. *Stem Cells* **2014**, *32*, 1254–1266. [CrossRef] [PubMed]

154. Akgun, I.; Unlu, M.C.; Erdal, O.A.; Ogut, T.; Erturk, M.; Ovali, E.; Kantarci, F.; Caliskan, G.; Akgun, Y. Matrix-induced autologous mesenchymal stem cell implantation versus matrix-induced autologous chondrocyte implantation in the treatment of chondral defects of the knee: A 2-year randomized study. *Arch. Orthop. Trauma Surg.* **2015**, *135*, 251–263. [CrossRef] [PubMed]
155. Fodor, P.B.; Paulseth, S.G. Adipose derived stromal cell (ADSC) injections for pain management of osteoarthritis in the human knee joint. *Aesthet. Surg. J.* **2016**, *36*, 229–236. [CrossRef] [PubMed]
156. Koh, Y.G.; Kwon, O.R.; Kim, Y.S.; Choi, Y.J.; Tak, D.H. Adipose-Derived mesenchymal stem cells with microfracture versus microfracture alone: 2-year follow-up of a prospective randomized trial. *Arthroscopy* **2016**, *32*, 97–109. [CrossRef] [PubMed]
157. Vangsness, C.T.; Farr, J.; Boyd, J.; Dellaero, D.T.; Mills, C.R.; LeRoux-Williams, M. Adult human mesenchymal stem cells delivered via intra-articular injection to the knee following partial medial meniscectomy: A randomized, double-blind, controlled study. *J. Bone Jt. Surg. Am.* **2014**, *96*, 90–98. [CrossRef] [PubMed]
158. Vega, A.; Martin-Ferrero, M.A.; del Canto, F.; Alberca, M.; Garcia, V.; Munar, A.; Orozco, L.; Soler, R.; Fuertes, J.J.; Huguet, M.; et al. Treatment of knee osteoarthritis with allogeneic bone marrow mesenchymal stem cells: A randomized controlled trial. *Transplantation* **2015**, *99*, 1681–1690. [CrossRef] [PubMed]
159. De Windt, T.S.; Vonk, L.A.; Slaper-Cortenbach, I.C.; van den Broek, M.P.; Nizak, R.; van Rijen, M.H.; de Weger, R.A.; Dhert, W.J.; Saris, D.B. Allogeneic Mesenchymal Stem Cells Stimulate Cartilage Regeneration and Are Safe for Single-Stage Cartilage Repair in Humans upon Mixture with Recycled Autologous Chondrons. *Stem Cells* **2017**, *35*, 256–264. [CrossRef] [PubMed]
160. De Windt, T.S.; Vonk, L.A.; Slaper-Cortenbach, I.C.M.; Nizak, R.; van Rijen, M.H.P.; Saris, D.B.F. Allogeneic MSCs and Recycled Autologous Chondrons Mixed in a One-Stage Cartilage Cell Transplantion: A First-in-Man Trial in 35 Patients. *Stem Cells* **2017**, *35*, 1984–1993. [CrossRef] [PubMed]
161. Baldari, S.; Di Rocco, G.; Piccoli, M.; Pozzobon, M.; Muraca, M.; Toietta, G. Challenges and Strategies for Improving the Regenerative Effects of Mesenchymal Stromal Cell-Based Therapies. *Int. J. Mol. Sci.* **2017**, *18*, 2087. [CrossRef] [PubMed]
162. Liang, X.; Ding, Y.; Zhang, Y.; Tse, H.F.; Lian, Q. Paracrine mechanisms of mesenchymal stem cell-based therapy: Current status and perspectives. *Cell Transpl.* **2014**, *23*, 1045–1059. [CrossRef] [PubMed]
163. Steinert, A.F.; Rackwitz, L.; Gilbert, F.; Noth, U.; Tuan, R.S. Concise review: The clinical application of mesenchymal stem cells for musculoskeletal regeneration: Current status and perspectives. *Stem Cells Transl. Med.* **2012**, *1*, 237–247. [CrossRef] [PubMed]
164. Gomez-Aristizabal, A.; Sharma, A.; Bakooshli, M.A.; Kapoor, M.; Gilbert, P.M.; Viswanathan, S.; Gandhi, R. Stage-specific differences in secretory profile of mesenchymal stromal cells (MSCs) subjected to early- vs. late-stage OA synovial fluid. *Osteoarthr. Cartil.* **2017**, *25*, 737–741. [CrossRef] [PubMed]
165. Farrell, M.J.; Fisher, M.B.; Huang, A.H.; Shin, J.I.; Farrell, K.M.; Mauck, R.L. Functional properties of bone marrow-derived MSC-based engineered cartilage are unstable with very longterm in vitro culture. *J. Biomech.* **2014**, *47*, 2173–2182. [CrossRef] [PubMed]
166. Perez-Silos, V.; Camacho-Morales, A.; Fuentes-Mera, L. Mesenchymal stem cells subpopulations: Application for orthopedic regenerative medicine. *Stem Cells Int.* **2016**, 3187491. [CrossRef] [PubMed]
167. Clause, K.C.; Liu, L.J.; Tobita, K. Directed stem cell differentiation: The role of physical forces. *Cell Commun. Adhes.* **2010**, *17*, 48–54. [CrossRef] [PubMed]
168. Gugjoo, M.B.; Amarpal; Sharma, G.T.; Aithal, H.P.; Kinjavdekar, P. Cartilage tissue engineering: Role of mesenchymal stem cells along with growth factors & scaffolds. *Indian J. Med. Res.* **2016**, *144*, 339–347. [CrossRef] [PubMed]
169. Vinardell, T.; Sheehy, E.J.; Buckley, C.T.; Kelly, D.J. A comparison of the functionality and in vivo phenotypic stability of cartilaginous tissues engineered from different stem cell sources. *Tissue Eng. Part A* **2012**, *18*, 1161–1170. [CrossRef] [PubMed]
170. Mak, J.; Jablonski, C.L.; Leonard, C.A.; Dunn, J.F.; Raharjo, E.; Matyas, J.R.; Biernaskie, J.; Krawetz, R.J. Intra-articular injection of synovial mesenchymal stem cells improves cartilage repair in a mouse injury model. *Sci. Rep.* **2016**, *6*, 23076. [CrossRef] [PubMed]
171. Sekiya, I.; Muneta, T.; Horie, M.; Koga, H. Arthroscopic Transplantation of Synovial Stem Cells Improves Clinical Outcomes in Knees with Cartilage Defects. *Clin. Orthop. Relat. Res.* **2015**, *473*, 2316–2326. [CrossRef] [PubMed]

172. Van Osch, G.J.; Brittberg, M.; Dennis, J.E.; Bastiaansen-Jenniskens, Y.M.; Erben, R.G.; Konttinen, Y.T.; Luyten, F.P. Cartilage repair: Past and future—Lessons for regenerative medicine. *J. Cell. Mol. Med.* **2009**, *13*, 792–810. [CrossRef] [PubMed]
173. Gomoll, A.H. Microfracture and augments. *J. Knee Surg.* **2012**, *25*, 9–15. [CrossRef] [PubMed]
174. Bonzani, I.C.; George, J.H.; Stevens, M.M. Novel materials for bone and cartilage regeneration. *Curr. Opin. Chem. Biol.* **2006**, *10*, 568–575. [CrossRef] [PubMed]
175. Kon, E.; Roffi, A.; Filardo, G.; Tesei, G.; Marcacci, M. Scaffold-based cartilage treatments: With or without cells? A systematic review of preclinical and clinical evidence. *Arthroscopy* **2015**, *31*, 767–775. [CrossRef] [PubMed]
176. Benthien, J.P.; Behrens, P. Autologous Matrix-Induced Chondrogenesis (AMIC): Combining Microfracturing and a Collagen I/III Matrix for Articular Cartilage Resurfacing. *Cartilage* **2010**, *1*, 65–68. [CrossRef] [PubMed]

11

Electronegative Low-Density Lipoprotein L5 Impairs Viability and NGF-Induced Neuronal Differentiation of PC12 Cells via LOX-1

Jiz-Yuh Wang [1,2,*], Chiou-Lian Lai [3,4], Ching-Tien Lee [5] and Chen-Yen Lin [1]

1 Graduate Institute of Medicine, College of Medicine, Kaohsiung Medical University, Kaohsiung 80708, Taiwan; k00511882@gmail.com
2 Department of Medical Research, Kaohsiung Medical University Hospital, Kaohsiung 80708, Taiwan
3 Department of Neurology, Faculty of Medicine, College of Medicine, Kaohsiung Medical University, Kaohsiung 80708, Taiwan; cllai@kmu.edu.tw
4 Department of Neurology, Kaohsiung Medical University Hospital, Kaohsiung 80756, Taiwan
5 Department of Nursing, Hsin-Sheng College of Medical Care and Management, Taoyuan 32544, Taiwan; chingtien1213@gmail.com
* Correspondence: jizyuhwang@cc.kmu.edu.tw

Abstract: There have been striking associations of cardiovascular diseases (e.g., atherosclerosis) and hypercholesterolemia with increased risk of neurodegeneration including Alzheimer's disease (AD). Low-density lipoprotein (LDL), a cardiovascular risk factor, plays a crucial role in AD pathogenesis; further, L5, a human plasma LDL fraction with high electronegativity, may be a factor contributing to AD-type dementia. Although L5 contributing to atherosclerosis progression has been studied, its role in inducing neurodegeneration remains unclear. Here, PC12 cell culture was used for treatments with human LDLs (L1, L5, or oxLDL), and subsequently cell viability and nerve growth factor (NGF)-induced neuronal differentiation were assessed. We identified L5 as a neurotoxic LDL, as demonstrated by decreased cell viability in a time- and concentration-dependent manner. Contrarily, L1 had no such effect. L5 caused cell damage by inducing ATM/H2AX-associated DNA breakage as well as by activating apoptosis via lectin-like oxidized LDL receptor-1 (LOX-1) signaling to p53 and ensuring cleavage of caspase-3. Additionally, sublethal L5 long-termly inhibited neurite outgrowth in NGF-treated PC12 cells, as evidenced by downregulation of early growth response factor-1 and neurofilament-M. This inhibitory effect was mediated via an interaction between L5 and LOX-1 to suppress NGF-induced activation of PI3k/Akt cascade, but not NGF receptor TrkA and downstream MAPK pathways. Together, our data suggest that L5 creates a neurotoxic stress via LOX-1 in PC12 cells, thereby leading to impairment of viability and NGF-induced differentiation. Atherogenic L5 likely contributes to neurodegenerative disorders.

Keywords: electronegative LDL; lectin-like oxidized LDL receptor-1 (LOX-1); nerve growth factor (NGF); neuronal differentiation; apoptosis

1. Introduction

Dementia is the most common neurodegenerative disorder afflicting the aged. Growing evidence suggests a strong and likely causal association of cardiovascular disease (CVD) with cognitive decline and Alzheimer's disease (AD) [1]. Actually, a high prevailing rate of often neglected cardiovascular problems is found in the AD population [1,2]. Epidemiological studies have established a strong relation between CVD and AD, but it remains unclear whether this relation is due to shared risk factors that independently influence disease progression, or if certain CVD risk factors contribute to AD pathogenesis by inducing neuronal damage or promoting the accumulation of plaques and tangles. Among CVD risk factors, elevated low-density lipoprotein (LDL) is reported to reduce cerebral perfusion, increase oxidative stress, and activate neuroinflammatory responses, all of which promote AD progression [3,4]. An association of high LDL with cognitive impairment and AD has been demonstrated; however, how plasma LDL induces dementia has yet to be clearly defined.

Hypercholesterolemia has been emphasized a risk factor for the development of AD [5,6]. Cholesterol is transported inside LDL particles in circulation, so high LDL-cholesterol (LDL-C) level may increase the individuals suffering from cognitive decline and dementia. Cholesterol-related studies suggest that there is a negative correlation between plasma LDL-C level and cognition [7,8], and that high LDL-C level is associated with faster cognitive degeneration in AD patients [9]. Moreover, LDL particles are known to cause mischief to both cardiovasculature and cerebrovasculature if they become oxidized and invade the endothelium. Oxidized LDL (oxLDL) can promote AD progression through inducing cerebrovascular dysfunction [10,11]. Thus, lowering LDL-C with statins has been an excellent strategy for reducing dementia risk [12].

One plausible mechanisms by which LDLs contribute to cognitive dysfunction and dementia progression is through the modification to electronegative LDL [LDL(−)], a class of naturally occurring atherogenic lipoproteins [13]. Similar to oxLDL, plasma LDL(−) is increased in patients with high CVD risk, including patients with hyperlipidemia, diabetes, severe renal disease, and nonalcoholic steatohepatitis [14]. Of note, L5 has the relatively highest electronegative charge among chromatographically resolved human LDL subfractions (L1–L5), and evidence has shown that L5 induces marked atherogenic changes and apoptosis in cultured vascular endothelial cells (ECs) [15]. Further, circulating L5 is moderately elevated in asymptomatic individuals with increased CVD risk, such as those with metabolic syndrome, hypercholesterolaemia and type 2 diabetes [16,17]. Nevertheless, to our knowledge, the role of L5 in neurodegenerative pathogenesis remains uncharacterized. Specifically, it remains uncertain whether L5 leakage into brain tissue under the situations of aberrant cerebrovasculature caused by cerebral amyloid angiopathy or increased blood-brain barrier (BBB) permeability induced by CVD-related vascular factors can directly induce neuronal dysfunction or death.

We hypothesized that L5 is neurotoxic, thereby leading to neurodegeneration. Thus, our purpose in this in vitro study was to examine whether L5 negatively impacts on neuron-like PC12 cell reactivities, such as cell viability and nerve growth factor (NGF)-induced differentiation. The related signaling cascades that L5 disturbs were assessed after the desired treatments. We found that L5 induces ataxia-telangiectasia mutated (ATM) protein/H2AX-associated DNA damage, causes cell apoptosis vià lectin-like oxidized LDL receptor-1 (LOX-1)/p53/caspase-3, and inhibits neurite outgrowth by interacting with LOX-1 and reducing NGF-stimulated Akt activation. Here, we present novel findings showing that L5 induces neurotoxicity directly, thereby identifying elevated plasma L5 as a possible causal link between hypercholesterolemia-related CVD and neurodegeneration, such as AD.

2. Results

2.1. L5 Shows a Cytotoxic Property and Reduces the Viability of PC12 Cells

To characterize the action of L5 on neuronal cell reactivity, both cell viability and NGF-induced neuronal differentiation were assessed in cultured neuron-like PC12 cells. Two controls were included in most experiments, L1 as a negative control and oxLDL as a positive control. Both L5 and L1 are naturally occurring lipoproteins in human circulation; in contrast to L5, L1 possesses the lowest electronegative charge among fractions and is regarded as non-cytotoxic [15,18]. OxLDL is a known toxic lipoprotein that plays a pivotal role in the progression of atheromatous plaque via mechanisms, including the destruction of the arterial wall and induction of vascular cell apoptosis [19,20].

We first examined whether L5 decreases the survival of PC12 cells by treating cultures with 0 to 50 μg/mL L1, L5, or oxLDL for 24 h, followed by MTT reduction assays (Figure 1A). Compared to the untreated control, L5 ≥ 30 μg/mL and oxLDL ≥ 10 μg/mL significantly reduced cell viability, while no such effects were observed in L1-treated cultures. Thus, we defined 30 μg/mL L5 as the threshold lethal concentration for PC12 cells. Next, cultures were exposed to 30 μg/mL of each LDL for times ranging from 0 to 48 h. Both L5 and oxLDL induced measurable cell death at 12 h and progressive cytotoxicity thereafter. In contrast, L1 entirely exerted no damaged effect on cell viability even after a 48 h exposure (Figure 1B). Regarding cell morphological changes in response to LDLs, a large amount of fragmented cell debris was detectable in L5- or oxLDL-treated cultures, but not in L1-treated cultures (Figure 1C). These results indicate that L5 induces both concentration- and time-dependent PC12 cell death.

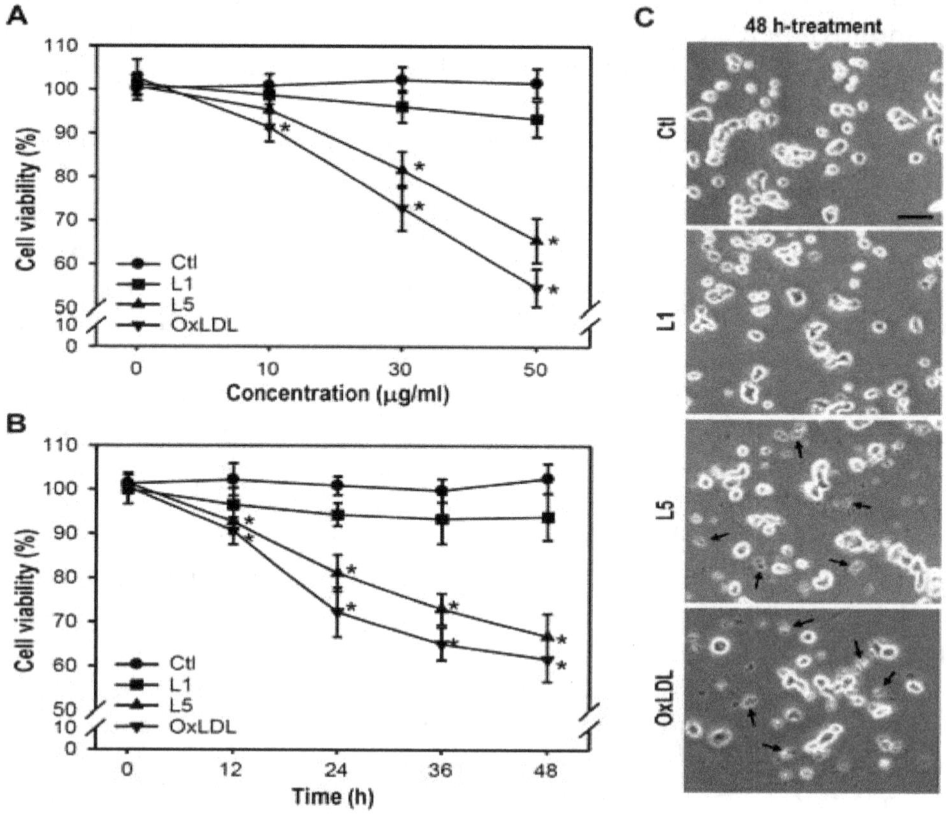

Figure 1. LDL fraction L5 shows a concentration- and time-dependent cytotoxicity to cultured PC12 cells. (**A**) Concentration-response relationships for L1 (negative control), L5, and oxLDL (positive control) were established. Indicated LDLs were applied for 24 h at various concentrations (0 to 50 μg/mL); (**B**) Time course was determined for L1, L5, and oxLDL cytotoxicity. Cultures were treated with the indicated LDL at 30 μg/mL for different times (0 to 48 h). In (**A**,**B**), the MTT reduction assay was applied to measure PC12 cell survival (viability) with untreated cells used as the control (Ctl). The number of live cells per well was calculated as a percentage of untreated control cell number. Each point is presented as the mean ± SEM from at least four independent experiments performed in triplicate. * $p < 0.05$ vs. Ctl at equal concentration (**A**) or at the same time point (**B**); and (**C**) Representative photos show an untreated culture and cultures treated with 30 μg/mL of the indicated LDL for 48 h. Fragmented cell debris (putative apoptotic bodies) are indicated by arrows. Scale bar = 50 μm.

2.2. L5 Induces Genotoxicity via ATM/H2AX Activation in PC12 Cells

Next, we assessed whether L5-induced cell death involves DNA damage, such as the formation of double-strand breaks (DSBs) in chromatin, using a neutral comet assay. Under the experimental conditions tested in our study, both L5 and oxLDL, but not L1, caused DSBs as evidenced by the appearance of migrating DNA fragments (reflected by the length of the comet tail) (Figure 2A). Further, compared to control cultures, clear comet tails were observed in cultures treated with L5 or oxLDL at 6 and 12 h (Figure 2B), indicating that L5 has a genotoxic property that leads to destruction of DNA structure.

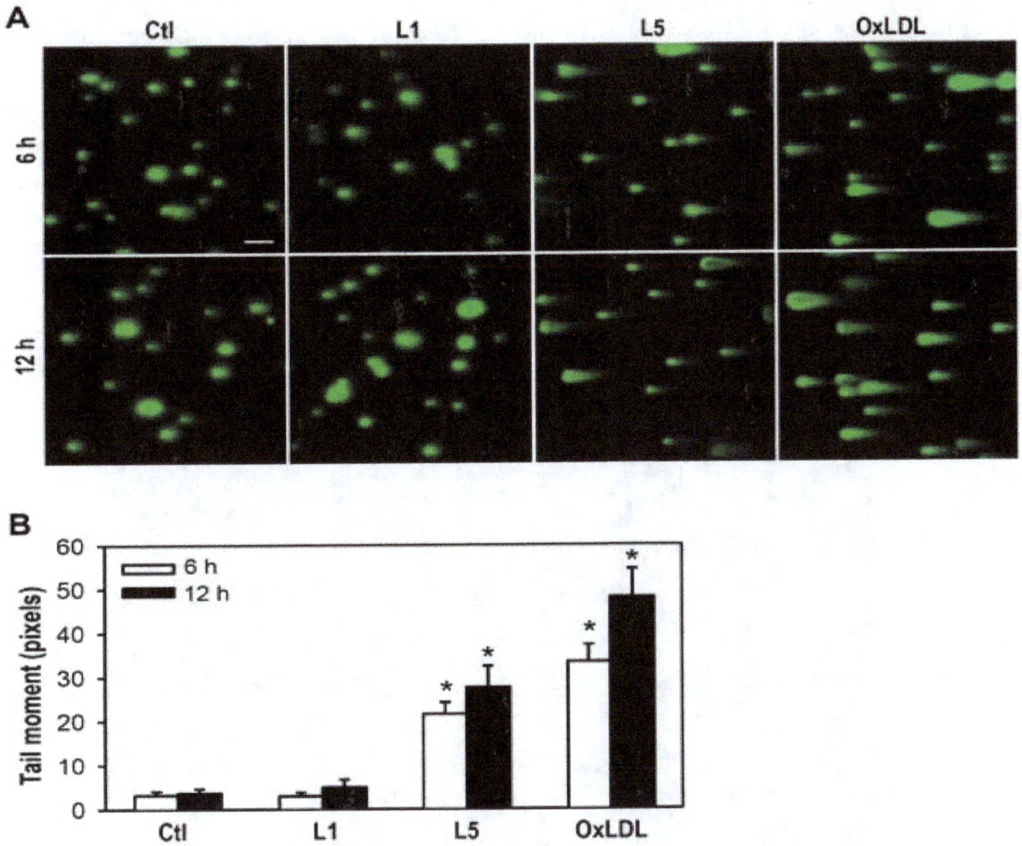

Figure 2. L5 induces DNA double-strand breaks (DSBs) in cultured PC12 cells. (**A**) Cultures treated with the indicated LDL (30 μg/mL) for 6 or 12 h were analyzed for DSBs using a neutral comet assay kit. Untreated cells were used as a control. Representative images from one of four independent experiments are presented. Scale bar = 50 μm; and (**B**) The comet tail moment used to determine DNA damage was quantified by COMETscore.v1.5 software. Data are presented as mean ± SEM from four independent experiments. * $p < 0.05$ vs. Ctl at the same time point. At least 200 cells were analyzed in each treatment group per experiment.

Studies have suggested that DSBs formation is closely correlated with activation of both ATM and H2AX [21]. Hence, we examined whether DSBs induction by L5 is associated with ATM/H2AX activation. Immunostaining revealed the formation of γH2AX (H2AX phosphorylation on serine 139), which positively corresponds to DNA DSBs. Both L5 and oxLDL induced γH2AX foci formation in the nucleus as evidenced by punctate immunofluorescence signals, while such γH2AX immunoreactivity was not observed in untreated control or L1-treated cultures (Figure 3A,B). To further verify L5-induced genotoxicity, ATM and H2AX activation were determined by western blotting. Consistent with immunostaining results, a rapid and marked increase in both pATM and γH2AX was observed after only 10 min of L5 treatment, but not L1 treatment (Figure 3C). Together with the data presented in Figure 2, these results suggest that L5 injures PC12 cells by inducing ATM/H2AX-associated DNA DSBs.

2.3. *L5 Induces Apoptotic Death of PC12 Cells via the LOX-1/p53/Caspase-3 Pathway*

Damage to genomic integrity is known to cause apoptosis [22,23], and indeed many of the debris fragments observed following L5 or oxLDL treatment resembled apoptotic bodies (Figure 1C). Accordingly, we examined whether L5 causes apoptotic death in PC12 cells and activates apoptosis-associated signal transduction pathways. Compared to control, L5 increased cleaved caspase-3 (a key apoptotic caspase) expression after 6 or 12 h of treatment while L1 had no such effect (Figure 4A); moreover, this apoptotic insult was evidently inhibited by the pan-caspase inhibitor Z-VAD-FMK (Figure 4B). Subsequently, p53 activity was examined due to its close association with apoptosis and activation upon cellular stresses such as DNA damage. Furthermore, p53 is a direct substrate of ATM [24]. ATM rapidly phosphorylates p53 at Ser15 during early phase of DNA damage response, thereby reducing the interaction of p53 with MDM2, a negative p53 regulator that inhibits accumulation of p53 by targeting it for ubiquitination and proteasomal degradation [25,26]. Compared to the control, L5-treated cultures (but not L1-treated cultures) exhibited phosphorylated p53 elevation after as little as 10 min of exposure (Figure 4C). Moreover, the p53 inhibitor pifithrin-α (PFT-α) electively reduced the cleaved caspase-3 level in L5-treated cultures without altering the L5-phosphorylated p53 level, indicating that p53-dependent apoptosis is a major mediator of L5-induced PC12 cell death (Figure 4D).

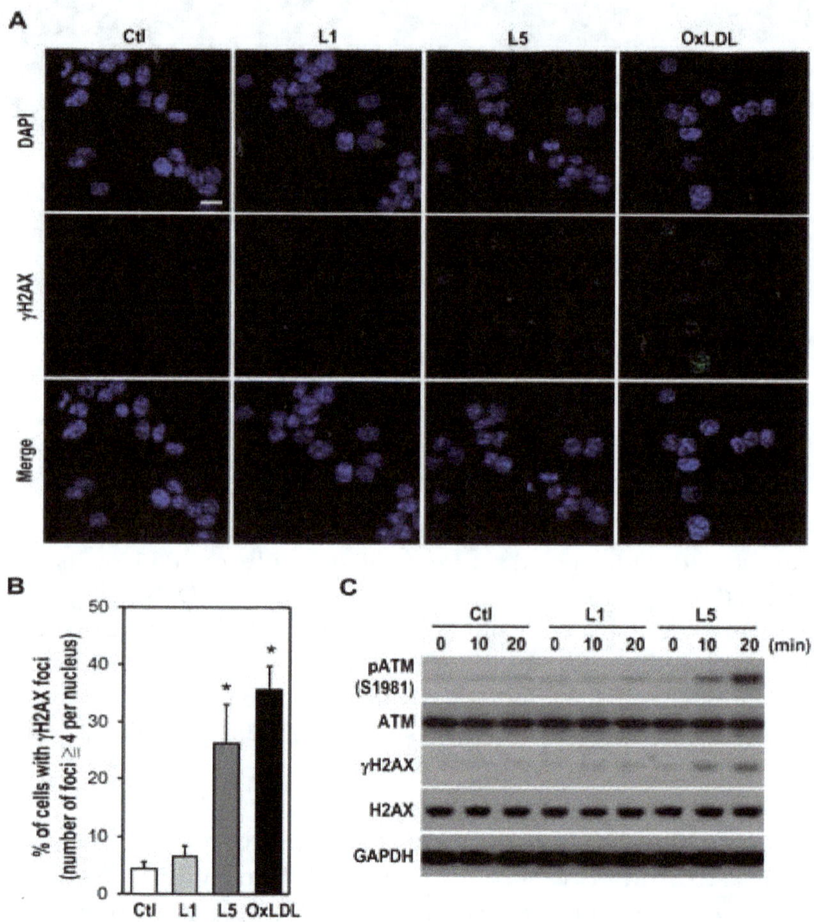

Figure 3. L5 induces ATM phosphorylation and formation of γH2AX foci in cultured PC12 cells. (**A**) Representative immunofluorescence images of γH2AX foci are shown. Cells grown on coverslips were treated with the indicated LDL (30 μg/mL) for 30 min. Untreated cells were used as a control. Immunostaining was performed using an antibody against γH2AX (green). Cells were counterstained with DAPI to recognize the nucleus (blue). Scale bar = 10 μm; (**B**) The histogram shows the quantification of (**A**). At least 20 randomly selected fields for each treatment group were examined. Cells with ≥ 4γH2AX foci per nucleus were regarded as positive and then scored. Value expressed as a percentage by calculating the number of positive cells (% of total). Data are presented as mean ± SEM from four independent experiments. * $p < 0.05$ vs. Ctl; and (**C**) After treating the cultures with L1 or L5 at 30 μg/mL for different times as indicated, western blotting was performed to detect pATM, ATM, γH2AX, and H2AX expression. GAPDH was a protein loading control. Representative blots selected from one of four independent experiments are presented.

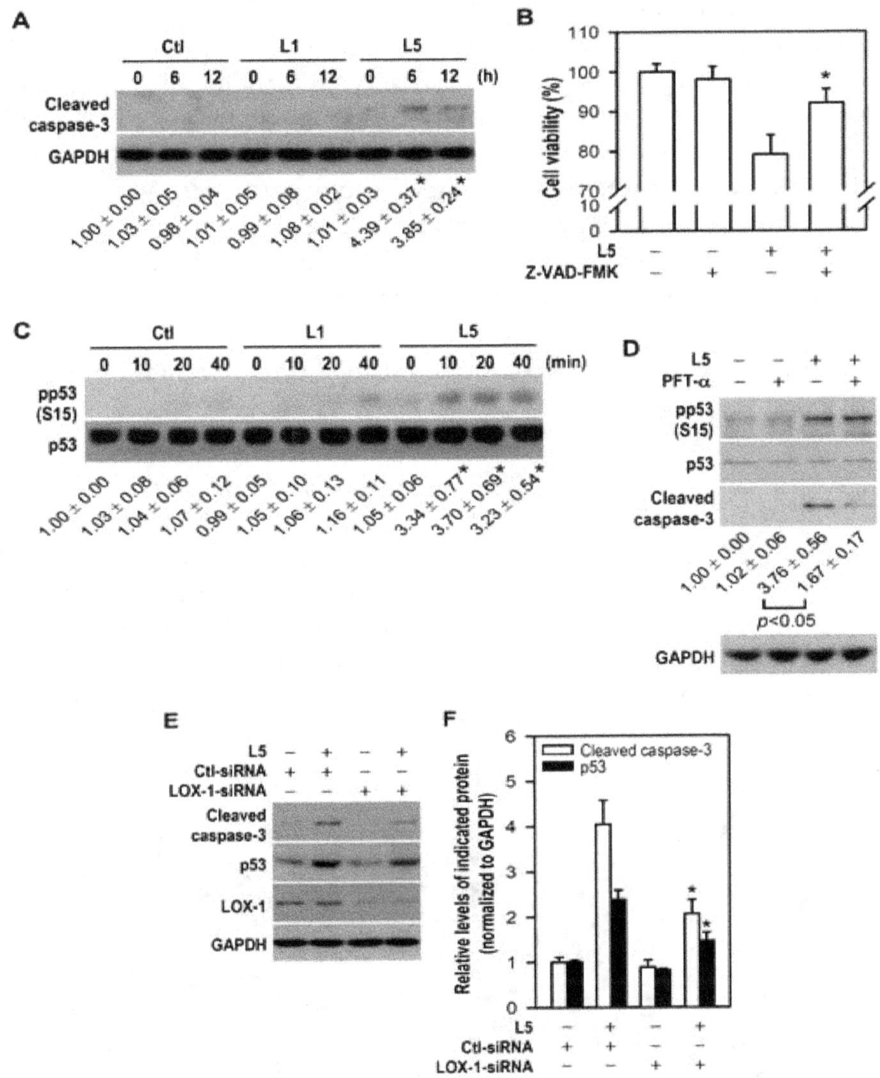

Figure 4. Reduced viability of L5-treated PC12 cells is associated with LOX-1 expression, p53 activation, and caspase-3 cleavage. (**A**) Cultures were treated with L1 or L5 (30 μg/mL) for the indicated times and then western blotting was used to detect cleaved caspase-3. Untreated cells were used as a control. GAPDH was a protein loading control. Quantitative values are expressed relative to untreated control at a time point of 0 h (assigned a value of 1); the means ± SEM from four independent experiments are shown below the representative blots. * $p < 0.05$ vs. Ctl at the same time point; (**B**) Cells were treated with or without L5 (30 μg/mL) for 12 h in the absence or presence of a pan-caspase inhibitor Z-VAD-FMK (20 μM). The histogram shows the cell viability of each treatment group relative to the untreated control (assigned a value of 100%). Data are presented as mean ± SEM from at least three independent experiments performed in triplicate. * $p < 0.05$ vs. L5 alone; (**C**) After the indicated treatments, western blotting was used to detect pp53 and p53 expression. Quantitative results of relative pp53 levels from four independent experiments are shown below the representative blots. * $p < 0.05$ vs. Ctl at the same time point; (**D**) Before sham or L5 (30 μg/mL) treatment for either 20 min or 12 h, cells were pretreated with or without PFT-α (10 μM) for 1 h. The expression of pp53 and p53 (at 20 min), and cleaved caspase-3 (at 12 h) was detected by western blotting. Relative quantitative results of cleaved caspase-3 from four independent experiments are shown below the representative blots; (**E**) One day after transfection with a scrambled siRNA (Ctl-siRNA) or a LOX-1-siRNA, cultures were treated with or without L5 for 12 h. Cleaved caspase-3, p53, and LOX-1 were detected by western blotting and representative blots are presented; and (**F**) Relative quantitative expression of cleaved caspase-3 and p53 in (**E**) is shown by a histogram. Data are from four independent experiments. * < 0.05 vs. Ctl-siRNA + L5.

To identify the upstream factors leading to activation of the p53/caspase-3 pathway, we first focused on possible receptors involved. It has been shown that L5 signals and is internalized through LOX-1, and that the binding complex of L5/LOX-1 plays a critical role in L5-induced apoptosis of vascular ECs [15]. Accordingly, we examined whether LOX-1 participates in L5-induced induction of p53/caspase-3-dependent apoptosis in PC12 cells. Compared to L5-treated cultures transfected with control small interfering RNA (Ctl-siRNA), silencing of endogenous LOX-1 by RNA interference using a LOX-1-siRNA not only downregulated LOX-1 protein expression, as determined by western blotting, but also markedly reduced both cleaved caspase-3 level and p53 accumulation in response to L5 (Figure 4E,F). Noteworthily, this reduced p53 accumulation might be primarily because LOX-1-siRNA disturbs L5-induced p53 phosphorylation and then MDM2-mediated p53 degradation occurs. This finding suggests that LOX-1 is required for L5-induced downstream activation of p53/caspase-3. Taken together, these results strongly suggest that LOX-1/p53/caspase-3 signaling mediates L5-induced PC12 cell apoptosis.

2.4. L5 Inhibits NGF-Induced Differentiation of PC12 Cells

Neurite outgrowth in PC12 cells in response to NGF stimulation is a widely used model to examine neuronal differentiation and development. In addition to assessing L5 effects on PC12 cell viability, we further examined whether L5 disturbs NGF-induced neuronal differentiation of PC12 cells. According to above results indicating that L5 < 30 μg/mL did not cause detectable PC12 cell death (Figure 1A), we defined 10 μg/mL as the sublytic concentration to assess the impact of L5 on PC12 cell differentiation induced by NGF.

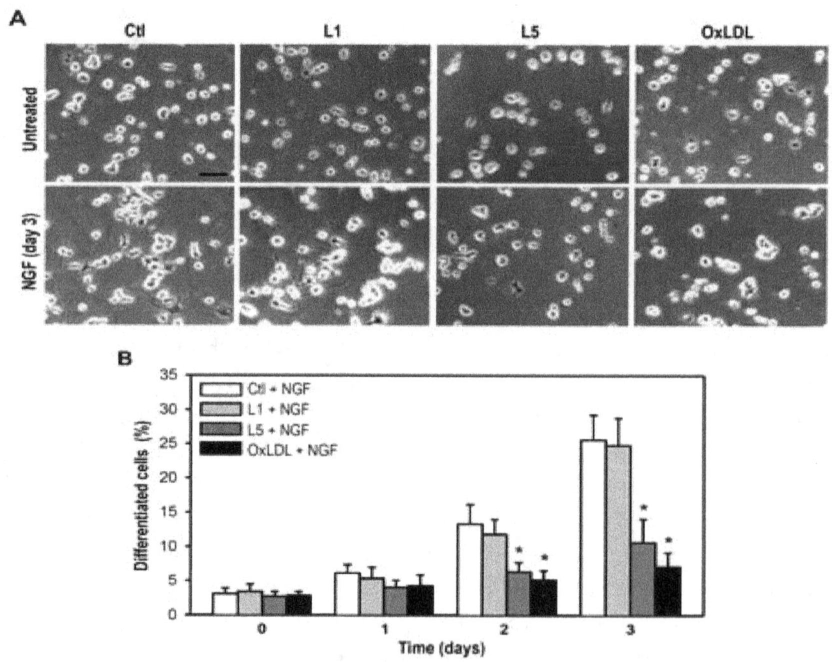

Figure 5. L5 inhibits NGF-induced neuronal differentiation of cultured PC12 cells. (**A**) Representative photos show PC12 cells treated with the indicated LDLs (10 μg/mL) in the absence or presence of NGF (50 ng/mL) for 3 days. Cells untreated with LDLs were used as a control. NGF-induced neuronal differentiation is indicated by the extent of neurite outgrowth. Scale bar = 50 μm; and (**B**) The percentage of neuronal differentiation in PC12 cells exposed to LDLs (10 μg/mL) plus NGF (50 ng/mL) for 1, 2, and 3 days was determined by calculating the number of cells (% of total) bearing neurites longer than one cell body in diameter. Ten randomly selected fields were examined and at least 300 cells were counted for each treatment group at each time point. Data are presented as mean ± SEM of one representative experiment; two other experiments revealed consistent results. * $p < 0.05$ vs. Ctl + NGF at the same time point.

As shown in Figure 5A, both L5 and oxLDL interfered with neurite outgrowth in PC12 cultures subjected to long-term NGF exposure, as evidenced by generally shorter neurites compared to control NGF-treated cultures on day 3 of treatment. As expected, cultured cells treated with L1 plus NGF displayed normal outgrowth of neurites. This finding implies that L5 at sublytic concentration is capable of disturbing NGF-induced neurite outgrowth. Indeed, both L5 and oxLDL but not L1 markedly lowered the proportion cells showing NGF-induced morphological differentiation (defined as cells with neurites longer than one soma in length) on days 2 and 3 of treatment compared to control cultures incubated with NGF (Figure 5B).

Early growth response factor-1 (Egr-1) is a NGF-responsive transcription factor and exerts long-term effects on neural cell growth, while neurofilament is critical for radial axon growth and determines axon caliber [27,28]. Therefore, we further determined the expression levels of both Egr-1 and neurofilament-medium (NF-M) under the conditions of NGF combined with distinct LDLs. The expression of Egr-1 was induced within 1 h after NGF addition, and this response was markedly reduced by both L5 and oxLDL but not by L1 (Figure 6A). Further, NGF induced an elevation in neurite growth-associated NF-M expression level, and again this response was evidently attenuated by L5 over a 4-day experimental period (Figure 6B). Thus, L5 appears to have a negative impact on neurodifferentiation-associated upregulation of Egr-1 and NF-M. Collectively, these data suggest that a sublytic concentration of L5 (10 μg/mL) remains still neurotoxic and impairs neuronal development by inhibiting NGF-induced differentiation.

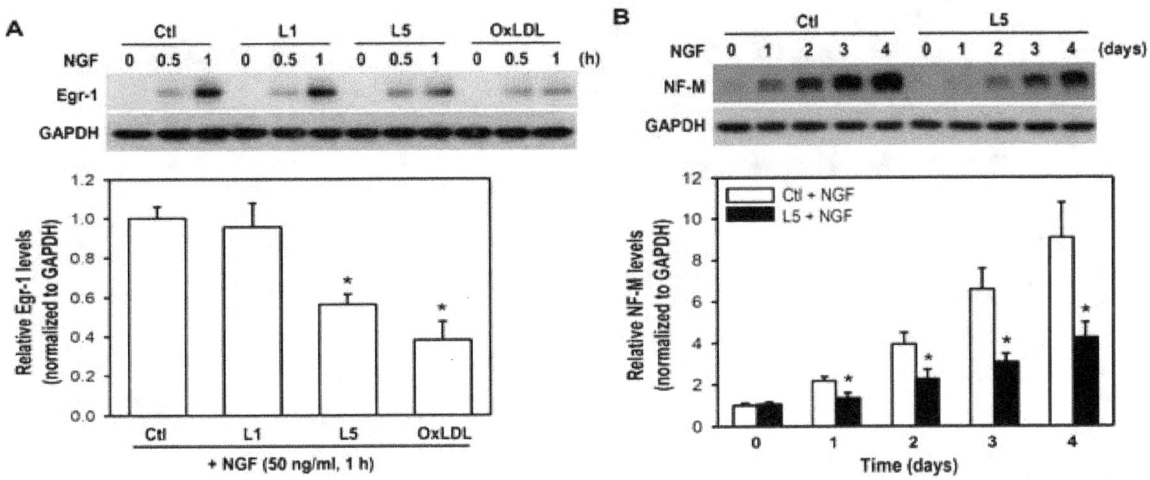

Figure 6. L5 inhibits NGF-induced upregulation of Egr-1 and NF-M. (**A**) Cultures were treated with or without the indicated LDLs (10 μg/mL) for 1 h, followed by NGF (50 ng/mL) addition for the indicated time periods. Cells untreated with LDLs were used as a control. Egr-1 expression was detected by western blotting (representative blot is shown). GAPDH was a protein loading control. The histogram shows relative Egr-1 expression values of each treatment group at a time point of 1 h. Data are presented as mean ± SEM from four independent experiments. * $p < 0.05$ vs. Ctl + NGF; and (**B**) Cultures were treated with L5 (10 μg/mL) for 1 h, followed by NGF (50 ng/mL) addition for another times (days) as indicated. Cells untreated with LDLs were used as a control. Western blotting was performed to detect NF-M expression (representative blot of NF-M is shown). The histogram shows relative NF-M levels between Ctl + NGF and L5 + NGF groups from day 0 to 4. Data are from four independent experiments. * $p < 0.05$ vs. Ctl + NGF on the same day.

2.5. L5 Weakens NGF-Induced Akt but Not TrkA and MAPKs Activation

We then examined the upstream signaling pathways responsible for L5 suppression of NGF-induced differentiation in PC12 cells. Given that many NGF effects are mediated by activation of its receptor TrkA and downstream signaling kinases such as MAPKs and PI3K/AKT, we examined whether L5 weakens NGF-induced TrkA phosphorylation and resultant activation of MAPKs

(ERK, JNK, and p38) and Akt in PC12 cultures. We first measured the phosphorylation status of several crucial residues within the tyrosine kinase domain of TrkA because autophosphorylation at these sites reflects TrkA activity or is required for activation of downstream kinase cascades [29]. In response to NGF stimulation, all tested tyrosine residues within TrkA including Tyr490, Tyr674/675, Tyr751, and Tyr785 were rapidly phosphorylated; however, no obvious difference in phosphorylation was found at any one of these tyrosine sites between cultures treated with NGF alone versus NGF plus L1, L5, or oxLDL (Figure 7A). This indicates that L5 has no influence on TrkA catalytic activity or on TrkA coupling to downstream Ras/MAPK, PI3K/Akt, and phospholipase Cγ. Further, no detectable difference was observed in the phosphorylation levels of ERK, JNK, and p38 between cultures treated with NGF alone and those treated with NGF plus L1, L5, or oxLDL. In contrast, NGF-induced Akt phosphorylation was markedly reduced in L5- and oxLDL-treated cultures at both 10 and 30 μg/mL compared to cultures treated with NGF alone, while such a repressive effect was not found in cultures incubated with L1 plus NGF (Figure 7B). These results suggest that L5 represses NGF-induced neuronal differentiation in PC12 cells by interfering with the TrkA/PI3K/Akt pathway.

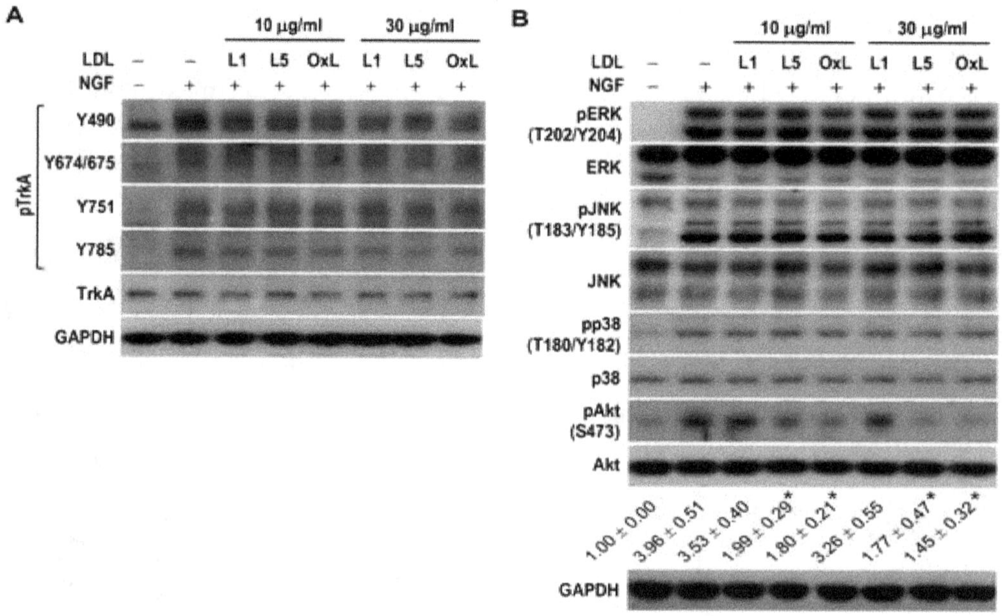

Figure 7. L5 decreases the level of phospho-Akt (pAkt), but not pTrkA and pMAPKs, in NGF-treated PC12 cells. (**A**) Cultures were treated with L1, L5, or oxLDL (OxL) at 10 or 30 μg/mL for 1 h, followed by NGF (50 ng/mL) addition for another 20 min. Untreated cells were used as a control. Western blotting was used to detect the expression of TrkA phosphorylated at various tyrosine sites and total TrkA protein. GAPDH was a protein loading control. Representative blots selected from one of four independent experiments are presented; and (**B**) Alternatively, western blotting was performed to detect pERK, ERK, pJNK, JNK, pp38, p38, pAkt, and Akt expression. Quantitative values of pAkt relative to the level of untreated control (assigned a value of 1) are expressed; the means ± SEM from four independent experiments are shown below the representative blots. * $p < 0.05$ vs. NGF alone.

2.6. LOX-1 Is Required for L5 Suppression of NGF-Induced Akt Phosphorylation

To verify abovementioned findings that NGF-induced Akt activation is reduced in L5-treated cultures, cultures were treated with NGF alone or NGF combined with L1 or L5 for brief periods and Akt phosphorylation/activation status was measured. As shown in Figure 8A, phosphorylated Akt became detectable within 10–40 min after the onset of NGF treatment, and this response was reduced in the presence of L5 but not L1. The suppressive effect of L5 on NGF-induced Akt phosphorylation reached significance at time points of 10, 20, and 40 min compared to control group treated with NGF (Ctl + NGF) (Figure 8B).

Results present in Figure 4 strongly suggest that LOX-1 is involved in PC12 cell apoptosis induced by L5. We also explored the possibility that LOX-1 participates in L5-induced suppression of neuronal differentiation in NGF-treated PC12 cells. Because NGF-stimulated Akt activation is impaired by L5, we examined if L5 weakens the TrkA/PI3K/Akt signal cascade via LOX-1. As shown in Figure 8C, NGF-induced stimulation of Akt phosphorylation was not reduced by L5 in cultures transfected with a LOX-1-siRNA, but was weakened by L5 in cultures transfected with a Ctl-siRNA. Therefore, these results suggest that L5 attenuates NGF-activated Akt via LOX-1, and that LOX-1 acts as a mediator coupling extrinsic L5 to intracellular PI3K/Akt pathway.

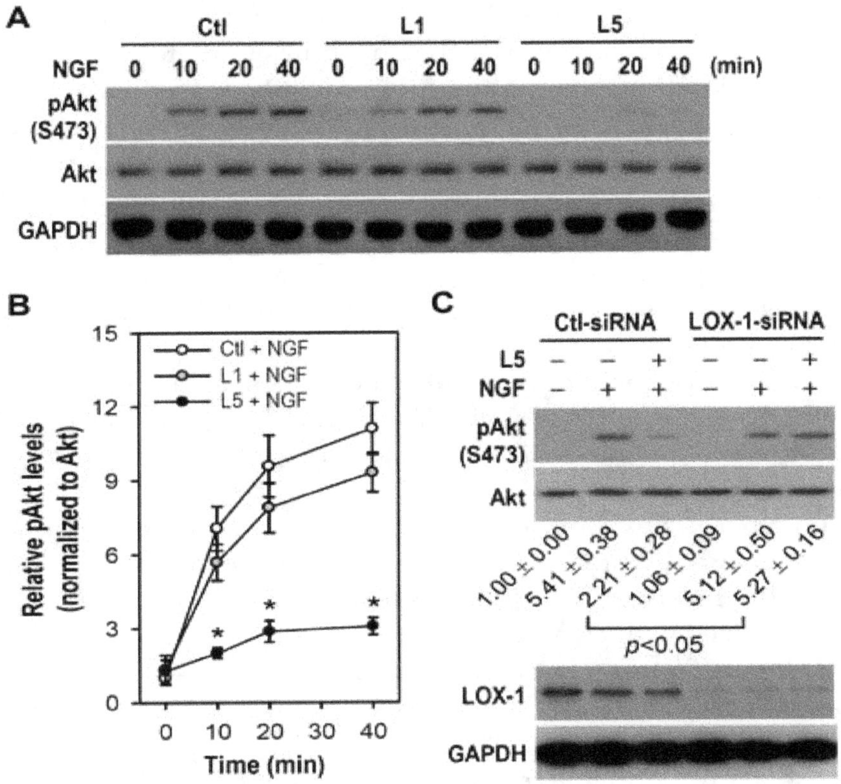

Figure 8. LOX-1 knockdown abolishes L5-induced Akt phosphorylation decline in NGF-treated PC12 cells. (**A**) Cultures were treated with L1 or L5 (10 μg/mL) for 1 h, followed by NGF (50 ng/mL) addition for the indicated time periods. Cells untreated with LDLs were used as a control. Western blotting was used to detect pAkt and Akt expression. GAPDH was a protein loading control. Representative blots selected from one of four independent experiments are presented; (**B**) According to the results in (**A**), quantitative analyses of relative pAkt levels were done in each treatment group. Data are presented as the mean ± SEM from four independent experiments. * $p < 0.05$ vs. Ctl + NGF at the same time point; and (**C**) One day after transfection with siRNA as indicated, cultures were treated with or without L5 (10 μg/mL) for 1 h and incubated in the absence or presence of NGF (50 ng/mL) for another 20 min. Western blotting was conducted to detect pAkt, Akt, and LOX-1 expression. Quantitative results of relative pAkt levels were obtained from four independent experiments and are shown below the representative blots.

3. Discussion

Frequent comorbidity of AD with CVD suggests that vascular problems contribute to cognitive decline and AD-associated dementia. High circulating LDL levels, a strong CVD risk factor, are associated with increased production of cerebrovascular amyloid β (Aβ) peptide and increased risk of AD [4]. Further, more studies also suggest that elevated blood cholesterol and triacylglycerol increase the likelihood of AD [6]. Cerebrovasculature damage induced by circulating LDL or other vascular mechanisms may enhance access of detrimental LDLs to brain parenchyma, resulting in neurotoxicity. Indeed, this study suggests that in a situation of BBB breach, L5 may directly impair neuronal viability and NGF effects, such as neurodifferentiation. Thus, it is a feasible strategy for prevention of AD and other forms of age-related cognitive impairment by aggressively targeting hypercholesterolemia.

Numerous studies have highlighted a negative role of L5 in the progression of CVDs, especially atherosclerosis, and thus L5 is regarded as a potent atherogenic LDL. It has been indicated that L5 is abundant in dyslipidemic but not normolipidemic human plasma, and hyperlipidemia is also a shared factor for AD [3]. Shen et al. found a functional link between pro-atherogenic lipoproteins and platelet-mediated thrombus formation in stroke, and pointed out that L5 is substantially elevated (40-fold higher than control subjects) in ischemic stroke patients [30]. Moreover, L5 can cause Aβ peptide secretion from platelets, which contributes to platelet hyper-reactivity and stroke complications [31]. These clinical results suggest the possibility of L5 directly impacting neurological functions, such as cognition, under the premise of impaired BBB. In the present work, we identify a negative role of L5 in basal viability and NGF-induced neuronal differentiation of PC12 cells, consistent with a neurotoxic effect in aging humans. Further investigations aimed at establishing the clinical relevance of plasma L5 to AD-related neurodegeneration are clearly warranted.

It is highly possible that plasma LDL penetrates the BBB due to a broken architecture of cerebral microvasculature during the progression of AD or CVD, which in turn leads to neuronal damage and neuroinflammation-related glial activation. In fact, apolipoprotein B (apoB) or LDL has been detected in cerebrospinal fluid (CSF) or/and central nervous system under pathological conditions. For example, apoB/LDL was found or obviously elevated in CSF collected from patients with subarachnoid hemorrhage, cerebrotendinous xanthomatosis, or tuberculous meningitis [32–34]. Plasma apoB was co-localized with cerebral Aβ in the plaques of transgenic AD mice as revealed by a 3-dimensional immunomicroscopy; further, plaque abundance in these mice positively correlated with apoB [35,36]. Moreover, BBB breakdown has been described in chronic CVDs, and peripheral inflammatory response is a cause of enhanced BBB permeability [37]. CVDs like arteriosclerosis and hypertension are characterized by increased production of pro-inflammatory cytokines in blood [38], and administration of pro-inflammatory cytokines such as TNF-α, IL-1β, and IL-6 to monolayers of cerebral ECs or pericyte/endothelial cell co-cultures leads to BBB disruption [39,40]. Clinical studies show that diseases compromising the vascular system, such as hypertension, hypercholesterolemia, and diabetes, are able to disrupt BBB integrity and increase the risk of AD [41]. Autopsy studies have also shown that vascular abnormalities, including endothelial damage-associated microangiopathy, were universally observed in AD brain tissue [42]. Together, these studies revealing the occurrence of BBB dysfunction in CVDs or encephalopathies set a stage for this study and suggest that L5 and other neurotoxic agents in plasma may directly access neurons via a damaged BBB.

Actually, L5 does not exist in healthy individuals with clinically normolipidemia; certainly, L5 does not appear in the brain under normally physiological conditions. However, plasma L5 likely extravasates directly into brain milieu in certain pathological cases, such as BBB dysfunction. Moreover, the L5 concentration (10 or 30 μg/mL) used in this study should not be present in humans with normal or pathological CNS states, but is approximately equal to or less than other in vitro studies examining the impact of L5 or LDL(−) on the pathogenic process of atherosclerosis. For example, Chu et al. used 50 μg/mL of L5 for 24 h to examine C-reactive protein expression in vascular ECs [43]. Estruch et al. assessed cytokine release in monocytes treated with LDL(−) at 150 μg apoB/mL [44]. Because in vitro L5 toxicity has a tendency towards a concentration- and time-dependency, we can reasonably consider that neurotoxicity is attainable in vivo if using lower L5 concentrations (<10 μg/mL) for longer treatment periods (a few weeks or months) under the premise of impaired BBB. To elucidate this thought, a long-term exposure to low plasma L5 levels will be applied to future animal studies using transgenic AD mice, and hypertensive or hypercholesterolemic rodents.

It is worthily noticed that the differential effects of L1 and L5 on PC12 cell viability and NGF-induced neuronal differentiation are mainly associated with activation of different cell surface receptors and intracellular signaling pathways. Several properties ascribed to L5, such as highly electronegative charge, higher aggregation potential, conformationally distinct apoB, and greater content in inflammatory lipids, suggest that L5 interacts with different receptors than L1. Due to this higher electronegativity than L1, it was thought that L5 binds to the LDL receptor (LDLR) with less affinity. Avogaro et al. observed that the more electronegative LDL subfraction exhibited a lower binding capacity for LDLR [45]. This finding is similar to Benitez et al. who found that LDLR affinity was three-fold lower for LDL(−) than for native LDL [46]. The low binding affinity of L5 to LDLR may be partly explained by high nonesterified fatty acid content [46], increased degree of aggregation [47], and abnormal conformation of apoB [48]. The consequence of this loss of LDLR affinity is a diminished L5 clearance from human circulation, allowing for further deleterious effects on vascular cells and neurons.

Regarding cell surface receptor for L5 binding, Chen and coworkers reported that L5, a highly pure form of LDL(−), is a ligand for LOX-1, but not normal LDLR. L5 recognizes, signals through, and is internalized by LOX-1, which has high affinity for negatively charged ligands, whereas the less electronegative LDL subfractions L1–L4 rely on the LDLR for biological effects [15,18]. In addition to L5, LOX-1 is also activated by oxLDL, reactive oxygen species (ROS), endothelin-1, angiotensin II, advanced glycation end products, and shear stress. Previous studies have demonstrated activation of diverse downstream signaling pathways upon binding of L5 to LOX-1. For example, L5 suppresses Akt phosphorylation via LOX-1 to impair Akt-mediated growth and survival signals in bovine aortic ECs [15]. The L5/LOX-1 complex also triggers ROS production to induce oxidative stress in human aortic ECs [43], and stimulates overexpression of various adhesion molecules and inflammatory chemokines, thus promoting monocyte adherence to vascular endothelium, an early pathogenic event for atherosclerosis [49]. L5 binding to LOX-1 induces the apoptosis of human aortic ECs via p38 MAPK/caspase-3 signaling [50]. L5/LOX-1-activated platelets switch on a signaling pathway including IκB kinase 2 and nuclear factor-κB activation, which is critical for stroke pathobiology [31]. Further, we found that L5 signals to ATM/H2AX and p53/caspase-3 cascades through LOX-1, resulting in PC12 cell DNA breaks and apoptosis. Based on these findings, we conclude that LOX-1 transmits damage signals from L5 but not L1, thereby accounting for the unique cytotoxic effects of L5 in PC12 cells.

Once DNA damage such as DSBs is elicited by genotoxic insults like radiation and free radicals, apoptosis may be activated if this damage is not repaired [22]. We identified L5 as a genotoxic agent that injures PC12 cells through DNA DSBs and apoptotic death, and further found out the intermediary signaling pathways. Several lines of evidence suggest that ATM is activated in response to DNA damage, which then promotes H2AX phosphorylation at DSB sites (manifested as nuclear foci) for initiation of DSB repair [21,22]. As expected, γH2AX foci formation was observed by immunofluorescence, and increased phosphorylation levels of both ATM and H2AX were revealed by western blotting after L5 stimulation. In addition, activated p53 exerts pro-apoptotic effects by transcriptionally activating genes involved in cell cycle arrest, inhibition of proliferation, and induction of senescence, all of which are conducive to the maintenance of genomic integrity following genotoxic insults [51]. Indeed, we found that L5 rapidly triggers p53 phosphorylation accompanied by caspase-3 activation and PC12 cell apoptosis. This finding was further verified by the p53 inhibitor PFT-α, which effectively lowered the cleaved caspase-3 level and inhibited apoptosis.

In this study, L5-induced PC12 cell apoptosis also relied on LOX-1 expression, as evidenced by the reduction of L5-elevated caspase-3 cleavage and p53 accumulation levels in cells transfected with LOX-1 siRNA. These results concur with those of Li et al. who reported that LOX-1 is mainly found in cortical neurons, and its upregulation is involved in neuronal apoptosis [52]. To mediate L5 cytotoxicity, we speculate that unknown intracellular transmitters triggered by L5/LOX-1 complex should signal to ATM/H2AX and p53/caspase-3 cascades, followed by DNA breaks and apoptotic death in PC12 cells. Of note, L5 but not L1 has been indicated to rapidly elicit ROS production via LOX-1 and functions similarly to oxLDL in inducing oxidative stress [43]. Moreover, ROS is able to directly evoke p53-dependent apoptosis in PC12 cells [53], and the accumulation of ROS caused by polyQ proteins activates ATM/ATR-dependent DNA damage response [54]. ATM acts upstream of p53 in a signal transduction pathway initiated by ionizing radiation and can directly activate/phosphorylate p53 in vivo [24]. Thus, it is possible that ROS serves as a stress signal transmitter that connects the L5/LOX-1 complex to ATM/H2AX and p53/caspase-3 pathways in our PC12 cell model. Further work is required to verify this inference.

Morphological differentiation of neurons is essential for cell-cell communication and information processing. Differentiation begins with neurite sprouting, followed by progressive elongation of axons and elaboration of dendrites. Regarding this, we found that L5 impaired NGF-induced neurite outgrowth through weakening Akt phosphorylation. Actually, PI3K/Akt cascade has been suggested to be critical for NGF-induced PC12 cell differentiation [55,56]. Moreover, LOX-1 knockdown abolished L5-mediated inhibition of Akt activation by NGF, indicating that L5 requires interaction with LOX-1 to inhibit NGF-elevated Akt activity. Given that NGF exerts trophic effects via TrkA binding, it was expected that L5/LOX-1 would interfere with NGF-induced neuronal differentiation by disrupting TrkA. TrkA phosphorylation at specific sites is required for activation of various kinase pathways (Tyr490 for Shc/Ras/MAPK, Tyr751 for PI3K/Akt, Tyr785 for PLCγ/PKC/MAPK) and elevated TrkA kinase activity (Tyr674/675) [29]. However, L5 had no effect on overall phosphotyrosine status after NGF stimulation or on NGF-induced ERK, JNK, and p38 activation. This illustrates that L5/LOX-1 selectively weakens intracellular PI3K/Akt signaling, but not TrkA receptor activity or downstream MAPK pathways. Our findings agree with previous evidence indicating that L5 executes its biological effects via PI3K/Akt. For example, L5 activates CXCR2/PI3K/NFκB signaling, indirectly inducing cardiomyocyte apoptosis [57]. In ECs and endothelial progenitor cells as well, the PI3k/Akt pathway is inhibited by L5/LOX-1 [15,58]. Although our findings indicate that L5/LOX-1 suppresses TrkA/PI3K/Akt-associated neuronal differentiation in PC12 cells, more detailed mechanisms are still unclear at the present stage. Profound studies are needed in the future.

In summary, our findings reveal, for the first time, the direct cytotoxicity of LDL(−), especially fraction L5, to neuron-like PC12 cells. We demonstrate that L5 concentration- and time-dependently reduces cell viability by inducing ATM/H2AX-associated DNA damage and LOX-1/p53/caspase-3-dependent apoptosis; moreover, sublytic concentration of L5 inhibits NGF-induced neuronal differentiation by LOX-1-mediated suppression of the PI3K/Akt cascade (Figure 9). High circulating LDL is strongly implicated in the pathophysiology of neurodegenerative disorders such as AD-type dementia. Therefore, lowering plasma LDL(−) and inhibiting electronegative modification of LDL should be considered primary prevention measures for cognitive impairment and AD.

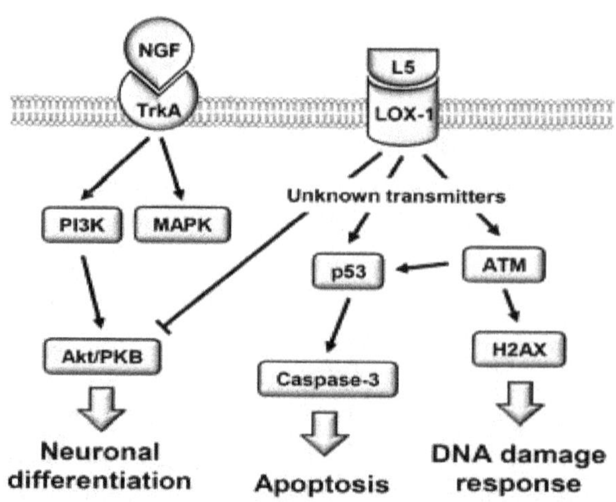

Figure 9. A schematic illustration shows the L5-induced cytotoxicity in PC12 cells. Through LOX-1 and unknown transmitters, L5 particle triggers ATM/H2AX-associated DNA damage response, activates p53/caspase 3-dependent apoptosis, and impairs NGF-induced neuronal differentiation (i.e., the suppression of NGF-activated PI3K/Akt cascade).

4. Materials and Methods

4.1. Chemicals, Antibodies, Kits and Reagents

All chemicals were from Sigma-Aldrich (Saint Louis, MO, USA) unless stated otherwise. Comet assay kits, reagents and slides were purchased from Trevigen (Gaithersburg, MD, USA). Antibodies, including phospho-ERK (pERK), pJNK, pp38, pAkt, pp53, pTrkA, ERK, JNK, p38, p53, ATM, H2AX, Egr-1, NF-M, TrkA, and cleaved caspase-3 were purchased from Cell Signaling Technology (Beverly, MA, USA). The pATM and γH2AX antibodies were obtained from Millipore (Billerica, MA, USA). Akt, LOX-1 and GAPDH antibodies, and siRNA were obtained from Santa Cruz Biotechnology (Santa Cruz, CA, USA). Alexa Fluor 488-conjugated antibody and Lipofectamine 2000 reagent were purchased from ThermoFisher Scientific (Waltham, MA, USA). Recombinant human β-NGF and caspase inhibitor Z-VAD-FMK were purchased from R & D System (Minneapolis, MN, USA). Horseradish peroxidase-conjugated anti-mouse and anti-rabbit IgG antibodies were purchased from Jackson ImmunoResearch Laboratories (West Grove, PA, USA). All cell culture reagents were obtained from Gibco-BRL/Invitrogen (Carlsbad, CA, USA).

4.2. Obtainment of Human Plasma LDL

Plasma LDL was obtained from blood samples of hypercholesterolemic patients (diagnosed by physicians) in Kaohsiung Medical University (KMU) Hospital. All participants provided written consent, and ethics committees (Institutional Review Board of KMU Hospital) reviewed and approved the consent procedure. The preparation of LDL particles was at Lipid Science and Aging Research Center (LSARC) of KMU, Kaohsiung, Taiwan. Initially, LDL isolation was done by sequential potassium bromide density centrifugation. The yielding LDL at a density of 1.019 to 1.063 g/mL was treated with 5 mM EDTA and nitrogen to avoid ex vivo oxidation. After removing salts by dialysis (20 mM Tris-HCl [pH 8.0], 0.5 mM EDTA and 0.01% NaN_3), LDL was further separated into subfractions of L1 to L5 according to electrical charge by using a fast protein liquid chromatography with a UnoQ12 column (Bio-Rad Laboratories, Inc., Hercules, CA, USA), as described previously [18,59]. OxLDL was prepared by incubating L5-free LDL (L1) with 5 μM $CuSO_4$ at 37 °C for 24 h. All LDL particles were sterilized by passing through 0.22 μm filters before using for cell experiments.

4.3. Cell Culture

Rat PC12 cells (American Type Culture Collection, Rockville, MD, USA) were grown as monolayer cultures and maintained in Dulbecco's modified Eagle's medium (DMEM) containing 10% horse serum, 5% heat-inactivated fetal bovine serum, and 1% penicillin/streptomycin. In order to induce morphological differentiation, cells (5×10^4 cells/mL) were first subcultured in multiwell culture plates previously coated with poly-L-lysine (0.1 mg/mL). One day later, cells were rinsed once with fresh DMEM, followed by NGF (50 ng/mL) treatment for the indicated time periods in low serum medium composed of DMEM, 1% horse serum, and 1% penicillin/streptomycin. The medium containing NGF was replaced every 2 days when long-term treatment was executed.

4.4. MTT Reduction Assay

For the determination of cell viability, a biochemical method based on 3-(4, 5-dimethylthianol-2-yl)-2, 5-diphenyltetrazolium bromide (MTT) reduction was used to assay the metabolic activity of cultured cells. Stock MTT solution (5 mg/mL) was added to all cell-containing wells and diluted to a final concentration of 0.5 mg/mL. After incubation at 37 °C for 2 h, the MTT-containing cell medium was removed. The purple formazan crystals yielded by the action of mitochondrial dehydrogenase was dissolved with dimethyl sulfoxide and quantified spectrophotometrically. The light absorbance values at 570 nm against a 630 nm reference wavelength (ΔOD; OD: optical density) were recorded. The cell survival percentage is calculated by the formula: (viable cells) % = (ΔOD of treated sample/ΔOD of untreated control) × 100. The untreated control well was assigned a percentage value of 100% cell survival.

4.5. siRNA Transfection

Cells were cultured in growth medium without antibiotics for 24 h prior to transfection. According to the manufacturer's protocol, transfection of siRNA duplex (100 pmol) in 6-well culture plates was performed using Lipofectamine 2000 reagent and Opti-MEM. After maintaining transfected cells for 6 h, the culture medium was replaced with fresh growth medium. Western blotting was used for determining the knockdown effect of siRNA on target protein. All siRNA oligos were designed and synthesized by Santa Cruz Biotechnology. Rat LOX-1 siRNA (sc-156076) is a pool of 3 target-specific 19–25 nt siRNAs. The specific sequences are as follows: (i) LOX-1 siRNA-1 sense, 5′-CUGUAAGCUACUACAUAGATT-3′ and antisense, 5′-UCUAUGUAGUAGCUUACAGTT-3′; (ii) LOX-1 siRNA-2 sense, 5′-CCAUUAUGCUAGAGGUAAUTT-3′ and antisense, 5′-AUUACCUCUAGCAUAAUGGTT-3′; (iii) LOX-1 siRNA-3 sense, 5′-CUAGAACAAACACCAAUCUTT-3′ and antisense, 5′-AGAUUGGUGUUUGUUCUAGTT-3′. Control siRNA (sc-37007) is a non-targeting 20–25 nt siRNA designed as a negative control and leads to no degradation of any known cellular mRNA. The manufacturer does not offer the sequence of scrambled control siRNA.

4.6. Comet Assay

A neutral comet assay (single cell gel electrophoresis assay) was used to detect DSBs, as per the manufacturer's instructions. After finishing electrophoresis, at least 50 randomly selected images were analyzed from each treatment group under a fluorescence microscope (Nikon ECLIPSE Ts2 microscope, Nikon, Inc., Melville, NY, USA) equipped with a fluorescein isothiocyanate filter set. Images were captured using a cooled CCD camera (Spot, Diagnostic Instruments, Sterling Heights, MI, USA). As an informative and reliable DNA damage parameter, the Olive tail moment, which is defined as the product of the amount of DNA in the tail (fraction of total DNA in the comet tail) and the mean distance of migration in the tail (comet tail length), was calculated. The quantifications of the comet tail length and olive tail moment were conducted using the COMETscore.v1.5 image processing software.

4.7. Immunofluorescence Detection of DNA DSBs

Cultures grown on coverslips were subjected to immunostaining. To detect DNA DSBs, cells were fixed in 4% paraformaldehyde, permeabilized with 0.3% Triton X-100 in phosphate buffered saline, and then incubated with 5% normal goat serum to block nonspecific binding. Subsequently, an antibody against phosphorylated H2AX (γH2AX, 1:200 dilution) was used overnight at 4 °C, followed by the corresponding secondary antibody conjugated to Alexa Fluor 488. The nuclei were observable by labelling with 4′, 6-diamidino-2-phenylindole (DAPI). After rinsing the labelled cells with phosphate buffered saline and mounting slides with an anti-fading aqueous medium, observation was carried out under a fluorescent microscope equipped with appropriate filters and a digital camera.

4.8. Western Blotting Analysis

Cells were collected and homogenized in ice-cold RIPA buffer as described previously [59]. After a 20-min incubation at 4 °C, cell extracts were centrifuged at 14,000× *g* for 10 min and protein concentration in the supernatant was determined with a Bio-Rad protein assay (Bio-Rad, Hercules, CA, USA). Cell lysates (40 μg/lane) were separated by electrophoresis through 8–12% SDS-polyacrylamide gels and then electroblotted to 0.45 μm PVDF membranes (Millipore, Bedford, MA, USA) using a semi-dry transfer apparatus (Hoefer Scientific Instruments, San Francisco, CA, USA). Membranes were blocked in 5% non-fat dry skim milk for 1 h at room temperature, followed by immunoblotting for desired proteins with the assist of specific primary a ntibodies and appropriate HRP-conjugated secondary antibodies. Protein bands developed on the X-ray film were visualized by an enhanced chemiluminescence kit (Amersham Biosciences, Piscataway, NJ, USA). Analyses of protein band densities were performed using an Image J software (NIH, Bethesda, MD, USA).

4.9. Statistical Analysis

Treatment group means were compared by ANOVA, followed by Dunnett's test or Bonferroni's *t*-test for pair-wise comparisons. Paired groups were compared by Student's *t*-test. All results are expressed as the mean ± standard error of the mean (SEM). Differences were considered significant when the probability value was less than 0.05 ($p < 0.05$). SigmaStat version 4.0 software (Jandel Scientific, San Diego, CA, USA) was used for all statistical analyses.

Acknowledgments: We are grateful to KMU-LSARC for providing us with LDL particles, including L1, L5, and oxLDL, and excellent technical assistances. This work was supported by grants (MOST 104-2314-B-037-069 owned by Jiz-Yuh Wang and MOST 104-2320-B-570-002 owned by Ching-Tien Lee from the Ministry of Science and Technology, Taipei, Taiwan; and grants (KMU-M106005 owned by Jiz-Yuh Wang and KMU-TP103D02 owned by Chiou-Lian Lai from KMU, Kaohsiung, Taiwan.

Author Contributions: Jiz-Yuh Wang designed and supervised experiments and wrote the paper. Ching-Tien Lee and Chen-Yen Lin performed experiments and data analysis. Chiou-Lian Lai contributed valuable suggestions and critically revised the manuscript for important intellectual content. Submission of the final manuscript was endorsed by all authors.

Abbreviations

AD	Alzheimer's disease
ApoB	Apolipoprotein B
ATM	Ataxia-telangiectasia mutated
BBB	Blood-brain barrier
CSF	Cerebrospinal fluid
CVD	Cardiovascular disease
DAPI	4′,6-Diamidino-2-phenylindole
DMEM	Dulbecco's modified Eagle's medium
DSBs	Double strand breaks
EC	Endothelial cell
Egr-1	Early growth response-1
ERK	Extracellular signal-regulated kinase
JNK	c-JUN NH2-terminal protein kinase
LDL	Low-density lipoprotein
LDL(−)	Electronegative low-density lipoprotein
LDL-C	LDL-cholesterol
LDLR	LDL receptor
LOX-1	Lectin-like oxidized low-density lipoprotein receptor-1
MAPKs	Mitogen-activated protein kinases
MTT	3-(4,5-Dimethylthianol-2-yl)-2,5 diphenyltetrazolium bromide
NGF	Nerve growth factor
NF-M	Neurofilament-medium
OxLDL	Oxidized LDL
PFT-α	Pifithrin-α

References

1. Stampfer, M.J. Cardiovascular disease and Alzheimer's disease: Common links. *J. Intern. Med.* **2006**, *260*, 211–223. [CrossRef] [PubMed]
2. Kalaria, R.N. Arteriosclerosis, apolipoprotein E, and Alzheimer's disease. *Lancet* **1997**, *349*, 1174. [CrossRef]

3. Luchsinger, J.A.; Mayeux, R. Cardiovascular risk factors and Alzheimer's disease. *Curr. Atheroscler. Rep.* **2004**, *6*, 261–266. [CrossRef] [PubMed]
4. Kuo, Y.M.; Emmerling, M.R.; Bisgaier, C.L.; Essenburg, A.D.; Lampert, H.C.; Drumm, D.; Roher, A.E. Elevated low-density lipoprotein in Alzheimer's disease correlates with brain abeta 1–42 levels. *Biochem. Biophys. Res. Commun.* **1998**, *252*, 711–715. [CrossRef] [PubMed]
5. Refolo, L.M.; Malester, B.; LaFrancois, J.; Bryant-Thomas, T.; Wang, R.; Tint, G.S.; Sambamurti, K.; Duff, K.; Pappolla, M.A. Hypercholesterolemia accelerates the Alzheimer's amyloid pathology in a transgenic mouse model. *Neurobiol. Dis.* **2000**, *7*, 321–331. [CrossRef] [PubMed]
6. Kivipelto, M.; Laakso, M.P.; Tuomilehto, J.; Nissinen, A.; Soininen, H. Hypertension and hypercholesterolaemia as risk factors for Alzheimer's disease: Potential for pharmacological intervention. *CNS Drugs* **2002**, *16*, 435–444. [CrossRef] [PubMed]
7. Lai, C.L.; Hsu, C.Y.; Liou, L.M.; Hsieh, H.Y.; Hsieh, Y.H.; Liu, C.K. Effect of cholesterol and CYP46 polymorphism on cognitive event-related potentials. *Psychophysiology* **2011**, *48*, 1572–1577. [CrossRef] [PubMed]
8. Taylor, V.H.; MacQueen, G.M. Cognitive dysfunction associated with metabolic syndrome. *Obes. Rev.* **2007**, *8*, 409–418. [CrossRef] [PubMed]
9. Helzner, E.P.; Luchsinger, J.A.; Scarmeas, N.; Cosentino, S.; Brickman, A.M.; Glymour, M.M.; Stern, Y. Contribution of vascular risk factors to the progression in Alzheimer disease. *Arch. Neurol.* **2009**, *66*, 343–348. [CrossRef] [PubMed]
10. Smith, C.C.; Stanyer, L.; Betteridge, D.J.; Cooper, M.B. Native and oxidized low-density lipoproteins modulate the vasoactive actions of soluble beta-amyloid peptides in rat aorta. *Clin. Sci.* **2007**, *113*, 427–434. [CrossRef] [PubMed]
11. Griffiths, H.; Irundika, D.; Lip, G.; Spickett, C.; Polidori, C. Oxidised LDL lipids, statins and a blood-brain barrier. *Free Radic. Biol. Med.* **2014**, *75*, S15–S16. [CrossRef] [PubMed]
12. Kuller, L.H. Statins and dementia. *Curr. Atheroscler. Rep.* **2007**, *9*, 154–161. [CrossRef] [PubMed]
13. Sanchez-Quesada, J.L.; Benitez, S.; Ordonez-Llanos, J. Electronegative low-density lipoprotein. *Curr. Opin. Lipidol.* **2004**, *15*, 329–335. [CrossRef] [PubMed]
14. Sanchez-Quesada, J.L.; Estruch, M.; Benitez, S.; Ordonez-Llanos, J. Electronegative LDL: A useful biomarker of cardiovascular risk? *Clin. Lipidol.* **2012**, *7*, 345–359. [CrossRef]
15. Lu, J.; Yang, J.H.; Burns, A.R.; Chen, H.H.; Tang, D.; Walterscheid, J.P.; Suzuki, S.; Yang, C.Y.; Sawamura, T.; Chen, C.H. Mediation of electronegative low-density lipoprotein signaling by LOX-1: A possible mechanism of endothelial apoptosis. *Circ. Res.* **2009**, *104*, 619–627. [CrossRef] [PubMed]
16. Chen, H.H.; Hosken, B.D.; Huang, M.; Gaubatz, J.W.; Myers, C.L.; Macfarlane, R.D.; Pownall, H.J.; Yang, C.Y. Electronegative LDLs from familial hypercholesterolemic patients are physicochemically heterogeneous but uniformly proapoptotic. *J. Lipid Res.* **2007**, *48*, 177–184. [CrossRef] [PubMed]
17. Chen, C.H.; Jiang, T.; Yang, J.H.; Jiang, W.; Lu, J.; Marathe, G.K.; Pownall, H.J.; Ballantyne, C.M.; McIntyre, T.M.; Henry, P.D.; et al. Low-density lipoprotein in hypercholesterolemic human plasma induces vascular endothelial cell apoptosis by inhibiting fibroblast growth factor 2 transcription. *Circulation* **2003**, *107*, 2102–2108. [CrossRef] [PubMed]
18. Ke, L.Y.; Engler, D.A.; Lu, J.; Matsunami, R.K.; Chan, H.C.; Wang, G.J.; Yang, C.Y.; Chang, J.G.; Chen, C.H. Chemical composition-oriented receptor selectivity of L5, a naturally occurring atherogenic low-density lipoprotein. *Pure Appl. Chem.* **2011**, *83*, 1731–1740. [CrossRef] [PubMed]
19. Lee, T.; Chau, L. Fas/Fas ligand-mediated death pathway is involved in oxLDL-induced apoptosis in vascular smooth muscle cells. *Am. J. Physiol. Cell Physiol.* **2001**, *280*, C709–C718. [PubMed]
20. Maziere, C.; Meignotte, A.; Dantin, F.; Conte, M.A.; Maziere, J.C. Oxidized LDL induces an oxidative stress and activates the tumor suppressor p53 in MRC5 human fibroblasts. *Biochem. Biophys. Res. Commun.* **2000**, *276*, 718–723. [CrossRef] [PubMed]
21. Burma, S.; Chen, B.P.; Murphy, M.; Kurimasa, A.; Chen, D.J. ATM phosphorylates histone H2AX in response to DNA double-strand breaks. *J. Biol. Chem.* **2001**, *276*, 42462–42467. [CrossRef] [PubMed]
22. Roos, W.P.; Kaina, B. DNA damage-induced cell death by apoptosis. *Trends Mol. Med.* **2006**, *12*, 440–450. [CrossRef] [PubMed]
23. Kaina, B. DNA damage-triggered apoptosis: Critical role of DNA repair, double-strand breaks, cell proliferation and signaling. *Biochem. Pharmacol.* **2003**, *66*, 1547–1554. [CrossRef]

24. Canman, C.E.; Lim, D.S.; Cimprich, K.A.; Taya, Y.; Tamai, K.; Sakaguchi, K.; Appella, E.; Kastan, M.B.; Siliciano, J.D. Activation of the ATM kinase by ionizing radiation and phosphorylation of p53. *Science* **1998**, *281*, 1677–1679. [CrossRef] [PubMed]
25. Shieh, S.Y.; Ikeda, M.; Taya, Y.; Prives, C. DNA damage-induced phosphorylation of p53 alleviates inhibition by MDM2. *Cell* **1997**, *91*, 325–334. [CrossRef]
26. Honda, R.; Tanaka, H.; Yasuda, H. Oncoprotein MDM2 is a ubiquitin ligase E3 for tumor suppressor p53. *FEBS Lett.* **1997**, *420*, 25–27. [CrossRef]
27. Beckmann, A.M.; Wilce, P.A. Egr transcription factors in the nervous system. *Neurochem. Int.* **1997**, *31*, 477–510. [CrossRef]
28. Al-Chalabi, A.; Miller, C.C. Neurofilaments and neurological disease. *Bioessays* **2003**, *25*, 346–355. [CrossRef] [PubMed]
29. Longo, F.M.; Massa, S.M. Small-molecule modulation of neurotrophin receptors: A strategy for the treatment of neurological disease. *Nat. Rev. Drug Discov.* **2013**, *12*, 507–525. [CrossRef] [PubMed]
30. Shen, M.Y.; Chen, F.Y.; Hsu, J.F.; Fu, R.H.; Chang, C.M.; Chang, C.T.; Liu, C.H.; Wu, J.R.; Lee, A.S.; Chan, H.C.; et al. Plasma L5 levels are elevated in ischemic stroke patients and enhance platelet aggregation. *Blood* **2016**, *127*, 1336–1345. [CrossRef] [PubMed]
31. Podrez, E.A.; Byzova, T.V. Prothrombotic lipoprotein patterns in stroke. *Blood* **2016**, *127*, 1221–1222. [CrossRef] [PubMed]
32. Kay, A.D.; Day, S.P.; Nicoll, J.A.; Packard, C.J.; Caslake, M.J. Remodelling of cerebrospinal fluid lipoproteins after subarachnoid hemorrhage. *Atherosclerosis* **2003**, *170*, 141–146. [CrossRef]
33. Salen, G.; Berginer, V.; Shore, V.; Horak, I.; Horak, E.; Tint, G.S.; Shefer, S. Increased concentrations of cholestanol and apolipoprotein B in the cerebrospinal fluid of patients with cerebrotendinous xanthomatosis. Effect of chenodeoxycholic acid. *N. Engl. J. Med.* **1987**, *316*, 1233–1238. [CrossRef] [PubMed]
34. Mu, J.; Yang, Y.; Chen, J.; Cheng, K.; Li, Q.; Wei, Y.; Zhu, D.; Shao, W.; Zheng, P.; Xie, P. Elevated host lipid metabolism revealed by iTRAQ-based quantitative proteomic analysis of cerebrospinal fluid of tuberculous meningitis patients. *Biochem. Biophys. Res. Commun.* **2015**, *466*, 689–695. [CrossRef] [PubMed]
35. Takechi, R.; Galloway, S.; Pallebage-Gamarallage, M.; Wellington, C.; Johnsen, R.; Mamo, J.C. Three-dimensional colocalization analysis of plasma-derived apolipoprotein B with amyloid plaques in APP/PS1 transgenic mice. *Histochem. Cell Biol.* **2009**, *131*, 661–666. [CrossRef] [PubMed]
36. Takechi, R.; Galloway, S.; Pallebage-Gamarallage, M.M.; Wellington, C.L.; Johnsen, R.D.; Dhaliwal, S.S.; Mamo, J.C. Differential effects of dietary fatty acids on the cerebral distribution of plasma-derived apo B lipoproteins with amyloid-beta. *Br. J. Nutr.* **2010**, *103*, 652–662. [CrossRef] [PubMed]
37. Yang, Y.; Rosenberg, G.A. Blood-brain barrier breakdown in acute and chronic cerebrovascular disease. *Stroke* **2011**, *42*, 3323–3328. [CrossRef] [PubMed]
38. Szczepanska-Sadowska, E.; Cudnoch-Jedrzejewska, A.; Ufnal, M.; Zera, T. Brain and cardiovascular diseases: Common neurogenic background of cardiovascular, metabolic and inflammatory diseases. *J. Physiol. Pharmacol.* **2010**, *61*, 509–521. [PubMed]
39. Kerkar, S.; Williams, M.; Blocksom, J.M.; Wilson, R.F.; Tyburski, J.G.; Steffes, C.P. TNF-alpha and IL-1beta increase pericyte/endothelial cell co-culture permeability. *J. Surg. Res.* **2006**, *132*, 40–45. [CrossRef] [PubMed]
40. de Vries, H.E.; Blom-Roosemalen, M.C.; van Oosten, M.; de Boer, A.G.; van Berkel, T.J.; Breimer, D.D.; Kuiper, J. The influence of cytokines on the integrity of the blood-brain barrier in vitro. *J. Neuroimmunol.* **1996**, *64*, 37–43. [CrossRef]
41. Zenaro, E.; Piacentino, G.; Constantin, G. The blood-brain barrier in Alzheimer's disease. *Neurobiol. Dis.* **2016**. [CrossRef] [PubMed]
42. Kalaria, R.N.; Hedera, P. beta-Amyloid vasoactivity in Alzheimer's disease. *Lancet* **1996**, *347*, 1492–1493. [PubMed]
43. Chu, C.S.; Wang, Y.C.; Lu, L.S.; Walton, B.; Yilmaz, H.R.; Huang, R.Y.; Sawamura, T.; Dixon, R.A.; Lai, W.T.; Chen, C.H.; et al. Electronegative low-density lipoprotein increases C-reactive protein expression in vascular endothelial cells through the LOX-1 receptor. *PLoS ONE* **2013**, *8*, e70533. [CrossRef] [PubMed]
44. Estruch, M.; Bancells, C.; Beloki, L.; Sanchez-Quesada, J.L.; Ordonez-Llanos, J.; Benitez, S. CD14 and TLR4 mediate cytokine release promoted by electronegative LDL in monocytes. *Atherosclerosis* **2013**, *229*, 356–362. [CrossRef] [PubMed]
45. Avogaro, P.; Bon, G.B.; Cazzolato, G. Presence of a modified low density lipoprotein in humans. *Arteriosclerosis* **1988**, *8*, 79–87. [CrossRef] [PubMed]

46. Benitez, S.; Villegas, V.; Bancells, C.; Jorba, O.; Gonzalez-Sastre, F.; Ordonez-Llanos, J.; Sanchez-Quesada, J.L. Impaired binding affinity of electronegative low-density lipoprotein (LDL) to the LDL receptor is related to nonesterified fatty acids and lysophosphatidylcholine content. *Biochemistry* **2004**, *43*, 15863–15872. [CrossRef] [PubMed]
47. Bancells, C.; Villegas, S.; Blanco, F.J.; Benitez, S.; Gallego, I.; Beloki, L.; Perez-Cuellar, M.; Ordonez-Llanos, J.; Sanchez-Quesada, J.L. Aggregated electronegative low density lipoprotein in human plasma shows a high tendency toward phospholipolysis and particle fusion. *J. Biol. Chem.* **2010**, *285*, 32425–32435. [CrossRef] [PubMed]
48. Bancells, C.; Benitez, S.; Ordonez-Llanos, J.; Oorni, K.; Kovanen, P.T.; Milne, R.W.; Sanchez-Quesada, J.L. Immunochemical analysis of the electronegative LDL subfraction shows that abnormal N-terminal apolipoprotein B conformation is involved in increased binding to proteoglycans. *J. Biol. Chem.* **2011**, *286*, 1125–1133. [CrossRef] [PubMed]
49. Abe, Y.; Fornage, M.; Yang, C.Y.; Bui-Thanh, N.A.; Wise, V.; Chen, H.H.; Rangaraj, G.; Ballantyne, C.M. L5, the most electronegative subfraction of plasma LDL, induces endothelial vascular cell adhesion molecule 1 and CXC chemokines, which mediate mononuclear leukocyte adhesion. *Atherosclerosis* **2007**, *192*, 56–66. [CrossRef] [PubMed]
50. Chen, W.Y.; Chen, F.Y.; Lee, A.S.; Ting, K.H.; Chang, C.M.; Hsu, J.F.; Lee, W.S.; Sheu, J.R.; Chen, C.H.; Shen, M.Y. Sesamol reduces the atherogenicity of electronegative L5 LDL in vivo and in vitro. *J. Nat. Prod.* **2015**, *78*, 225–233. [CrossRef] [PubMed]
51. Symonds, H.; Krall, L.; Remington, L.; Saenz-Robles, M.; Lowe, S.; Jacks, T.; van Dyke, T. p53-dependent apoptosis suppresses tumor growth and progression in vivo. *Cell* **1994**, *78*, 703–711. [CrossRef]
52. Li, Y.; Duan, Z.; Gao, D.; Huang, S.; Yuan, H.; Niu, X. The new role of LOX-1 in hypertension induced neuronal apoptosis. *Biochem. Biophys. Res. Commun.* **2012**, *425*, 735–740. [CrossRef] [PubMed]
53. Zhou, L.J.; Zhu, X.Z. Reactive oxygen species-induced apoptosis in PC12 cells and protective effect of bilobalide. *J. Pharmacol. Exp. Ther.* **2000**, *293*, 982–988. [PubMed]
54. Giuliano, P.; De Cristofaro, T.; Affaitati, A.; Pizzulo, G.M.; Feliciello, A.; Criscuolo, C.; De Michele, G.; Filla, A.; Avvedimento, E.V.; Varrone, S. DNA damage induced by polyglutamine-expanded proteins. *Human Mol. Genet.* **2003**, *12*, 2301–2309. [CrossRef] [PubMed]
55. Kim, Y.; Seger, R.; Suresh Babu, C.V.; Hwang, S.Y.; Yoo, Y.S. A positive role of the PI3-K/Akt signaling pathway in PC12 cell differentiation. *Mol. Cells* **2004**, *18*, 353–359. [PubMed]
56. Read, D.E.; Gorman, A.M. Involvement of Akt in neurite outgrowth. *Cell Mol. Life Sci.* **2009**, *66*, 2975–2984. [CrossRef] [PubMed]
57. Lee, A.S.; Wang, G.J.; Chan, H.C.; Chen, F.Y.; Chang, C.M.; Yang, C.Y.; Lee, Y.T.; Chang, K.C.; Chen, C.H. Electronegative low-density lipoprotein induces cardiomyocyte apoptosis indirectly through endothelial cell-released chemokines. *Apoptosis* **2012**, *17*, 1009–1018. [CrossRef] [PubMed]
58. Tang, D.; Lu, J.; Walterscheid, J.P.; Chen, H.H.; Engler, D.A.; Sawamura, T.; Chang, P.Y.; Safi, H.J.; Yang, C.Y.; Chen, C.H. Electronegative LDL circulating in smokers impairs endothelial progenitor cell differentiation by inhibiting Akt phosphorylation via LOX-1. *J. Lipid Res.* **2008**, *49*, 33–47. [CrossRef] [PubMed]
59. Yu, L.E.; Lai, C.L.; Lee, C.T.; Wang, J.Y. Highly electronegative low-density lipoprotein L5 evokes microglial activation and creates a neuroinflammatory stress via Toll-like receptor 4 signaling. *J. Neurochem.* **2017**, *142*, 231–245. [CrossRef] [PubMed]

12

Functional Cognitive Disorder: Diagnostic Challenges and Future Directions

Catherine Pennington [1,2,*], Harriet Ball [1] and Marta Swirski [1]

1 ReMemBr Group, University of Bristol, Bristol Brain Centre, Southmead Hospital, Southmead Road, BS10 5NB Bristol, UK; harriet.ball@bristol.ac.uk (H.B.); Marta.swirski@nbt.nhs.uk (M.S.)
2 Centre for Dementia Prevention, University of Edinburgh, 9A Bioquarter, 9 Little France Road, Edinburgh EH16 4UX, UK
* Correspondence: c.pennington@nhs.net

Abstract: Functional cognitive disorder describes patients with persistent, troublesome subjective cognitive complaints that are inconsistent with a recognized disease process, and where significant discrepancies are found between subjective and objectively observed cognitive functioning. The etiology is heterogeneous and potentially related to underlying psychological factors. Making a diagnosis of functional cognitive disorder can be challenging and there is the potential for misdiagnosis of early-stage neurodegeneration. We compared neuropsychological findings in three groups: functional cognitive disorder (FCD), mild cognitive impairment (MCI), and healthy controls. Participants were recruited from the ReMemBr Group Clinic, North Bristol NHS Trust, and via Join Dementia Research. Both the FCD and MCI groups showed elevated prospective and retrospective memory symptom scores. Performance on the Montreal cognitive assessment was equivalent in the FCD and MCI groups, both being impaired compared with the controls. The FCD group was younger than those with MCI. We discuss challenges and controversies in the diagnosis of functional cognitive disorder, alongside illustrative cases and proposals for areas of research priority.

Keywords: functional cognitive disorder; neurodegeneration; mild cognitive impairment; functional neurological disorder cognition

---

1. Introduction

Functional cognitive disorder (FCD) describes patients presenting with significant subjective cognitive symptoms that are out of keeping with their observed level of cognitive functioning and not compatible with a recognizable neurodegenerative, psychiatric, or systemic primary cause [1]. In order to make a diagnosis of FCD, a marked discrepancy between self-reported cognitive symptomatology and observed or reported cognitive functioning must be present. This internal inconsistency in symptoms is evident on comparison of symptom severity with performance on neuropsychological testing or everyday "real world' cognitive ability. For example, above average performance on list learning tasks, or continued work in a skilled profession without difficulty, is inconsistent with a self-report of complete inability to recall any new information over a short time period. The etiology is heterogeneous and likely to be related to underlying psychological factors. FCD is a relatively recently described clinical entity and exists within an expanding spectrum of cognitive diagnoses, which range in severity from subjective cognitive decline (SCD) through to severe dementia. FCD is distinguished from SCD by the presence of significant inconsistency between subjective and objectively observed cognitive functioning, a greater severity of self-reported symptomatology, and resistance to reassurance that observed cognitive functioning is intact. Diagnosing FCD currently relies on expert opinion from a specialist in cognitive disorders. The optimal diagnostic criteria and management strategies for FCD are still areas of debate, and longitudinal studies of prognosis and rate of diagnostic change are lacking. Particular areas of interest are the potential for misdiagnosis of early-stage neurodegeneration, or multifactorial cognitive impairment. The prevalence of FCD is still under investigation and will vary depending on the population being studied. A review of patients attending a tertiary referral cognitive disorders clinic found a third of those aged 60 years or less to have a functional diagnosis [2]. SCD is extremely common, particularly in aging populations. A German LIFE study found that 53% of adults aged 40–79 years reported subjective memory concerns [3], whilst a USA survey identified cognitive concerns in 11.1% of adults over 45 years [4]. The SCD literature has suffered from variable terminology and definitions, which makes estimating true prevalence and incidence difficult.

Some individuals may manifest cognitive symptomatology due to a combination of etiological factors, corresponding to the concept of "functional overlay" seen in systematic and functional neurological conditions, whereby core symptoms caused by an underlying structural disease process are complicated by additional functional features [5]. A dual diagnosis of both epilepsy and psychogenic nonepileptic seizures is not uncommon [6], and individuals with chronic conditions such as multiple sclerosis may manifest additional functional symptoms, which can be misattributed [7]. In the context of cognitive symptoms, there are significant challenges around confirming diagnosis, potential for diagnostic evolution over time, and overlapping conditions. In a clinical setting, rapid access to detailed neuropsychological testing (including effort testing) is often limited, as is the use of CSF biomarkers and advanced imaging techniques, such as amyloid PET. Therefore, the distinction between neurodegenerative and functional or alternative causes for cognitive symptoms frequently depends on a combination of self-report, collateral history, and clinician opinion. The picture is further complicated by memory complaints being a common experience for healthy older adults, and psychiatric symptoms potentially being an early feature of neurodegenerative disease [8]. Therefore, careful exploration of symptom severity, evaluation of discrepancies between self-reported and observed cognitive ability, consideration of potential contributing psychological factors, beliefs or mental health symptoms, and search for evidence of neurodegenerative, toxic, or metabolic causes of cognitive decline are required when considering a diagnosis of FCD. Additionally, a correct diagnosis of FCD does not mean an individual is immune from developing future neurodegeneration.

Here, we discuss issues around prognosis, misdiagnosis, and functional overlay symptoms in FCD. We report data and illustrative cases from a recent study of FCD and MCI patients drawn from a specialist cognitive clinic.

2. Methods

Participants with FCD or MCI were recruited from a specialist cognitive disorders clinic (ReMemBr Group, North Bristol Trust). Diagnoses were reached after clinical assessment by a consultant neurologist and clinically appropriate neuroimaging and neuropsychological assessment. The diagnoses of participants recruited from the clinic were reviewed at a multidisciplinary meeting comprising three cognitive neurologists and a consultant neuropsychologist. One patient in the FCD group did not attend for subsequent clinical follow-up, and one MCI participant was recruited from Join Dementia Research. All other FCD and MCI participants attended for additional clinical follow-up in the cognitive disorders clinic.

A diagnosis of FCD was made in patients displaying significant discrepancies between self-reported and observed cognitive functioning (on neuropsychological assessment and/or everyday functioning). Exclusion criteria were evidence of neurodegeneration, toxic or metabolic causes of cognitive decline, major psychiatric disorder, or active systemic disease that could impact cognition.

Diagnoses of MCI were made based on a clinical history of mild cognitive symptoms, consisting of preserved everyday cognitive functioning and mildly impaired performance on neuropsychological testing. Only patients with MCI felt to have a neurodegenerative cause (based on investigation findings and clinical history) were included in the present study. People with toxic or metabolic causes of cognitive decline, major psychiatric disorder, or significant systemic disease that could impact cognition were excluded from this group. One additional participant with MCI was recruited from the

Join Dementia Research database; their case notes were reviewed by a cognitive neurologist (C.P.) to confirm the diagnosis. Healthy controls (HC) were recruited from a local database of adult research volunteers and the Join Dementia Research database. Controls self-identified as having no significant cognitive complaints. We did not exclude persons with mild mood or anxiety symptoms that (in the opinion of the cognitive neurology team) would not be expected to impact cognition.

Participants underwent neuropsychological testing, and demographic data were collected. This included the Montreal Cognitive Assessment (MoCA) [9], the Test of Premorbid Functioning—UK version (ToPF) [10], and the Prospective and Retrospective Memory Questionnaire (PRMQ) [11]. The MoCA is a 30-point brief cognitive assessment, with one further bonus point awarded to adults with formal education of 12 years or less. The PRMQ is a brief questionnaire asking respondents to answer 16 questions about minor everyday memory errors, using a 5-point Likert scale (from "never" to "very often"). Half of the questions refer to prospective memory, and half to retrospective. The responses are assigned values from 5 for "very often" to 1 for "never" and summed, and total scores are a minimum of 16 and maximum of 80. The ToPF provides an estimate of premorbid IQ, based on knowledge of the pronunciation of irregularly spelt words. Subjects are asked to read words with irregular grapheme–phoneme association aloud from a stimulus card. The words increase in difficulty, and the task is finished and a score assigned when errors in pronunciation occur.

The project was given Research Ethics Committee approval by the South West—Cornwall and Plymouth Research Ethics Committee, REC reference 15/SW/0298 and IRAS project ID: 188539. All participants provided informed consent. The study was funded by the BRACE charity.

Statistical analysis was undertaken using IBM SPSS Statistics version 22 and Stata version 15.1. Group comparisons were undertaken using 1-way ANOVA, or alternative tests where data did not meet assumptions for parametric data.

3. Results

A total of 21 people with FCD, 17 with MCI, and 25 HC participated in the main study. In the FCD group, all but two participants had structural neuroimaging (CT, MRI, or both). In the MCI group, all the participants had structural imaging, and six had additional functional imaging (HMPAO SPECT or DAT). The group demographics are shown in Table 1, and analysis of group differences on the PRMQ are shown in Table 2.

Table 1. Group demographics and cognitive functioning (mean values; significant p values in bold).

	FCD	MCI	HC	FCD vs. HC p Value	FCD vs. MCI p Value	MCI vs. HC p Value
Female:Male	10:11	8:9	18:7		0.15*	
Age (years)	58.3	72.1	60.8	0.30	**<0.01**	**<0.01**
Years of Education	13.8	14.4	14.7		0.61 *	
MoCA	23.9	23.3	27.8	**<0.01**	0.52	**<0.01**
ToPF	46.5	55.1	57.2	**<0.01**	**0.04**	0.87

* No significant difference across samples found; therefore, multiple comparisons not performed. Gender: Pearson's Chi-square = 3.7, $p = 0.15$; Age: Kruskal-Wallis test. Chi-square = 12.7, df = 2, $p < 0.01$; Years of education: one-way ANOVA. F = 0.5, df = 60, 2, $p = 0.61$; MoCA: Kruskal–Wallis test. Chi-square = 19.0, df = 2, $p < 0.01$; ToPF: Kruskal–Wallis test. Chi-square = 7.6, df =2, $p = 0.02$.

3.1. Case Studies

An additional two patients were recruited into the study and completed informed consent and study procedures. A subsequent case review was performed on study completion, and diagnostic uncertainty was raised in both cases. They are presented separately from the main study cohort, to illustrate potential diagnostic difficulties and change in the cognitive clinic population.

Table 2. Mean scores on the Prospective and Retrospective Memory Questionnaire.

	FCD	MCI	HC	FCD vs. HC *p* Value	FCD vs. MCI *p* Value	MCI vs. HC *p* Value
Prospective memory (raw score)	29.2	27.6	18.6	**<0.01**	0.72	**<0.01**
Retrospective memory (raw score)	25.2	25.4	16.4	**<0.01**	1.00	**<0.01**
Total T score (Prospective + Retrospective)	33.3	35.1	54.7			

Higher raw scores indicate greater self-reported memory symptoms. Lower T scores indicate greater symptomatology. T scores have a mean of 50 and SD of 10; therefore, both FCD and MCI were both approximately 2 SD below population norms. T scores were obtained using tables in Crawford et al. 2003 (Crawford et al., 2003). Analyses were repeated as an ANCOVA (controlling for age), obtaining consistent results. One-way ANOVA with Tukey post-hoc comparisons. Prospective memory raw score, $F(2,60) = 19.91$, $p < 0.01$. Effect size η^2 0.40 Retrospective memory raw score, $F(2,60) = 16.5$, $p < 0.01$. Effect size η^2 0.35.

3.1.1. Case 1

A person in their sixties presented following several years of behavioral and cognitive changes. Symptom onset began around the time of a job change and an uncomplicated elective operation with subsequent opiate prescription. There was no evidence of excessive or dependent opiate use, and cognitive symptoms did not remit on the gradual cessation of opiates. The individual was less able to manage a complex occupation and had reduced empathy and extraversion. Episodic word finding difficulties were reported, exacerbated by fatigue. Symptoms improved during holiday periods.

Examination was notable for mild extrapyramidal signs. HMPAO SPECT showed frontal hypoperfusion. Negative investigations included blood tests for genetic and autoimmune causes of neurodegeneration.

On neuropsychological testing, the participant passed tests of performance validity. Most scores were in the average range, and a minority of subsets were in the low-average range. On subjective questionnaires, memory was self-rated as good, whereas their spouse rated it as significantly impaired. Depression, anxiety, and stress self-report scores were in the average range. An initial diagnosis of MCI was made.

On follow-up, MoCA scores showed an improving pattern (Figure 1). Neuropsychological testing was repeated after a one-year interval, and during this assessment, anxiety was evident. The patient also showed catastrophic interpretation of normal memory lapses. Cognitive performance results were stable or improved. A neuropsychiatric opinion highlighted exaggerated interpretation of normal memory lapses, and a revised diagnosis was made of SCD, and possible functional overlay. The individual remains under follow-up, and the trajectory of improved neuropsychology now points away from neurodegenerative processes.

3.1.2. Case 2

A person in their fifties was referred for investigation of cognitive symptoms and extensive vascular change on MRI of the brain. Two years earlier, the individual had experienced a critical illness requiring ITU stay. Following this, they had initially been able to return to previous employment but reported cognitive slowing, word-finding difficulties, and problems remembering appointments. These symptoms and stress resulted in a subsequent decision to cease work. The individual reported lack of motivation, depression and anxiety, and progressive cognitive symptoms. Their partner felt that the cognitive symptoms had been static since ceasing work. The clinical picture was complicated by poor sleep, chronic pain and opiate use, and alcohol intake. They were a current cigarette smoker, had a family history of cardiovascular disease in a first-degree relative, and dementia in second-degree relatives.

Neurological examination demonstrated jerky saccadic movements, limb weakness related to previous surgery, and chronic pain. There were no pyramidal or extrapyramidal signs. A brain MRI showed small vessel ischemic change out of proportion to age, which showed mild progression on follow-up imaging a year later. Blood tests for vasculitis and inflammatory conditions (including CADASIL genetics) were unrevealing.

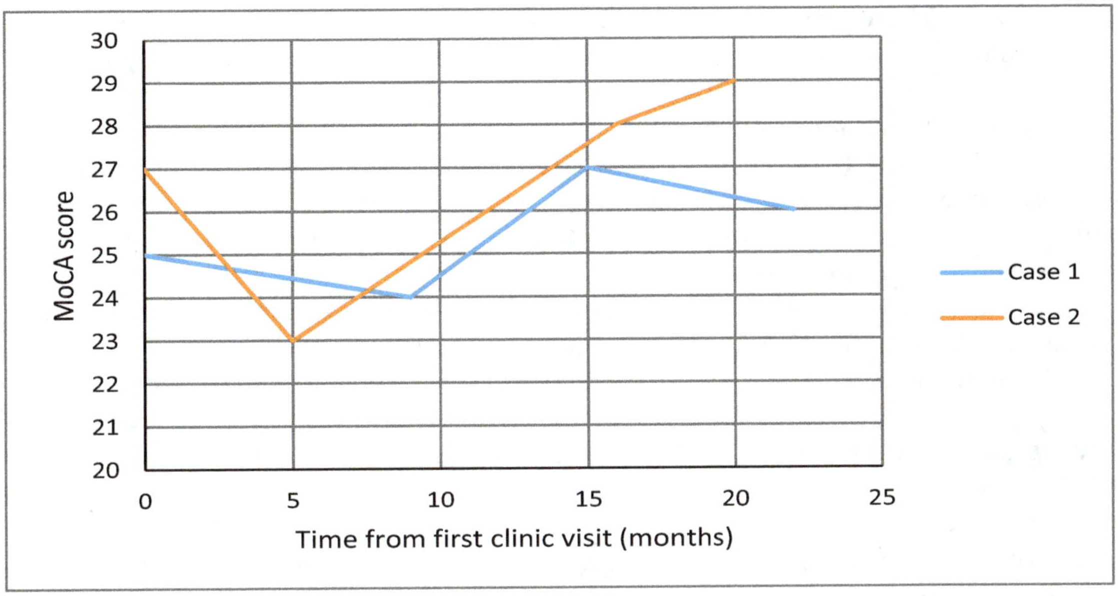

Figure 1. Serial Montreal Cognitive Assessment (MoCA) scores (bonus point included if appropriate) for illustrative cases one and two.

On neuropsychological testing, they passed tests of performance validity. Scores were low average or borderline impaired on several subsets (in particular, on word list recall, alongside average performance on short story recall). Depression and anxiety screening questionnaire scores were elevated. There were inconsistencies between self-reports of progressive cognitive symptoms in the absence of evidence of progressive cognitive decline on clinical review, and the collateral history of cognitive stability. Significant contributing adverse psychological factors were present that were felt to be impacting cognition, in conjunction with toxic and metabolic factors and vascular disease. A diagnosis of multifactorial MCI was ultimately made, and management included optimizing vascular risk factors, referral for psychological therapies, and support to attempt to reduce opiate use.

4. Discussion

In this case series of adults with FCD and neurodegenerative MCI, we found those with FCD to report an equivalent burden of cognitive symptomatology to people with MCI. Total PRMQ T scores were 33.3 in the FCD group and 35.1 in the MCI group, approximately 1.6 SD below the normative population mean [11]. This finding is in line with previous literature on functional neurological disorder, where self-ratings of disability by patients with functional symptoms are as severe or worse than those with organic neurological disease [12]. Performance on the MoCA was also indistinguishable between FCD and MCI, as both groups showed significantly impaired scores compared with the controls.

The FCD group showed lower performance on the ToPF, compared with the controls and the MCI group. The ToPF is designed to estimate premorbid cognitive abilities but is known to potentially be vulnerable to the impact of neurodegeneration and nonorganic underperformance [13]. Martin et al. examined links between performance validity test results and the ToPF, finding those failing validity tests were more likely to have a lower ToPF score than demographically predicted. People with FCD frequently show an invalid pattern of performance on neuropsychological testing [2], and it is possible that the ToPF results in the present FCD group may not accurately reflect their true premorbid baseline.

Limitations of this study include a lack of "gold standard" diagnostic criteria for FCD. Diagnostic criteria are still in evolution, and clinician judgement remains the mainstay of diagnosis. The ReMemBr Group cognitive clinic receives complex referrals from primary and secondary care; therefore, there is likely to be referral bias towards less straightforward diagnostic scenarios, which may have influenced the nature of the participants recruited in the present study. A common problem across cognitive research is a tendency for research participants to be of above population norm levels of education and socioeconomic status. Therefore, we would not consider our study sample to be truly representative of the local population, and it is possible that significant cultural differences may impact how FCD manifests and is diagnosed. Larger studies of more diverse populations in different world regions are needed to further our understanding of FCD.

Cognitive disorders are traditionally thought to reflect a binary, unidirectional process. They are present or absent, progress along a trajectory of increasing severity, and with the exception of rare, treatable causes of cognitive decline, they do not remit. This very linear view of cognition is increasingly at odds with evidence from large studies of populations with MCI, where a significant percentage of affected individuals revert to normal or near-normal cognition over time [14]. Those who improve retain an increased future risk of MCI or dementia compared to those who have not previously been diagnosed with MCI, and thus, they may move between diagnostic categories more than once during their cognitive journey [15,16]. Individuals with SCD are also highly heterogeneous. The SCIENCe cohort study subdivided people with SCD into those with preclinical Alzheimer's disease (AD; based on CSF or PET amyloid positivity), those with very mild psychiatric symptoms, and the remainder of individuals with features of neither [17]. A classification of preclinical AD was associated with older age and Apolipoprotein E4 status. Those with psychiatric features reported a greater degree of cognitive symptomatology than those with preclinical AD. Other studies of the long-term prognosis of SCD have identified a variety of potential clinical trajectories, including symptom remittance. Those with persistent symptoms reported over a number of time points appear to be at greater risk of progression to MCI or dementia, whilst those who intermittently report cognitive symptoms are not at increased risk, compared to people who have never reported cognitive symptoms [18]. Clearly, in the instances of SCD and MCI, diagnostic status is often a dynamic concept.

Our case reports highlight the potential for cognitive multimorbidity and diagnostic change over time. Case 1 was initially diagnosed with MCI, but this was revised on clinical follow up to SCD, with a possible element of functional overlay. Potential "red flags" for future cognitive decline are present in this case, based on the abnormal HMPAO SPECT, and cognitive changes being noted by close informants. Symptoms reported by significant others is regarded as a pointer towards neurodegeneration, as opposed to self-reported symptoms [19]. Contrarily, the improvement in MoCA performance would go against a neurodegenerative process, and the observed tendency to catastrophic thinking is a positive feature of functional symptoms. Given the diagnostic ambiguity, it could be argued that this patient might benefit from advanced neurodegenerative biomarker analysis with amyloid or tau imaging, and CSF analysis. However, these tests are not yet widely available in the UK NHS, and there is potential for iatrogenic harm by over-investigation, either through physical complications or adverse psychological consequences.

The diagnosis of FCD depends on expert clinician opinion, with the use of targeted clinical investigations. The clinical picture in FCD is of a significant burden of persistent cognitive symptoms, which cause patient distress and worry, but objective cognitive deficits are inconsistent with self-reported symptoms—this may be based on neuropsychological assessment, or self or collateral reports of activities requiring a high level of cognitive functioning. The discrepancy between symptoms and behavior is key to the diagnosis of FCD, and additional positive features are resistance to reassurance, repeated medical consultations, and failure of performance validity tests.

Case 2 illustrates the multifactorial nature of cognitive changes experienced by many patients, and the potential for functional symptoms to overlay other cognitive pathologies. The patient had been exposed to significant serious systemic morbidity, had evidence of neuronal injury on neuroimaging, in addition to ongoing issues with psychoactive medications, alcohol, and sleep pathology. There were also significant mental health symptoms, and the clinical impression was of functional symptoms contributing to the cognitive picture. It is extremely challenging to unpick the contributions of these different factors. A pragmatic management strategy should aim to improve potentially reversible factors, such as sleep, mental health, and cognitive toxin intake. Longitudinal follow-up is often needed, as the pattern of cognitive change (or lack thereof) is of diagnostic value, particularly to avoid missing neurodegeneration in complex individuals. The possibility of mental health symptoms arising as part of a dementia prodrome should be considered, particularly in older adults and those without a past history of mental health disorders.

Findings from our case series comparison of groups with FCD, MCI, and healthy controls show that PRMQ scores were equivalent in both the FCD and MCI groups, as was MoCA performance. This is despite expert opinion that those in the FCD group reported cognitive symptoms that were disproportionate to their observed cognitive functioning. Therefore, the PRMQ may not capture sufficiently detailed self-reported symptoms to be used diagnostically. The presence of a major discrepancy between subjective and objective cognition remains the mainstay of FCD diagnosis. More detailed exploration of neuropsychological features of FCD is warranted to seek out potential condition specific features that can aid in diagnosis. The potential for a diagnosis of FCD to change over time has not yet been explored, and there are little data available on the long-term prognosis. The optimal extent of investigations and follow-up is also unresolved. A deep phenotyping study of FCD will shortly open at the University of Edinburgh [20]. It is hoped that this and other future studies will establish clear diagnostic criteria for FCD and provide insight into causative mechanisms and avenues for potential therapeutic developments. Clinicians and researchers should be mindful of the potential for both diagnostic overlap and diagnostic change over time.

Author Contributions: C.P.—study design, data analysis, manuscript writing and editing; H.B.—data analysis and manuscript editing; M.S.—participant recruitment and evaluation.

Acknowledgments: We would like to thank all the study participants for their support of this work. Additionally, we would like to acknowledge recruitment support from the Join Dementia Research platform. Join Dementia Research is funded by the Department of Health and delivered by the National Institute for Health Research in partnership with Alzheimer Scotland, Alzheimer's Research UK and Alzheimer's Society.

References

1. Pennington, C.; Hayre, A.; Newson, M.; Coulthard, E. Functional Cognitive Disorder: A Common Cause of Subjective Cognitive Symptoms. *J. Alzheimer's Dis.* **2015**, *48*, S19–S24. [CrossRef] [PubMed]
2. Stone, J.; Pal, S.; Blackburn, D.; Reuber, M.; Thekkumpurath, P.; Carson, A. Functional (Psychogenic) Cognitive Disorders: A Perspective from the Neurology Clinic. *J. Alzheimer's Dis.* **2015**, *49*, S5–S17. [CrossRef] [PubMed]
3. Luck, T.; Roehr, S.; Rodriguez, F.S.; Schroeter, M.L.; Witte, A.V.; Hinz, A.; Mehner, A.; Engel, C.; Loeffler, M.; Thiery, J.; et al. Memory-related subjective cognitive symptoms in the adult population: Prevalence and associated factors - results of the LIFE-Adult-Study. *BMC Psychol.* **2018**, *21*, 6. [CrossRef] [PubMed]
4. Taylor, C.A.; Bouldin, E.D.; McGuire, L.C. Subjective cognitive decline among adults aged ≥45 years—United States, 2015–2016. *Morb. Mortal. Wkly. Rep.* **2018**, *67*, 754–757. [CrossRef] [PubMed]
5. Stone, J.; Reuber, M.; Carson, A. Functional symptoms in neurology: Mimics and chameleons. *Pract. Neurol.* **2013**, *13*, 104–113. [CrossRef] [PubMed]
6. Kutlubaev, M.A.; Xu, Y.; Hackett, M.L.; Stone, J. Dual diagnosis of epilepsy and psychogenic nonepileptic seizures: Systematic review and meta-analysis of frequency, correlates, and outcomes. *Epilepsy Behav.* **2018**, *89*, 70–78. [CrossRef] [PubMed]
7. Merwick, A.; Sweeney, B. Functional symptoms in clinically definite MS–pseudo-relapse syndrome. *Int. MS J.* **2008**, *15*, 47–51. [PubMed]
8. Stella, F.; Radanovic, M.; Balthazar, M.L.F.; Canineu, P.R.; De Souza, L.C.; Forlenza, O.V. Neuropsychiatric Symptoms in the Prodromal Stages of Dementia. *Curr. Opin. Psychiatry.* **2014**, *27*, 230–235. [CrossRef] [PubMed]
9. Nasreddine, Z.S.; Phillips, N.A.; Bédirian, V.; Charbonneau, S.; Whitehead, V.; Collin, I.; Cummings, J.; Certkow, H. The Montreal Cognitive Assessment, MoCA: A brief screening tool for mild cognitive impairment. *J. Am. Geriatr. Soc.* **2005**, *53*, 695–699. [CrossRef] [PubMed]

10. Pearson. Test of Premorbid Functioning, UK Version. Administration, Scoring and Techniques Manual. Available online: https://www.pearsonclinical.co.uk/Psychology/AdultCognitionNeuropsychologyandLanguage/AdultGeneralAbilities/TOPF/TestofPremorbidFunctioning.aspx (accessed on 20 September 2019).
11. Crawford, J.R.; Smith, G.; Maylor E a Della Sala, S.; Logie, R.H. The Prospective and Retrospective Memory Questionnaire (PRMQ): Normative data and latent structure in a large non-clinical sample. *Memory* **2003**, *11*, 261–275. [CrossRef] [PubMed]
12. Carson, A.; Stone, J.; Hibberd, C.; Murray, G.; Duncan, R.; Coleman, R.; Warlow, C.; Roberts, R.; Pelosi, A.; Cavanagh, J.; et al. Disability, distress and unemployment in neurology outpatients with symptoms "unexplained by organic disease". *J. Neurol. Neurosurg. Psychiatry* **2011**, *82*, 810–813. [CrossRef] [PubMed]
13. Martin, P.K.; Schroeder, R.W.; Wyman-Chick, K.A.; Hunter, B.P.; Heinrichs, R.J.; Baade, L.E. Rates of Abnormally Low TOPF Word Reading Scores in Individuals Failing Versus Passing Performance Validity Testing. *Assessment* **2018**, *25*, 640–652. [CrossRef] [PubMed]
14. Ganguli, M.; Jia, Y.; Hughes, T.F.; Snitz, B.E.; Chang, C.C.H.; Berman, S.B.; Sullivan KIlyas Kamboh, M. Mild Cognitive Impairment that Does Not Progress to Dementia: A Population-Based Study. *J. Am. Geriatr. Soc.* **2019**, *67*, 232–238. [CrossRef] [PubMed]
15. Aerts, L.; Heffernan, M.; Kochan, N.A.; Crawford, J.D.; Draper, B.; Trollor, J.N.; Brodaty, H. Effects of MCI subtype and reversion on progression to dementia in a community sample. *Neurology* **2017**, *88*, 2225–2232. [CrossRef] [PubMed]
16. Koepsell, T.D.; Monsell, S.E. Reversion from mild cognitive impairment to normal or near-Normal cognition; Risk factors and prognosis. *Neurology* **2012**, *79*, 1591–1598. [CrossRef] [PubMed]
17. Slot, R.E.R.; Verfaillie, S.C.J.; Overbeek, J.M.; Timmers, T.; Wesselman, L.M.P.; Teunissen, C.E.; Bols, A.; Bouwman, F.; Prins, N.; Barkhof, F.; et al. Subjective Cognitive Impairment Cohort (SCIENCe): Study design and first results. *Alzheimer's Res. Ther.* **2018**, *10*, 1–13. [CrossRef] [PubMed]
18. Roehr, S.; Villringer, A.; Angermeyer, M.C.; Luck, T.; Riedel-Heller, S.G. Outcomes of stable and unstable patterns of subjective cognitive decline—Results from the Leipzig Longitudinal Study of the Aged (LEILA75+). *BMC Geriatr.* **2016**, *16*, 1–8. [CrossRef] [PubMed]
19. Valech, N.; Mollica, M.A.; Olives, J.; Tort, A.; Fortea, J.; Lleo, A.; Belen, S.; Molinuevo, J.; Rami, L. Informant's Perception of Subjective Cognitive Decline Helps to Discriminate Preclinical Alzheimer's Disease from Normal Aging. *J. Alzheimer's Dis.* **2015**, *48*, S87–S98. [CrossRef] [PubMed]
20. McWhirter, L.; Ritchie, C.W.; Carson, A.J.; Stone, J. Improving Diagnosis in Cognitive Disorders. 2019. Available online: https://www.protocols.io/view/improving-diagnosis-in-cognitive-disorders-z97f99n/abstract (accessed on 28 September 2019).

13

Comparing the Diagnostic Accuracy of Two Cognitive Screening Instruments in Different Dementia Subtypes and Clinical Depression

Rónán O'Caoimh [1,2,*] and D. William Molloy [1]

1 Centre for Gerontology and Rehabilitation, University College Cork, St Finbarr's Hospital, Douglas road, T12 XH60 Cork City, Ireland
2 Department of Geriatric Medicine, Mercy University Hospital, Grenville Place, T12 WE28 Cork City, Ireland
* Correspondence: rocaoimh@hotmail.com or rocaoimh@muh.ie

Abstract: Short but accurate cognitive screening instruments are required in busy clinical practice. Although widely-used, the diagnostic accuracy of the standardised Mini-Mental State Examination (SMMSE) in different dementia subtypes remains poorly characterised. We compared the SMMSE to the Quick Mild Cognitive Impairment (*Qmci*) screen in patients (n = 3020) pooled from three memory clinic databases in Canada including those with mild cognitive impairment (MCI) and Alzheimer's, vascular, mixed, frontotemporal, Lewy Body and Parkinson's dementia, with and without co-morbid depression. Caregivers (n = 875) without cognitive symptoms were included as normal controls. The median age of patients was 77 (Interquartile = ±9) years. Both instruments accurately differentiated cognitive impairment (MCI or dementia) from controls. The SMMSE most accurately differentiated Alzheimer's (AUC 0.94) and Lewy Body dementia (AUC 0.94) and least accurately identified MCI (AUC 0.73), vascular (AUC 0.74), and Parkinson's dementia (AUC 0.81). The *Qmci* had statistically similar or greater accuracy in distinguishing all dementia subtypes but particularly MCI (AUC 0.85). Co-morbid depression affected accuracy in those with MCI. The SMMSE and *Qmci* have good-excellent accuracy in established dementia. The SMMSE is less suitable in MCI, vascular and Parkinson's dementia, where alternatives including the *Qmci* screen may be used. The influence of co-morbid depression on scores merits further investigation.

Keywords: dementia; mild cognitive impairment; screening; accuracy; standardised mini-mental state examination; quick mild cognitive impairment screen

---

1. Introduction

Although short cognitive screening instruments (CSIs) such as the Mini-Mental State Examination (MMSE) [1] and its standardised version, the SMMSE [2,3] are widely used in clinical practice and research studies, their accuracy and hence suitability for use in detecting different dementia subtypes is poorly characterised [4]. Numerous studies including recent systematic reviews show that the MMSE has poor accuracy and that an alternative instrument should be used to identify those with mild cognitive impairment (MCI) [5], a prodromal state characterised by cognitive deficits without loss of social or occupation function and before the onset of dementia [6]. Other instruments such as the Memory Alteration Test [7], the Quick Mild Cognitive Impairment (*Qmci*) screen [8] and Montreal Cognitive Assessment (MoCA) [9] are recommended as alternatives [5,10]. The MMSE has a "floor" effect such that a score of zero does not always support dementia and a "low ceiling" effect such that a normal score does not always mean normal cognition [11]. It is also influenced by age and education meaning that it is poorly sensitive when used among older and less educated adults [12,13]. It also has poor reliability, which led to the development of the SMMSE. Despite these issues, the MMSE remains the most widely used CSI in clinical practice [14].

Given that the MMSE and SMMSE cover a limited number of cognitive domains [2,3], their diagnostic accuracy in different types of dementia is unclear. The SMMSE lacks a subtest measuring executive function, which suggests that it is less useful in those with Parkinson's disease cognitive impairment [15] and is overly weighted towards language skills, making it less useful in frontotemporal dementia [16]. Compared with other short CSIs such as the MoCA, the MMSE has poor accuracy in detecting vascular cognitive impairment, which is often characterised by impaired attention, executive and visuospatial dysfunction, all poorly assessed with the MMSE subtests [17]. Similarly, the pentagon task may lack accuracy in post-stroke, frontotemporal and subcortical dementias [18].

Low mood and depression may also impact on cognition and may precede onset of cognitive decline, affecting executive function, memory, and attention [19,20]. While evidence suggests that depression in MCI is associated with disease progression, the effects of depression on cognitive screening are poorly characterised [21]. Limited data suggests that mood may negatively influence MMSE scores, underestimating true performance [22]. The extent to which depression affects the results of the MMSE and other CSIs and their subtests is however, poorly understood and the extent to which different dementia subtype scores are influenced by the presence of comorbid depression is not known.

Although several studies have compared the diagnostic accuracy of the newer and shorter *Qmci* screen and shown it is better able to differentiate MCI from mild dementia and normal cognition than the SMMSE [8,13], to date, this has only been examined in those with Alzheimer's and vascular type dementia. The objective of this study is therefore to explore the performance (diagnostic accuracy) of these instruments across a broad range of different dementia subtypes, and in patients with MCI and those with and without depression. More broadly, this also serves to investigate the extent to which CSI's perform differently in these settings.

2. Methods

2.1. Data Collection

This study compared the SMMSE and the *Qmci* screen in patients (n = 3020) obtained from three geriatric and memory clinics in Canada over the decade between 1999 and 2010. Data were collected and analysed retrospectively from two clinic databases and a randomised controlled clinical trial dataset: The Geriatric Assessment Tool (GAT) [23], the *Qmci* screen original validation [8], and the Doxycycline and Rifampicin for Alzheimer's Disease (DARAD) Trial databases [24]. Recruitment processes from all three studies have been published previously [8,23,24]. In summary, the GAT is a customised software application that automates clinicians' outpatient reviews [23]. These data were collected in outpatient geriatric and memory clinics in two university hospitals in Ontario, Canada between 1999 and 2010. It contains approximately 8000 individual assessments from 1749 people aged 41–104 years. The *Qmci* screen validation database includes patients referred for assessment of cognition aged ≥55 years and recruited from four memory clinics in Ontario Canada [8]. The DARAD was a multi-centre, blinded, randomised trial conducted between 2006 and 2010, comparing the effect of rifampicin and doxycycline to placebo on the progression of AD [24]. The DARAD database includes patients ≥50 years with mild to moderate AD recruited from 14 centres across Canada. All three studies were led by the same principle investigator (D.W.M) and each participant underwent similar comprehensive work-up including laboratory investigations, neuropsychological assessment and neuroimaging where appropriate [23,24]. Ethical approval was obtained in advance for all three studies and participants provided informed written consent.

2.2. Participants

Participants were included in this analysis if both their SMMSE and *Qmci* screen scores were available. Participant selection is presented in Figure 1. MCI was diagnosed in patients presenting with subjective and objective memory loss, without loss of function. This was consistent with Petersen's criteria, where patients present with subjective memory complaints, objective abnormal memory function but preservation of activities of daily living and have no evidence of dementia [25]. Dementia was diagnosed using the Diagnostic and Statistical Manual of Mental Disorders (4th-edition) [26]. Mood was screened using the geriatric depression scale-short form with scores ≥5 assessed clinically for depression [27]. All participants were English literate. Those with MCI, predominantly amnestic type (aMCI), and patients with Alzheimer's disease (AD), vascular dementia (VaD), frontotemporal dementia (FTD), Lewy body dementia (LBD) and Parkinson's disease dementia (PDD), meeting established clinical criteria, with and without a history of comorbid depression, were included. Patients without cognitive impairment and with depression as the primary symptom were excluded. Persons attending with patients without memory loss (mainly caregivers) were recruited by convenience sampling as normal controls (n = 875).

2.3. Outcome Measures

The SMMSE is a standardised form of the MMSE developed to improve inter-rater reliability and reduced administration time by using explicit administration and scoring guidelines [2,3]. Scored out of 30 points, a score of 25/30 or more suggests that the individual may have normal cognition. Below this, scores can indicate mild (21–24 points), moderate (10–20 points) and severe cognitive impairment (≤9 points), though a cut-off of <24/30 optimises sensitivity [2,3]. It covers several cognitive domains including orientation, registration, delayed (verbal) recall, attention (concentration and calculation), language (including writing, reading and naming), command following, and visuospatial (construction) subtests [2,3]. The *Qmci* screen is a more recently developed short CSI, designed to separate MCI from mild dementia [8]. Scored from 100 points it incorporates six subtests across five cognitive domains including orientation, working memory, sematic memory (verbal fluency-categories), visuo-spatial (clock drawing) and two tests of episodic memory: Delayed recall and logical memory (immediate verbal recall of short a story) [28]. It has an optimal cut-off score for cognitive impairment of <62/100 [13,29]. It has been validated against the MoCA and different neuropsychological tests and is published in multiple languages [30–34]. While data on total scores were available for both CSIs, data on subtests were only available for the *Qmci* screen as these were not collected as part of the DARAD trial [24].

2.4. Analysis

Data were analysed using SPSS 24.0. Data from the three data sets (original *Qmci* screen validation database, GAT and DARAD datasets) were pooled and analysed using simple descriptive statistics. Data were non-normally distributed and were analysed with non-parametric tests. The Mann–Whitney U test was used to compare distributions between variables. Receiver operating characteristic (ROC) curve analysis was used to determine diagnostic accuracy from the area under the curve (AUC). AUC scores range from 0.5–1.0; 0.5 equates to chance alone and 1.0 perfect predictive accuracy. Scores from 0.50–0.59 indicate no or very poor accuracy, 0.60–0.69 poor, 0.70–0.79 fair, 0.80–0.89 good and 0.90–1.0 excellent to perfect accuracy [35]. All AUC values are presented with 95% confidence intervals (CI) and where specified were compared using the DeLong method [36]. Optimal cut-off points were calculated using Youden's Index.

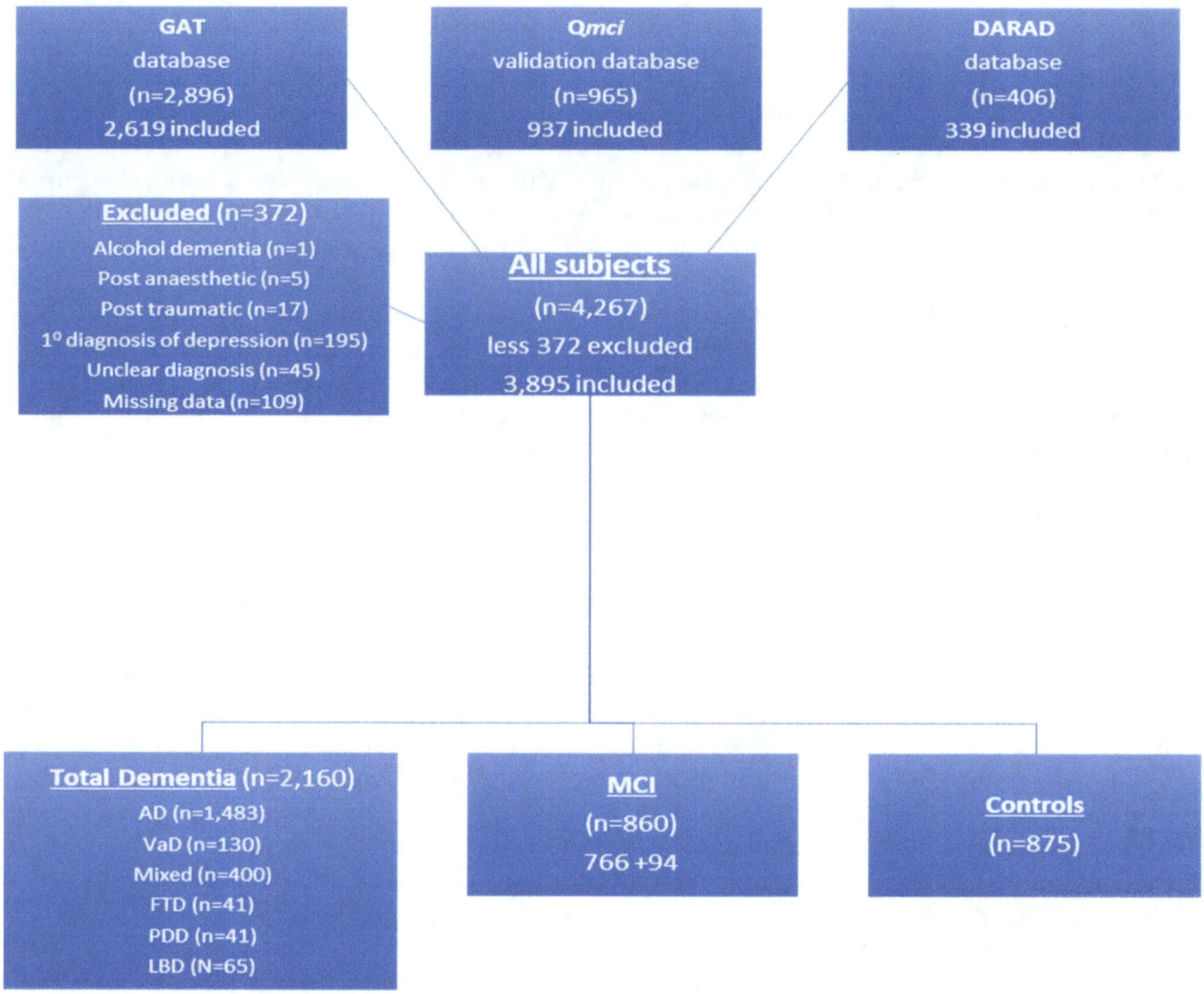

Figure 1. Flow chart presenting the recruitment of participants pooled from three data sets: The Geriatric Assessment Tool (GAT), Quick Mild Cognitive Impairment (*Qmci*) Screen and Doxycycline and Rifampicin for Alzheimer's Disease (DARAD) trial databases; it includes the number of controls, those with mild cognitive impairment (MCI) and specific dementia subtypes: Alzheimer's disease (AD), vascular dementia (VaD), mixed dementia, frontotemporal dementia (FTD), Parkinson's disease dementia (PDD) and Lewy body dementia (LBD) subtypes.

3. Results

In all, 3020 patients were available for analysis. A further 875 normal controls were included. The majority of participants had dementia ($n = 2160$) of which AD was the most common subtype ($n = 1483$), followed by mixed (AD-VaD) ($n = 400$) and VaD ($n = 130$). The median age of patients presenting with cognitive symptoms (MCI/dementia) was 77 years, interquartile range (IQR) ±9 compared to a median age of 69 (±14) years for normal controls, $p < 0.001$. In all, 51% of patients were male compared to 43% of controls, $p < 0.001$. Patients had completed a median of 12 (±5) years in education, similar to controls (13 ± 4), albeit statistically significantly lower, $p < 0.001$. The median SMMSE scores were 23/30 (±8) for dementia, 28/30 (±4) for MCI and 29/30 (±2) for controls. Median *Qmci* screen scores were 38/100 (±26) for dementia, 56/100 (±20) for MCI and 74/100 (±15) for controls. Differences in gender were seen between diagnosis with the percentage of males ranging from as high as 73% in those with VaD to as low as 41% in those with dementia and comorbid depression. Characteristics of participants including patients and controls are presented in Table 1.

Table 1. Characteristics of participants from the Quick Mild Cognitive Impairment (*Qmci*) Screen validation, Doxycycline And Rifampicin for Alzheimer's Disease study and Geriatric Assessment Tool databases, divided according to diagnosis: Depression, controls, mild cognitive impairment (MCI) and dementia including their Standardised Mini-Mental State Examination (SMMSE) and *Qmci* screen scores; comparison of SMMSE and *Qmci* screen score accuracy in differentiating each diagnosis from controls.

Diagnosis	$N = X$	Age (Median & IQR)	Education (Median & IQR)	Gender (% Male)	SMMSE (Median & IQR)	*Qmci* (Median & IQR)	SMMSE AUC NC v CI (95% Confidence Intervals)	*Qmci* AUC NC v CI (95% Confidence Intervals)	$p = x$
Total (All including co-morbid depression & MCI)	3020	77 (81 − 72 = 9)	12 (14 − 9 = 5)	1537/2997 * (51%)	25 (28 − 20 = 8)	43 (56 − 29 = 27)	0.87 (0.85–0.88)	0.93 (0.92–0.94)	$z = 11.6$ $p < 0.001$
Dementia (All including co-morbid depression)	2160	77 (82 − 73 = 9)	12 (14 − 9 = 5)	1087/2145 * (51%)	23 (26 − 18 = 8)	38 (50 − 24 = 26)	0.92 (0.91–0.93)	0.96 (0.95–0.96)	$z = -8.6$ $p < 0.001$
Dementia (All excluding co-morbid depression)	1879	78 (82 − 74 = 8)	11 (14 − 9 = 5)	971/1864 * (52%)	23 (26 − 18 = 8)	37 (49 − 24 = 25)	0.92 (0.91–0.93)	0.96 (0.95–0.97)	$z = -8.3$ $p < 0.001$
AD	1483	78 (83 − 74 = 9)	12 (14 − 9 = 5)	651/1475 * (44%)	23 (25.5 − 18 = 7.5)	37 (48 − 23 = 25)	0.94 (0.93–0.95)	0.97 (0.96–0.97)	$z = -5.9$ $p < 0.001$
VaD	130	74 (79 − 69 = 10)	12 (14 − 10 = 4)	95 (73%)	27 (29 − 25 = 4)	53 (64 − 40 = 24)	0.74 (0.68–0.79)	0.87 (0.84–0.91)	$z = -6.3$ $p < 0.001$
Mixed (AD/VaD)	400	77 (81 − 74 = 7)	11 (13 − 9 = 4)	256/393 * (65%)	22 (27 − 19 = 8)	36 (51 − 23 = 28)	0.91 (0.89–0.93)	0.95 (0.94–0.96)	$z = -5.7$ $p < 0.001$
AD, VaD and Mixed	2013	78 (82 − 74 = 4)	12 (14 − 9 = 5)	1002/1998 * (50%)	23 (26 − 18 = 8)	38 (50 − 24 = 26)	0.92 (0.91–0.93)	0.96 (0.95–0.97)	$z = 8.4$ $p < 0.001$
FTD	41	69 (71 − 62 = 9)	12 (14 − 10 = 4)	25/41 (61%)	23 (27 − 19 = 8)	42 (52 − 28 = 24)	0.90 (0.85–0.96)	0.96 (0.94–0.98)	$z = -2.5$ $p = 0.01$
PDD	41	75 (77 − 71 = 6)	12 (12 − 9.5 = 2.5)	28/41 (68%)	26 (29 − 21 = 8)	46 (61 − 32 = 29)	0.81 (0.72–0.90)	0.92 (0.88–0.95)	$z = -3.1$ $p = 0.002$
LBD	65	78 (82 − 73 = 9)	10 (14 − 8 = 6)	32/65 (49%)	24 (27 − 18 = 9)	37 (54 − 24 = 30)	0.94 (0.92–0.97)	0.94 (0.91–0.97)	$z = 0.11$ $p = 0.91$
MCI	860	75 (80 − 70 = 10)	12 (14 − 10 = 4)	450/852 * (53%)	28 (29 − 25 = 4)	56 (66 − 46 = 20)	0.73 (0.71–0.75)	0.85 (0.83–0.87)	$z = -10.8$ $p < 0.001$
Co-morbid depression	281	75 (81 − 70 = 11)	12 (14 − 10 = 4)	116/281 (41%)	25 (27 − 21 = 6)	44 (56 − 30 = 26)	0.88 (0.86–0.91)	0.93 (0.91–0.95)	$z = -4.2$ $p < 0.001$
MCI with co-morbid depression	94	73 (75 − 68 = 7)	12 (14 − 9 = 5)	50/92 * (54%)	26 (29 − 23 = 6)	52 (62 − 40 = 22)	0.79 (0.73–0.85)	0.90 (0.86–0.93)	$z = -4.4$ $p < 0.001$
MCI without co-morbid depression	766	76 (80 − 70 = 10)	12 (14 − 10 = 4)	400/760 * (53%)	28 (29 − 26 = 3)	57 (66 − 46 = 20)	0.72 (0.70–0.75)	0.84 (0.82–0.86)	$z = -10.4$ $p < 0.001$
Controls	875	70 (76 − 62 = 14)	13 (16 − 12 = 4)	372/875 (43%)	29 (30 − 28 = 2)	74 (81 − 66 = 15)	NA	NA	NA

AUC = area under the curve, AD = Alzheimer's disease, CI = cognitive impairment, FTD = frontotemporal dementia, IQR = interquartile range, LBD = Lewy body dementia, PDD = Parkinson's dementia, VaD = vascular dementia; NA = Not applicable; * Missing data.

Both instruments accurately differentiated cognitive impairment (MCI or dementia) from normal, although the *Qmci* screen was statistically more accurate than the SMMSE (AUC of 0.93 versus 0.87, respectively, $p < 0.001$). The SMMSE, at a cut-off of <24/30, had a sensitivity of 42%, specificity of 99% with a positive predictive value of 99% and negative predictive value of 33%. The *Qmci* screen had a sensitivity of 83% and specificity of 87% with a positive predictive value of 96% and negative predictive value of 60% at its published optimal cut-off score (<62/100). Using Youden's Index, the optimal cut-off scores for the SMMSE was 28/30, which gave a sensitivity of 75% and specificity of 88%. The optimal cut-off for the *Qmci* screen was <62. The SMMSE most accurately differentiated AD (AUC 0.94, 95% CI: 0.93–0.95) and LBD (AUC 0.94, 95% CI: 0.92–0.97) and least accurately identified MCI (AUC 0.73, 95% CI: 0.71–0.75), VaD (AUC 0.74, 95% CI: 0.68–0.79) and PDD (AUC 0.81, 95% CI: 0.72–0.90). The *Qmci* screen had statistically greater accuracy in distinguishing all dementia subtypes except LBD ($p = 0.91$). The *Qmci* screen was more accurate than the SMMSE in separating PDD and FTD from controls, albeit sample sizes were small. As expected, the *Qmci* screen had the greatest diagnostic accuracy for identifying MCI (AUC 0.85, 95% CI: 0.83-0.87) from normal controls, which was statistically significantly greater than the SMMSE (AUC 0.73, 95% CI: 0.71–0.75), $p < 0.001$. ROC curves demonstrating the accuracy of both instruments in each type of dementia, in MCI and in those with and without depression are presented in Figure 2a–l.

(**a**)

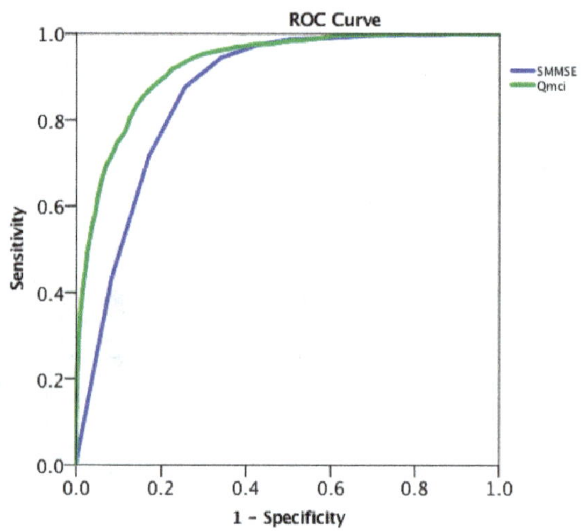

(**b**)

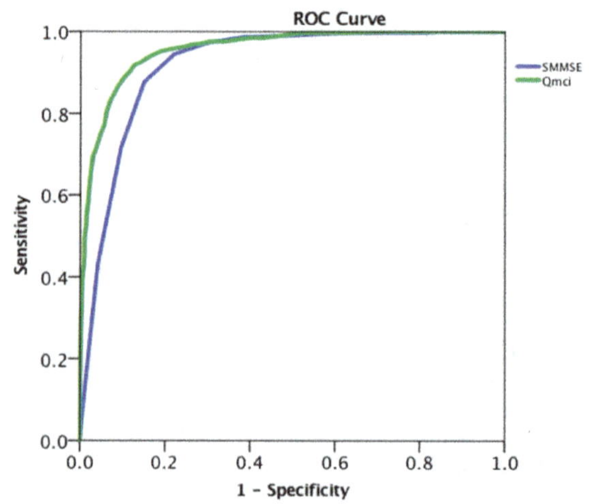

(**c**)

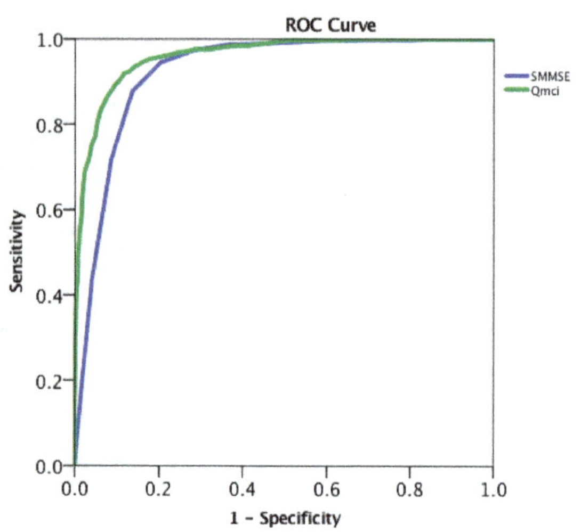

(**d**)

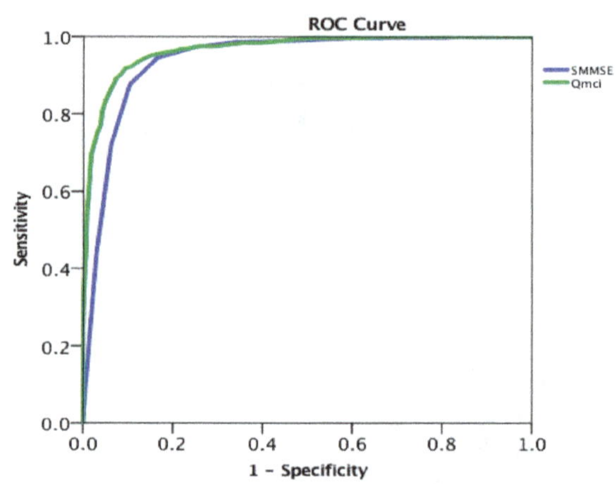

Figure 2. *Cont.*

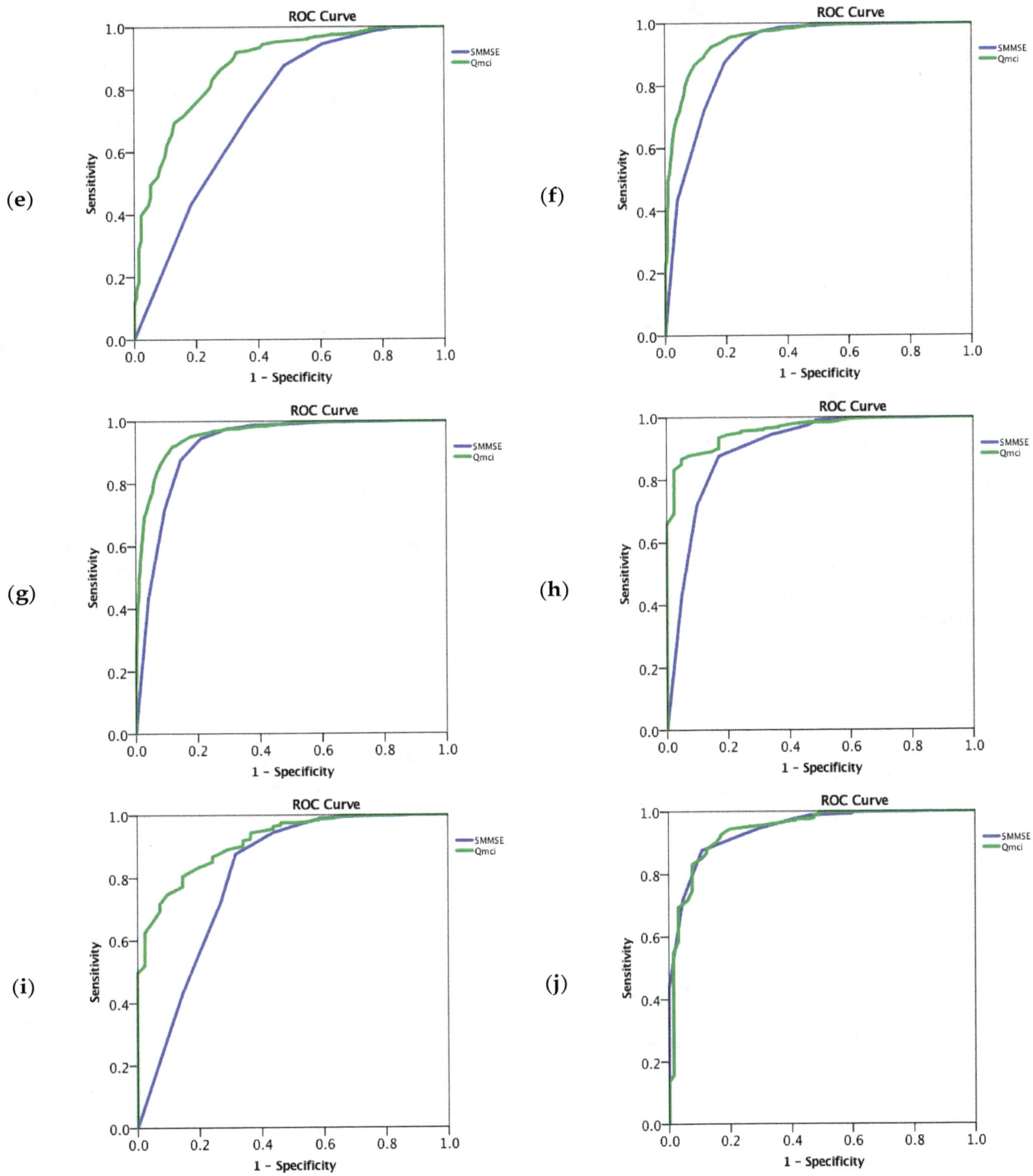

Figure 2. *Cont.*

(k)

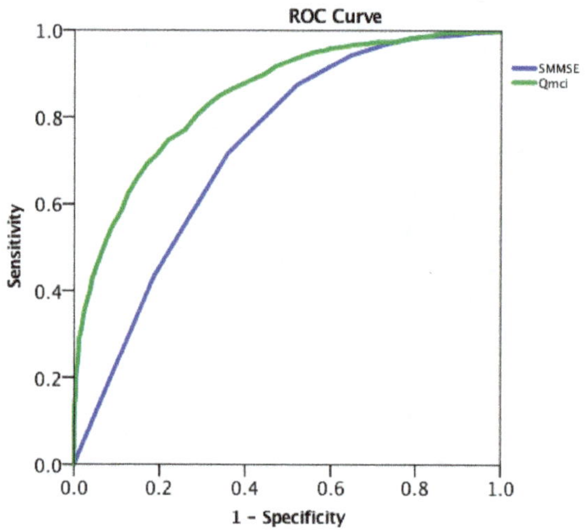

(l)

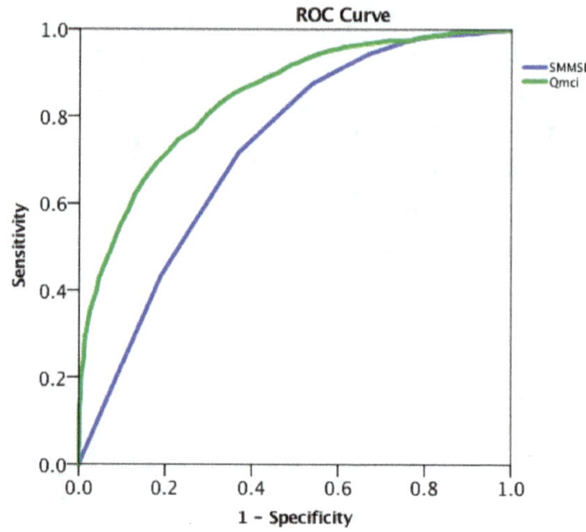

Figure 2. Receiver operating characteristic curves (**a**–**l**) comparing the accuracy of the Quick Mild Cognitive Impairment (Q*mci*) Screen and the Standardised Mini-Mental State Examination in differentiating normal controls (*n* = 875) from those with mild cognitive impairment (MCI), different dementia subtypes and comorbid depression for participants included within the Q*mci* screen validation, Doxycycline And Rifampicin for Alzheimer's Disease study and Geriatric Assessment Tool databases. (**a**). All patients (*n* = 3020); (**b**). All patients with dementia (*n* = 2160); (**c**). Dementia excluding depression (*n* = 1879); (**d**). Alzheimer's dementia (*n* = 1483); (**e**). Vascular dementia (*n* = 130); (**f**). Mixed dementia (*n* = 400); (**g**). Alzheimer's, vascular, mixed dementia (*n* = 2013); (**h**). Frontotemporal dementia (*n* = 41) (**i**). Parkinson's disease dementia (*n* = 41); (**j**). Lewy body dementia (*n* = 65); (**k**). All MCI (*n* = 860); (**l**) MCI excluding depression (*n* = 766).

The median subtest scores and AUC scores derived from ROC curves according to diagnosis are presented in Tables 2 and 3, respectively.

Table 2. Median scores for the Quick Mild Cognitive Impairment (*Qmci*) Screen subtests divided according to diagnosis: Depression, mild cognitive impairment (MCI) and dementia.

Diagnosis	*N* = X	Orientation (Median and IQR)	Registration (Median and IQR)	Clock Drawing (Median and IQR)	Delayed Recall (Median and IQR)	Verbal Fluency (Median and IQR)	Logical Memory (Median and IQR)	*Qmci* Total (Median and IQR)
Total (All)	3020	8 (10 – 6 = 4)	5 (5 – 4 = 1)	12 (14 – 5 = 9)	4 (12 – 0 = 12)	5 (7 – 3 = 4)	8 (12 – 4 = 8)	43 (56 – 29 = 27)
Dementia (All including co-morbid depression)	2160	7 (9 – 5 = 4)	5 (5 – 3 = 2)	11 (14 – 3 = 11)	4 (8 – 0 = 8)	5 (7 – 3 = 4)	8 (12 – 4 = 8)	38 (50 – 24 = 26)
Dementia (All excluding co-morbid depression)	1879	7 (9 – 5 = 4)	5 (5 – 3 = 2)	11 (13 – 3 = 10)	0 (8 – 0 = 8)	4 (6 – 3 = 3)	8 (12 – 4 = 8)	37 (49 – 24 = 25)
AD	1483	7 (9 – 5 = 4)	5 (5 – 3 = 2)	11 (13 – 3 = 10)	0 (8 – 0 = 8)	4 (6 – 3 = 3)	8 (12 – 4 = 8)	37 (48 – 23 = 25)
VaD	130	9 (10 – 7 = 3)	5 (5 – 4 = 1)	14 (15 – 11 = 4)	8 (12 – 0 = 12)	7 (9 – 4 = 5)	10 (14 – 8 = 6)	53 (64 – 40 = 24)
Mixed (AD/VaD)	400	7 (10 – 5 = 5)	5 (5 – 3 = 2)	10 (14 – 2 = 12)	0 (8 – 0 = 8)	5 (7 – 3 = 4)	8 (12 – 4 = 8)	35.5 (51 – 23 = 28)
AD, VaD and Mixed	2013	7 (9 – 5 = 4)	5 (5 – 3 = 2)	11 (14 – 3 = 11)	0 (8 – 0 = 8)	5 (7 – 3 = 4)	8 (12 – 4 = 8)	38 (50 – 24 = 26)
FTD	41	9 (10 – 6 = 4)	5 (5 – 3 = 2)	12 (13 – 5 = 8)	4 (8 – 0 = 8)	4 (7 – 3 = 4)	8 (12 – 4 = 8)	43 (55 – 30 = 25)
PDD	41	9.5 (10 – 7 = 3)	5 (5 – 4 = 1)	12.5 (15 – 7 = 8)	8 (12 – 0 = 12)	5.5 (7 – 4 = 3)	10 (14 – 8 = 6)	46 (61 – 32 = 29)
LBD	65	8 (10 – 6 = 4)	5 (5 – 3 = 2)	7 (12 – 1 = 11)	8 (12 – 0 = 12)	4 (6 – 3 = 3)	8 (10 – 4 = 6)	37 (54 – 24 = 30)
MCI	860	10 (10 – 8 = 2)	5 (5 – 5 = 0)	14 (15 – 12 = 3)	12 (16 – 4 = 12)	7 (9 – 5 = 4)	12 (16 – 8 = 8)	56 (66 – 46 = 20)
Co-morbid depression	281	8 (10 – 6 = 4)	5 (5 – 4 = 1)	11 (14 – 4 = 10)	4 (12 – 0 = 12)	6 (8 – 3 = 5)	10 (14 – 4 = 10)	44 (56 – 30 = 26)
MCI with co-morbid depression	94	9 (10 – 7 = 3)	5 (5 – 4 = 1)	13 (15 – 10 = 5)	8 (12 – 4 = 8)	8 (8 – 4 = 4)	12 (14 – 8 = 6)	51.5 (62 – 40 = 22)
MCI without co-morbid depression	766	10 (10 – 8 = 2)	5 (5 – 5 = 0)	14 (15 – 12 = 3)	12 (16 – 4 = 12)	7 (9 – 5 = 4)	12 (16 – 8 = 8)	57 (66 – 46 = 20)
Controls	875	10 (10 – 10 = 0)	5 (5 – 5 = 0)	15 (15 – 14 = 1)	16 (20 – 12 = 8)	10 (13 – 8 = 5)	18 (22 – 14 = 8)	74 (81 – 66 = 15)

AD = Alzheimer's disease, FTD = frontotemporal dementia, LBD = Lewy body dementia, PDD = Parkinson's dementia, VaD = vascular dementia (IQR = interquartile range).

Table 3. Comparison of the accuracy of the Quick Mild Cognitive Impairment (*Qmci*) Screen subtests in differentiating each diagnosis from controls (n = 875): Depression, mild cognitive impairment (MCI) and dementia.

Diagnosis	*N* = X	Orientation AUC (95% CI)	Registration AUC (95% CI)	Clock Drawing AUC (95% CI)	Delayed Recall AUC (95% CI)	Verbal Fluency AUC (95% CI)	Logical Memory AUC (95% CI)	*Qmci* Total AUC (95% CI)
Total (All)	3020	0.81 (0.79–0.82)	0.62 (0.60–0.64)	0.80 (0.79–0.82)	0.86 (0.85–0.87)	0.85 (0.84–0.87)	0.87 (0.85–0.88)	0.93 (0.92–0.94)
Dementia (All including co-morbid depression)	2160	0.86 (0.85–0.87)	0.65 (0.63–0.67)	0.85 (0.83–0.86)	0.90 (0.89–0.91)	0.89 (0.88–0.90)	0.89 (0.88–0.91)	0.96 (0.95–0.96)
Dementia (All excluding co-morbid depression)	1879	0.87 (0.85–0.88)	0.66 (0.64–0.68)	0.85 (0.84–0.87)	0.90 (0.89–0.92)	0.90 (0.88–0.91)	0.90 (0.89–0.91)	0.96 (0.95–0.97)
AD	1483	0.88 (0.87–0.90)	0.66 (0.64–0.68)	0.85 (0.84–0.87)	0.91 (0.90–0.93)	0.91 (0.89–0.92)	0.91 (0.89–0.92)	0.97 (0.96–0.97)
VaD	130	0.71 (0.66–0.77)	0.56 (0.50–0.61)	0.72 (0.67–0.77)	0.80 (0.75–0.84)	0.80 (0.77–0.84)	0.81 (0.77–0.85)	0.87 (0.84–0.91)
Mixed (AD/VaD)	400	0.84 (0.82–0.87)	0.65 (0.61–0.68)	0.85 (0.82–0.87)	0.90 (0.88–0.92)	0.89 (0.87–0.91)	0.89 (0.87–0.91)	0.95 (0.94–0.96)
AD, VaD & Mixed	2013	0.86 (0.85–0.88)	0.65 (0.63–0.67)	0.84 (0.83–0.86)	0.90 (0.89–0.91)	0.90 (0.88–0.91)	0.90 (0.88–0.91)	0.96 (0.95–0.97)
FTD	41	0.78 (0.69–0.87)	0.63 (0.53–0.73)	0.88 (0.81–0.94)	0.90 (0.87–0.95)	0.85 (0.78–0.92)	0.88 (0.83–0.93)	0.96 (0.94–0.98)
PDD	41	0.71 (0.61–0.81)	0.68 (0.58–0.77)	0.73 (0.63–0.82)	0.84 (0.77–0.91)	0.85 (0.79–0.91)	0.83 (0.77–0.88)	0.92 (0.88–0.95)
LBD	65	0.82 (0.74–0.88)	0.66 (0.58–0.74)	0.92 (0.87–0.96)	0.84 (0.79–0.90)	0.89 (0.85–0.93)	0.86 (0.81–0.92)	0.94 (0.91–0.97)
MCI	860	0.68 (0.65–0.70)	0.54 (0.51–0.57)	0.69 (0.67–0.72)	0.76 (0.74–0.78)	0.76 (0.74–0.78)	0.80 (0.77–0.81)	0.85 (0.83–0.87)
Co-morbid depression	281	0.80 (0.77–0.84)	0.62 (0.57–0.66)	0.81 (0.78–0.84)	0.86 (0.84–0.89)	0.84 (0.82–0.87)	0.84 (0.82–0.87)	0.93 (0.91–0.95)
MCI with co-morbid depression	94	0.75 (0.69–0.82)	0.59 (0.52–0.65)	0.75 (0.70–0.81)	0.82 (0.78–0.87)	0.80 (0.76–0.85)	0.80 (0.75–0.84)	0.90 (0.86–0.93)
MCI without co-morbid depression	766	0.67 (0.64–0.69)	0.53 (0.50–0.56)	0.69 (0.66–0.71)	0.75 (0.73–0.77)	0.76 (0.73–0.78)	0.80 (0.76–0.81)	0.84 (0.82–0.86)

AD = Alzheimer's disease, FTD = frontotemporal dementia, LBD = Lewy body dementia, PDD = Parkinson's dementia, VaD = vascular dementia; AUC = area under the curve; CI = confidence intervals.

ROC curves comparing the subtests of the *Qmci* screen are presented in Figure 3a–l. The highest median score for the clock drawing subtest was found in those with VaD (14/15), the lowest was in LBD (7/15). The logical memory subtest was the most accurate of the *Qmci* screen subtests for most dementia subtypes and MCI (AUC 0.80, 95% CI: 0.77–0.81). Orientation was accurate for AD (AUC 0.88, 95% CI:) but had particularly low accuracy in VaD (AUC 0.71, 95% CI: 0.66–0.71), FTD (AUC 0.78, 95% CI: 0.69–0.87), PDD (AUC 0.71, 95% CI: 0.61–0.81) and MCI (AUC 0.68, 95% CI: 0.65–0.70). Clock drawing had the highest accuracy for identifying PDD (AUC 0.92, 95% CI: 0.87–0.96). Word registration had the lowest accuracy for all dementia subtypes and MCI.

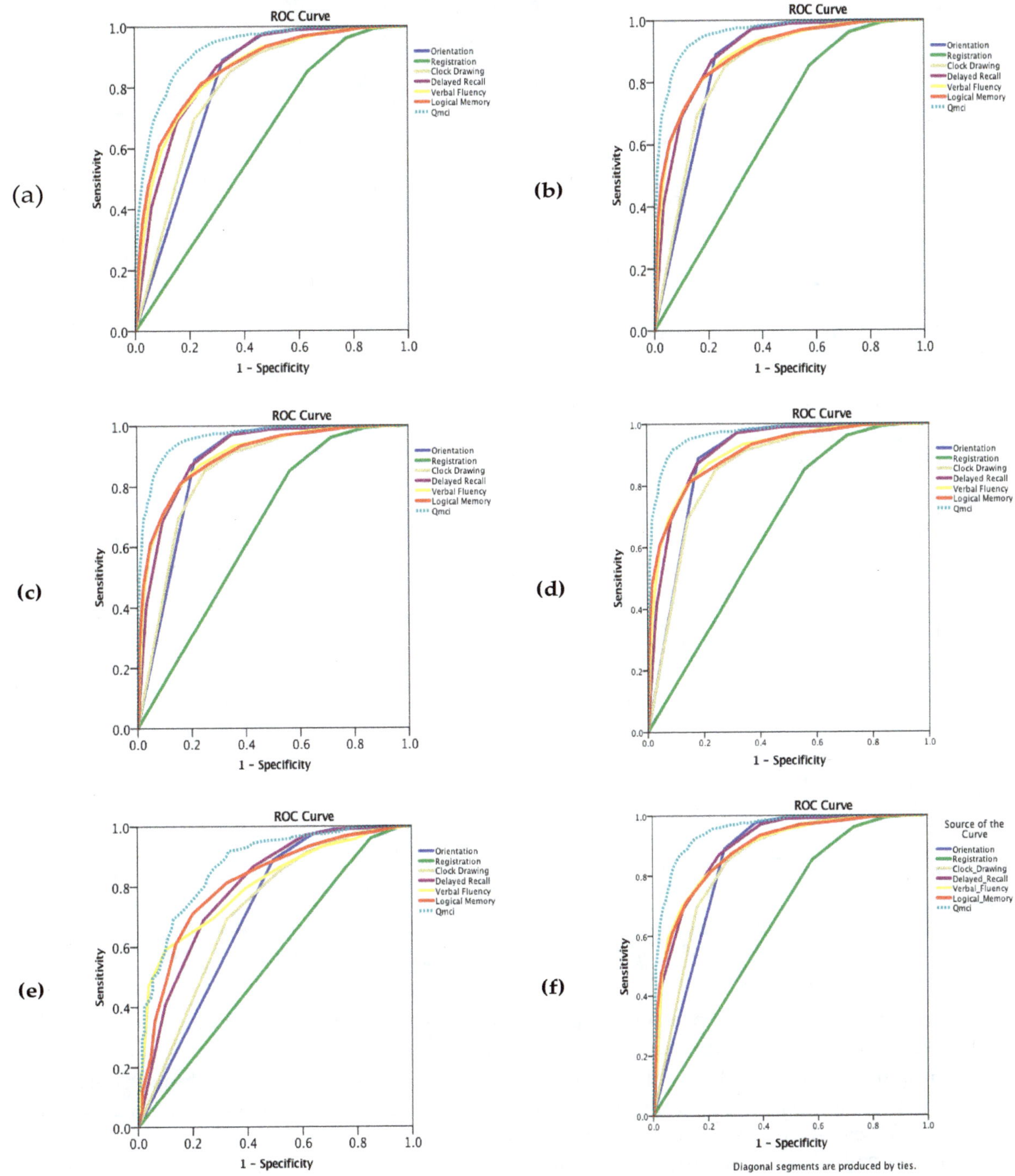

Figure 3. *Cont.*

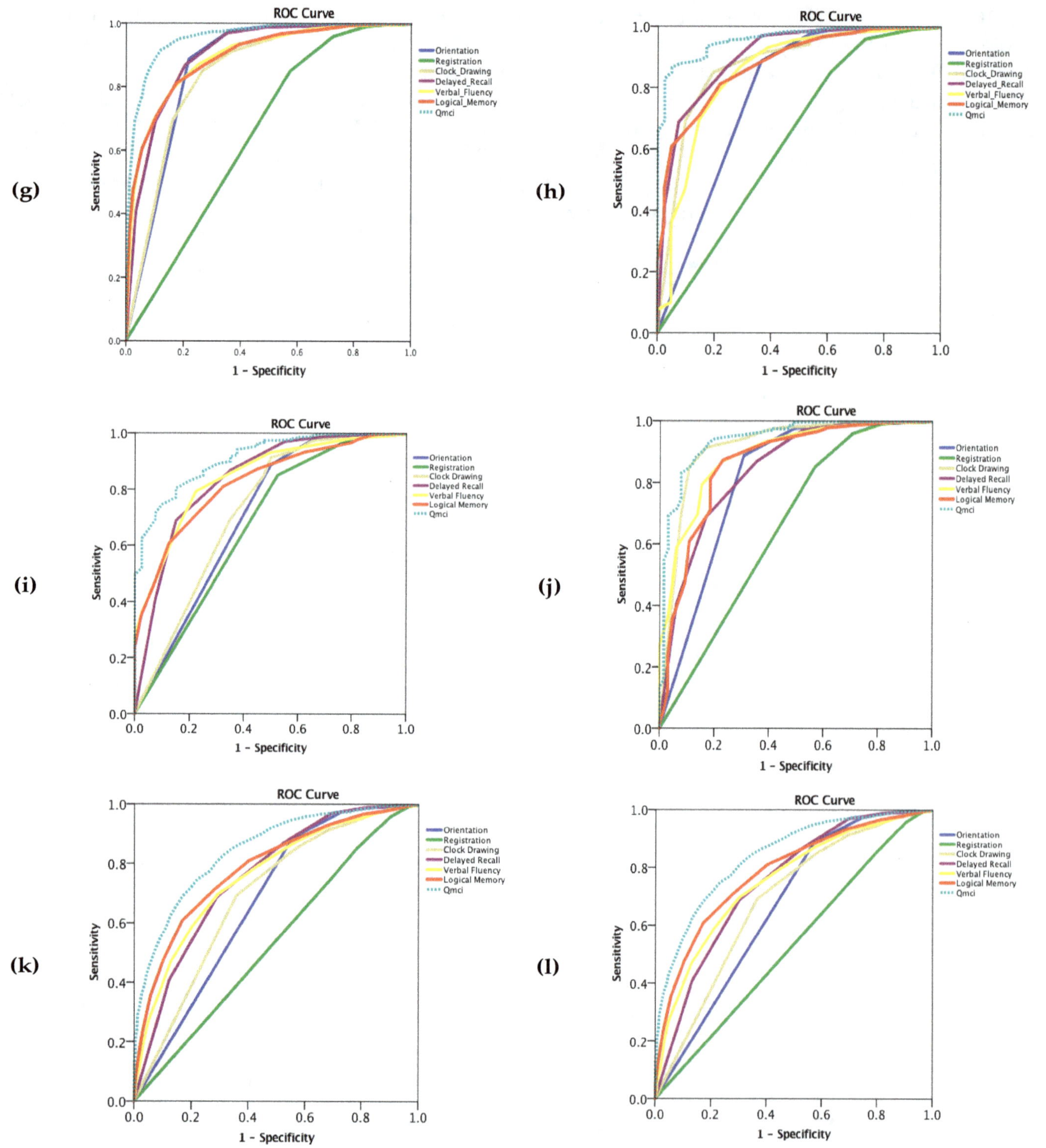

Figure 3. Receiver operating characteristic curves (**a**–**l**) comparing the accuracy of the Quick Mild Cognitive Impairment (Q*mci*) subtests in differentiating normal controls (n = 875) from those with mild cognitive impairment (MCI), different dementia subtypes and comorbid depression for participants included within the Q*mci* screen validation, Doxycycline and Rifampicin for Alzheimer's Disease study and Geriatric Assessment Tool databases. (**a**). All patients (n = 3020); (**b**). All patients with dementia (n = 2160); (**c**). Dementia excluding depression (n = 1879); (**d**). Alzheimer's dementia (n = 1483); (**e**). Vascular dementia (n = 130; (**f**). Mixed dementia (n = 400); (**g**). Alzheimer's, vascular, mixed dementia (n = 2013); (**h**). Frontotemporal dementia (n = 41); (**i**). Parkinson's disease dementia (n = 41); (**j**). Lewy body dementia (n = 65); (**k**). All MCI (n = 860); (**l**). MCI excluding depression (n = 766).

Those diagnosed with dementia and co-morbid depression were younger ($z = -5.9$, $p < 0.001$) and more likely to be female ($X^2 = 11.4$, $p < 0.001$) than those without comorbid depression. There was no statistically significant difference in the number of years in education ($z = -1.3$, $p = 0.21$). Those diagnosed with dementia (all subtypes excluding MCI) with co-morbid depression ($n = 281$) had statistically significantly higher median *Qmci* screen and SMMSE scores than those without ($n = 1879$) depression: Median *Qmci* screen scores of 44 versus 37, respectively ($z = -4.771$, $p < 0.001$) and median SMMSE scores of 25 versus 23, respectively ($z = -5.627$, $p < 0.001$). Contrasting this, comparison of median scores for MCI with and without depression showed that scores were significantly lower for those with co-morbid depression for both the *Qmci* screen, (52 and 57 respectively, $z = -2.927$, $p = 0.003$) and SMMSE (26 and 28 respectively, $z = -3.302$, $p = 0.001$). Co-morbid depression lowered the diagnostic accuracy of both instruments for dementia but improved the accuracy in those with MCI. All *Qmci* screen subtest scores were less accurate for MCI among those patients with co-morbid depression.

4. Discussion

This study compares the diagnostic accuracy of the SMMSE and *Qmci* screen in different dementia subtypes using a large sample of patients pooled from three different datasets using AUC values as a global measure of diagnostic accuracy. The results show that the SMMSE and *Qmci* screen are both accurate CSIs when used to identify dementia in patients presenting with cognitive symptoms to geriatric and memory clinics compared with normal controls. Overall, the *Qmci* screen had high sensitivity and specificity in separating normal controls from those with cognitive impairment (MCI or dementia with or with co-morbid depression). The SMMSE had poor sensitivity, albeit excellent specificity at its widely-used cut-off. These results would be expected as the *Qmci* screen contains more challenging tests of episodic memory [28], which are better able to differentiate MCI from mild dementia [8,29]. The SMMSE is overly weighted towards tests of orientation (one-third of its points), which is best able to identify established dementia [28]. Further, while a cut-off of <24/30 is widely applied for the SMMSE, recent studies suggest that higher cut-offs between 26 [37] and 29 [13], closer to that found here, are more accurate and produce a better balance between sensitivity and specificity. As with its' original validation study [8,28], this analysis confirms the *Qmci* screen is more accurate overall and that its logical memory subtest is its most accurate for separating MCI from normal controls. It also had high levels of accuracy for most dementia subtypes and patients with and without co-morbid depression. The SMMSE, while it had good to excellent accuracy in differentiating most dementia subtypes from normal controls, was less accurate in identifying MCI [8], and had only fair accuracy in identifying VaD (AUC of 0.74) from controls, supporting previous studies in these conditions, where an alternative instrument is suggested [17]. Similarly, while the SMMSE's accuracy in detecting PDD from normal controls was good (AUC 0.81), it performed relatively poorly compared to the *Qmci* screen, supporting evidence that it is less suitable due to both floor and ceiling effects in those with movement disorders [18,38]. The study also examined the subtests of the *Qmci* screen and their differential accuracy in separating those with MCI and dementia from normal controls. As was found in the initial validation, logical memory was most accurate in identifying MCI [28]. Clock drawing was most accurate in detecting LBD but the accuracy for PDD was relatively lower. Clock drawing is often grossly abnormal in LBD, particularly for copying rather than drawing clocks [39]. Differences between LBD and PDD were unexpected and it is likely that small numbers influenced the results. Orientation was only accurate for AD and mixed dementia having poor accuracy for other dementia subtypes and MCI.

In this study, co-morbid depression had a significant impact on CSI scores; those with dementia and depression scored significantly higher on both the SMMSE and *Qmci* screen than those without. This was unexpected as other studies [22] suggest that impaired attention and other cognitive deficits associated with low mood negatively impact on scores. Nevertheless, co-morbid depression did lower the diagnostic accuracy of both instruments for differentiating dementia from normal controls.

The opposite effect was seen for MCI; those with co-morbid depression scored less well on both CSIs, which had higher diagnostic accuracy for these patients. This suggests that comorbid depression may influence CSIs in different ways depending on the diagnostic stage of cognitive impairment. Depression may also have a greater clinical effect at earlier stages of disease progression with evidence that depressive symptoms increase the risk for converting from MCI to dementia, particularly amnestic type to AD [21,40].

The strength of this study is derived from its large sample size and careful pooling of data derived from similar data sets collected by the same principal investigator. This study also has limitations. Pooling data from discrete, albeit related, datasets with different populations may have created bias. Some data on gender were missing and subtest data for the SMMSE were not available across all three datasets, which limited the analysis. The number of patients with atypical or less common dementia subtypes was small and may be unrepresentative of the true performance of the instruments in that subtype, leading to bias. The data collection began in 1999 when the awareness of LBD was low, potentially resulting in misclassification bias. Likewise, only patients with AD or those with AD, VaD and mixed dementia were included in the DARAD and the *Qmci* validation databases respectively. In addition, the prevalence of cognitive impairment (MCI/dementia) was high among those attending these geriatric and memory clinics potentially leading to spectrum bias. Further, this study was a retrospective review of patients with no detailed information available regarding the type of depressive symptoms. Similarly, it was not possible to assess MCI subtypes in this study, though the majority of patients in the GAT database reported amnestic type symptoms, suggesting that most had aMCI. Finally, the statistical analysis was limited to using AUC scores as a global measure of diagnostic accuracy and further research is now planned to explore the psychometric properties of these instruments in different dementia subtypes and to identify the optimal cut-off scores.

In summary, this study reaffirms that both the SMMSE and *Qmci* screen are useful in separating patients with dementia from normal controls. It confirms the superior accuracy of the *Qmci* screen in MCI. It also shows that different short screens have significantly different accuracy in different dementia subtypes, suggesting that pre-screen/pre-test suspicion of a possible diagnosis (MCI or specific dementia subtype) based upon history and examination should direct the choice of instrument to be used when performing cognitive screening. This is important as time is limited in clinical practice and short CSIs can only include a limited number of domains, resulting in a time-accuracy trade-off supporting the need for careful selection a priori [41]. The results also suggest that a history of depression may affect the accuracy of cognitive screens, particularly in those with MCI in which it lowers median scores but increased the diagnostic accuracy of CSIs. The opposite effect was seen in dementia. This shows the importance of asking about depression when undertaking cognitive screening [20] and that the effect of comorbid depression on cognitive screening scores merits further investigation. Understanding the optimal cut-offs for these instruments and other short CSIs is also important, so that not only the most appropriate instrument is used in the right setting but also the correct cut-off score is applied. To date, no condition-specific cut-off scores for the SMMSE or *Qmci* screen are available, highlighting that this is an area requiring more research. Further study is also required to confirm these findings and compare with sensitive and specific instruments such as the MoCA and the Mini-Addenbrooke's Cognitive Examination [42].

Author Contributions: R.O. and D.W.M. conceived and designed the study; D.W.M. collected the data; R.O. analyzed the data; R.O. wrote the initial draft of the paper. R.O. and D.W.M. reviewed the submitted and revised drafts.

Acknowledgments: Yang Gao for his role in data preparation and analysis of these datasets.

References

1. Folstein, M.F.; Folstein, S.E.; McHugh, P.R. "Mini-Mental State". A practical method for grading the cognitive state of patients for the clinician. *J. Psychiatry Res.* **1975**, *12*, 189–198. [CrossRef]
2. Molloy, D.W.; Alemayehu, E.; Roberts, R. Reliability of a Standardized Mini-Mental State Examination compared with the traditional Mini-Mental State Examination. *Am. J. Psychiatry* **1991**, *148*, 102–105. [CrossRef] [PubMed]
3. Molloy, D.W.; Standish, T.I.M. A guide to the Standardized Mini-Mental State Examination. *Int. Psychogeriatry* **1997**, *9*, 87–94. [CrossRef]
4. Woodford, H.J.; George, J. Cognitive assessment in the elderly: A review of clinical methods. *QJM Int. J. Med.* **2007**, *100*, 469–484. [CrossRef] [PubMed]
5. Breton, A.; Casey, D.; Arnaoutoglou, N.A. Cognitive tests for the detection of mild cognitive impairment (MCI), the prodromal stage of dementia: Meta-analysis of diagnostic accuracy studies. *Int. J. Geriatr. Psychiatry* **2019**, *34*, 233–242. [CrossRef] [PubMed]
6. Albert, M.S.; DeKosky, S.T.; Dickson, D.; Dubois, B.; Feldman, H.H.; Fox, N.C.; Snyder, P.J. The diagnosis of mild cognitive impairment due to Alzheimer's disease: Recommendations from the national institute on aging-Alzheimer's association workgroups on diagnostic guidelines for Alzheimer's disease. *Alzheimers Dement.* **2011**, *7*, 270–279. [CrossRef]
7. Rami, L.; Molinuevo, J.L.; Sanchez-Valle, R.; Bosch, B.; Villar, A. Screening for amnestic mild cognitive impairment and early Alzheimer's disease with M@T (Memory Alteration Test) in the primary care population. *Int. J. Geriatr. Psychiatry* **2007**, *22*, 294–304. [CrossRef]
8. O'Caoimh, R.; Gao, Y.; McGlade, C.; Healy, L.; Gallagher, P.; Timmons, S.; Molloy, D.W. Comparison of the Quick Mild Cognitive Impairment (Qmci) screen and the SMMSE in screening for mild cognitive impairment. *Age Ageing* **2012**, *41*, 624–629. [CrossRef]
9. Nasreddine, Z.S.; Phillips, N.A.; Bédirian, V.; Charbonneau, S.; Whitehead, V.; Collin, I.; Cummings, J.L.; Chertkow, H. The Montreal Cognitive Assessment, MoCA: A brief screening tool for mild cognitive impairment. *J. Am. Geriatr. Soc.* **2005**, *53*, 695–699. [CrossRef]
10. Mitchell, A.J. A Meta-Analysis of the Accuracy of the Mini-Mental State Examination in the Detection of Dementia and Mild Cognitive Impairment. *J. Psychiatry Res.* **2009**, *43*, 411–431. [CrossRef]
11. Mitchell, A.J.; Shiri-Feshki, M. Rate of progression of mild cognitive impairment to dementia-meta-analysis of 41 robust inception cohort studies. *Acta Psychiatry Scand.* **2009**, *119*, 252–265. [CrossRef] [PubMed]
12. Crum, R.M.; Anthony, J.C.; Bassett, S.S.; Folstein, M.F. Population-based norms for the Mini-Mental State Examination by age and educational level. *J. Am. Med. Assoc.* **1993**, *269*, 2386–2391. [CrossRef]
13. O'Caoimh, R.; Gao, Y.; Svendovski, A.; Gallagher, P.; Eustace, J.; Molloy, D.W. Comparing approaches to optimize cut-off scores for short cognitive screening instruments in mild cognitive impairment and dementia. *J. Alzheimers Dis.* **2017**, *57*, 123–133. [CrossRef] [PubMed]
14. Velayudhan, L.; Ryu, S.H.; Raczek, M.; Philpot, M.; Lindesay, J.; Critchfield, M.; Livingston, G. Review of brief cognitive tests for patients with suspected dementia. *Int. Psychogeriatry* **2014**, *26*, 1247–1262. [CrossRef] [PubMed]
15. Nazem, S.; Siderowf, A.D.; Duda, J.E.; Have, T.T.; Colcher, A.; Horn, S.S.; Moberg, P.J.; Wilkinson, J.R.; Hurtig, H.I.; Stern, M.B.; et al. Montreal Cognitive Assessment performance in patients with Parkinson's disease with "normal" global cognition according to mini-mental state examination score. *J. Am. Geriatr. Soc.* **2009**, *57*, 304–308. [CrossRef] [PubMed]
16. Osher, J.E.; Wicklund, A.H.; Rademaker, A.; Johnson, N.; Weintraub, S. The Mini-Mental State Examination in behavioral variant frontotemporal dementia and primary progressive aphasia. *Am. J. Alzheimer's Dis.* **2008**, *22*, 468–473. [CrossRef] [PubMed]
17. Ghafar, M.Z.A.A.; Miptah, H.N.; O'Caoimh, R. Cognitive screening instruments to identify vascular cognitive impairment: A systematic review. *Int. J. Geriatr. Psychiatry* **2019**, *34*, 1114–1127. [CrossRef]
18. Bak, T.H.; Rogers, T.T.; Crawford, L.M.; Hearn, V.C.; Mathuranath, P.S.; Hodges, J.R. Cognitive bedside assessment in atypical parkinsonian syndromes. *J. Neurol. Neurosurg. Psychiatry* **2005**, *76*, 420–422. [CrossRef]
19. Russo, M.; Mahon, K.; Burdick, K. Measuring cognitive functions in MDD: Emerging assessment tools. *Depress. Anxiety* **2015**, *32*, 262–269. [CrossRef]

20. Richardson, L.; Adams, S. Cognitive deficits in patients with depression. *J. Nur. Pract.* **2018**, *14*, 437–443. [CrossRef]
21. Van der Mussele, S.; Fransen, E.; Struyfs, H.; Luyckx, J.; Mariën, P.; Saerens, J.; Somers, N.; Goeman, J.; De Deyn, PP.; Engelborghs, S. Depression in Mild Cognitive Impairment is associated with Progression to Alzheimer's Disease: A Longitudinal Study. *J. Alzheimers Dis.* **2014**, *42*, 1239–1250. [CrossRef] [PubMed]
22. Anderson, T.M.; Sachdev, P.S.; Brodaty, H.; Trollor, J.N.; Andrews, G. Effects of sociodemographic and health variables on Mini-Mental State Exam scores in older Australians. *Am. J. Ger. Psychiatry* **2007**, *15*, 467–476. [CrossRef] [PubMed]
23. Gao, Y.; O'Caoimh, R.; Healy, L.; Kerins, D.M.; Eustace, J.; Guyatt, G.; Sammon, D.; Molloy, D.W. Effects of centrally acting ACE inhibitors on the rate of cognitive decline in dementia. *BMJ Open* **2013**, *3*, e002881. [CrossRef] [PubMed]
24. Molloy, D.W.; Standish, T.I.; Zhou, Q.; Guyatt, G. DARAD Study Group. A multicenter, blinded, randomized, factorial controlled trial of doxycycline and rifampin for treatment of Alzheimer's disease: The DARAD trial. *Int. J. Geriatr. Psychiatry* **2013**, *28*, 463–470. [CrossRef] [PubMed]
25. Petersen, R.C.; Smith, G.E.; Waring, S.C.; Ivnik, R.J.; Tangalos, E.G.; Kokmen, E. Mild cognitive impairment: Clinical characterization an outcome. *Arch. Neurol.* **1999**, *56*, 303–308. [CrossRef]
26. American Psychiatric Association. *Diagnostic and Statistical Manual of Mental Disorders*, 4th ed.; American Psychiatric Association: Washington, DC, USA, 1994.
27. Yesavage, J.A. Geriatric Depression Scale. *Psychopharmacol. Bull.* **1988**, *24*, 709–711.
28. O'Caoimh, R.; Gao, Y.; Gallagher, P.F.; Eustace, J.; McGlade, C.; Molloy, D.W. Which part of the Quick Mild Cognitive Impairment screen (Qmci) discriminates between normal cognition, mild cognitive impairment and dementia? *Age Ageing* **2013**, *42*, 324–330. [CrossRef]
29. O'Caoimh, R.; Timmons, S.; Molloy, D.W. Screening for Mild Cognitive Impairment: Comparison of "MCI Specific" Screening Instruments. *J. Alzheimer's Dis.* **2016**, *51*, 619–629. [CrossRef]
30. O'Caoimh, R.; Svendrovski, A.; Johnston, B.C.; Gao, Y.; McGlade, C.; Eustace, J.; Timmons, S.; Guyatt, G.; Molloy, D.W. The Quick Mild Cognitive Impairment screen correlated with the Standardized Alzheimer's Disease Assessment Scale–cognitive section in clinical trials. *J. Clin. Epidemiol.* **2014**, *67*, 87–92. [CrossRef]
31. Bunt, S.; O'Caoimh, R.; Krijnen, W.P.; Molloy, D.W.; Goodijk, G.P.; Van der Schans, C.P.; Hobbelen, H.J.S.M. Validation of the Dutch version of the quick mild cognitive impairment screen (Qmci-D). *BMC Geriatr.* **2015**, *15*, 115. [CrossRef]
32. Yavuz, B.B.; Varan, H.D.; O'Caoimh, R.; Kizilarslanoglu, M.C.; Kilic, M.K.; Molloy, D.W.; Dogrul, R.T.; Karabulut, E.; Svendrovski, A.; Sagir, A.; et al. Validation of the Turkish Version of the Quick Mild Cognitive Impairment Screen. *Am. J. Alzheimer's Dis.* **2017**, *32*, 145–156. [CrossRef] [PubMed]
33. Iavarone, A.; Carpinelli Mazzi, M.; Russo, G.; D'Anna, F.; Peluso, S.; Mazzeo, P.; De Luca, V.; De Michele, G.; Iaccarino, G.; Abete, P.; et al. The Italian version of the Quick Mild Cognitive Impairment (Qmci-I) screen: Normative study on 307 healthy subjects. *Aging Clin. Exp. Res.* **2018**, *31*, 353–360. [CrossRef] [PubMed]
34. Morita, A.; O'Caoimh, R.; Murayama, H.; Molloy, D.W.; Inoue, S.; Shobugawa, Y.; Fujiwara, T. Validity of the Japanese Version of the Quick Mild Cognitive Impairment Screen. *Int. J. Environ. Res. Public Health* **2019**, *16*, 917. [CrossRef] [PubMed]
35. Metz, C.E. Basic principles of ROC curve analysis. *Sem. Nucl. Med.* **1979**, *8*, 283–298. [CrossRef]
36. DeLong, E.R.; DeLong, D.M.; Clarke-Pearson, D.L. Comparing the areas under two or more correlated receiver operating characteristic curves: A nonparametric approach. *Biometrics* **1988**, *44*, 837–845. [CrossRef] [PubMed]
37. Kvitting, A.S.; Fällman, K.; Wressle, E.; Marcusson, J. Age-Normative MMSE Data for Older Persons Aged 85 to 93 in a Longitudinal Swedish Cohort. *J. Am. Geriatr. Soc.* **2019**, *67*, 534–538. [CrossRef] [PubMed]
38. Biundo, R.; Weis, L.; Bostantjopoulou, S.; Stefanova, E.; Falup-Pecurariu, C.; Kramberger, M.G.; Geurtsen, G.J.; Antonini, A.; Weintraub, D.; Aarsland, D. MMSE and MoCA in Parkinson's disease and dementia with Lewy bodies: A multicenter 1-year follow-up study. *J. Neural Transm.* **2016**, *123*, 431–438. [CrossRef] [PubMed]
39. Gnanalingham, K.K.; Byrne, E.J.; Thornton, A.; Sambrook, M.A.; Bannister, P. Motor and cognitive function in Lewy body dementia: Comparison with Alzheimer's and Parkinson's diseases. *J. Neur. Neurosurg. Psychiatry* **1997**, *62*, 243–252. [CrossRef] [PubMed]

40. Kida, J.; Nemoto, K.; Ikejima, C.; Bun, S.; Kakuma, T.; Mizukami, K.; Asada, T. Impact of depressive symptoms on conversion from mild cognitive impairment subtypes to Alzheimer's disease: A community-based longitudinal study. *J. Alzheimer's Dis.* **2016**, *51*, 405–415. [CrossRef] [PubMed]
41. Larner, A.J. MACE versus MoCA: Equivalence or superiority? Pragmatic diagnostic test accuracy study. *Int. Psychogeriatr.* **2017**, *29*, 931–937. [CrossRef] [PubMed]
42. Larner, A.J. Speed versus accuracy in cognitive assessment when using CSIs. *Prog. Neurol. Psychiatry* **2015**, *19*, 21–24. [CrossRef]

14

Aged Mouse Cortical Microglia Display an Activation Profile Suggesting Immunotolerogenic Functions

Tanja Zöller [1], Abdelraheim Attaai [1,2,3], Phani Sankar Potru [4], Tamara Ruß [4] and Björn Spittau [1,4,*]

1 Institute for Anatomy and Cell Biology, Department of Molecular Embryology, Faculty of Medicine, University of Freiburg, Freiburg 79104, Germany; tanja.zoeller@googlemail.com (T.Z.); abdelraheim.attaai@anat.uni-freiburg.de (A.A.)
2 Faculty of Biology, University of Freiburg, Freiburg 79104, Germany
3 Department of Anatomy and Histology, Faculty of Veterinary Medicine, Assiut University, Assiut 71526, Egypt
4 Institute of Anatomy, University of Rostock, Rostock 18057, Germany; PhaniSankar.Potru@med.uni-rostock.de (P.S.P.); TamaraHeike.Russ@med.uni-rostock.de (T.R.)
* Correspondence: bjoern.spittau@med.uni-rostock.de

Abstract: Microglia are the resident immune cells of the central nervous system (CNS) and participate in physiological and pathological processes. Their unique developmental nature suggests age-dependent structural and functional impairments that might contribute to neurodegenerative diseases. In the present study, we addressed the age-dependent changes in cortical microglia gene expression patterns and the expression of M1- and M2-like activation markers. Iba1 immunohistochemistry, isolation of cortical microglia followed by fluorescence-activated cell sorting and RNA isolation to analyze transcriptional changes in aged cortical microglia was performed. We provide evidence that aging is associated with decreased numbers of cortical microglia and the establishment of a distinct microglia activation profile including upregulation of *Ifi204*, *Lilrb4*, *Arhgap*, *Oas1a*, *Cd244* and *Ildr2*. Moreover, flow cytometry revealed that aged cortical microglia express increased levels of Cd206 and Cd36. The data presented in the current study indicate that aged mouse cortical microglia adopt a distinct activation profile, which suggests immunosuppressive and immuno-tolerogenic functions.

Keywords: microglia; aging; cerebral cortex; neuroinflammation

1. Introduction

Aging has been described as one of the major risk factors for development, onset and progression of several diseases, including cancer, cardiovascular pathologies, as well as neurodegenerative disorders [1]. In the central nervous system (CNS), age-dependent changes are believed to foster the development of neuropathologies including Alzheimer's disease (AD) and Parkinson's disease (PD). The high incidence of neurodegenerative diseases in elderly individuals has been linked to dysregulated functions of innate immune responses mediated by CNS-resident microglia [2]. Microglia develop from yolk sac progenitors in a PU.1- and interferon regulatory factor 8 (Irf8)-dependent manner [3] and further colonize the embryonic CNS parenchyma by chemotactic attraction driven by neuron-derived IL34 [4]. Sensing of neuronal IL-34 is mediated by colony stimulating factor-1 receptor (CSF1R), which is essential for microglia homing and migration towards the developing CNS [5].

After induction of a microglia-specific gene expression pattern [6] in a transforming growth factor β1 (TGFβ1)-dependent mechanism [7] and the establishment of the blood-brain barrier (BBB), microglia turnover in the adult CNS involves microglia proliferation and apoptosis [8], but not replacement by bone-marrow-derived progenitor cells [9,10]. This self-renewal capacity causing high proliferative activity of microglia has been hypothesized to result in telomere shortening and subsequent senescence of aged microglia [11]. However, it appears that microglia in aged mice do not develop telomere shortening, and only transgenic approaches, such as those described in the DNA repair-deficient *Ercc1* mutant mice, display accelerated aging associated with microglial senescence, dystrophy and functional impairments [12,13]. However, it has been reported that aged microglia exhibit enhanced expression of inflammatory markers tumor necrosis factor α (Tnfα), Il1β and Il6 after challenge with lipopolysaccharide (LPS), indicating an increased response of aged microglia [14], which is caused by age-dependent priming of microglia. Toll-like receptors Tl2, Tlr3, Tlr4 [15], as well as high-mobility group box 1 (Hmgb1) [16], have been described to be important mediators of microglia priming. Holtman et al. [17] recently identified a highly conserved gene expression profile of primed microglia, which significantly differed from gene expression patterns observed after LPS-driven acute microglia activation. Interestingly, RNA sequencing from aged total brain microglia revealed increased expression of genes involved in microglia-mediated neuroprotective effects [18].

In the present study, we addressed the age-dependent changes of cortical microglia in 24 months old C57BL/6 mice and observed decreased microglia numbers, enhanced expression of genes related to innate immune responses, and increased numbers of $Cd206^{+}$ and $Cd36^{+}$ microglia. Our data indicate that aging is associated with changes in microglia gene expression, which points towards activation of alternative markers and genes involved in immunosuppressive functions and immune toleration.

2. Results

2.1. Decreased Numbers of Cortical $Iba1^{+}$ Microglia in Aged Mice

In order to address age-dependent changes in cortical thickness and total microglia numbers in the frontal cortex of C57BL/6JRj mice, 50 μm vibratome sections were stained against the microglia marker ionized calcium binding adaptor molecular 1 (Iba1). Figure 1A displays the area used for analysis of cortical thickness. No obvious differences in cortical thickness were observed between young (Figure 1B) and aged (Figure 1C) mice. Moreover, quantification of thicknesses and statistical analyses also revealed no significant differences between young and aged mice (Figure 1D). Interestingly, quantification of cortical microglia ($Iba1^{+}$) numbers revealed significant reduction of $Iba1^{+}$ microglia in aged mice. Figure 1F displays microglia from young mice, showing normal ramifications with fine processes and homogenous distributions throughout the cortex (Figure 1F). However, aged cortical microglia presented a reduced branching pattern and an uneven distribution compared to microglia in young mice (Figure 1G). These data indicate that aging is associated with a reduction of cortical microglia numbers, which tend to cluster and thereby show an uneven distribution pattern.

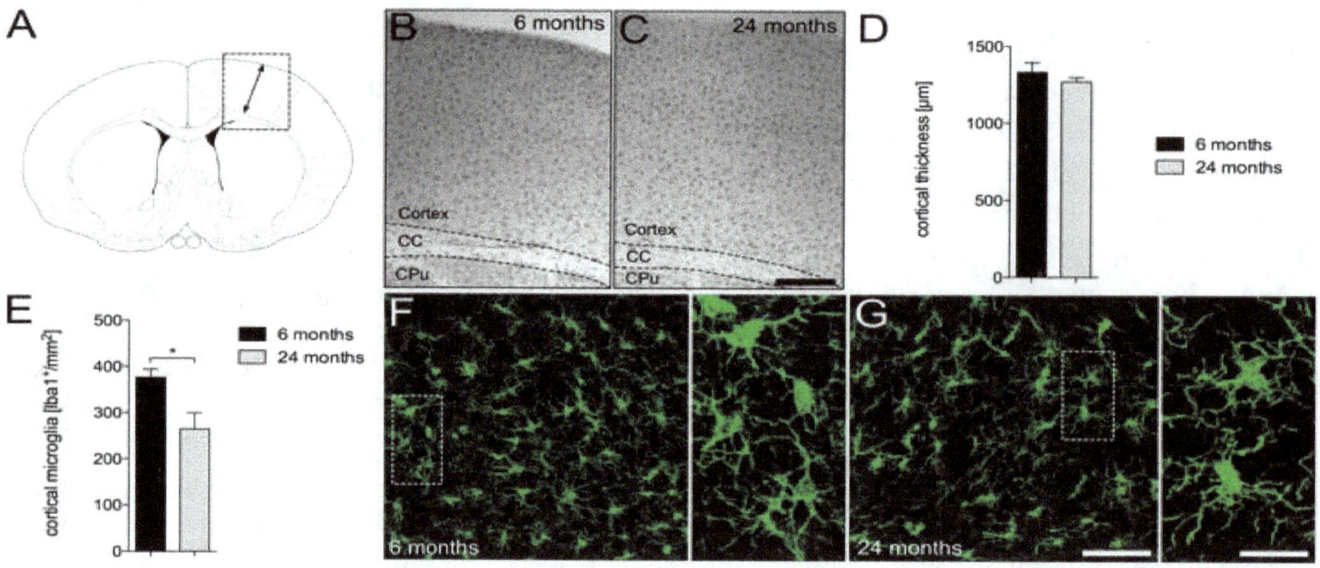

Figure 1. Age-dependent changes in cortical microglia. (**A**) Orientation scheme monitoring cortical areas for evaluation. Arrows mark the area for cortical thickness measurements. Representative images of Iba1$^+$ microglia in cortices from 6-month-old (**B**) and 24-month-old mice (**C**). Scale bar represents 300 µm. Quantifications of cortical thickness (**D**) and cortical Iba1$^+$ microglia numbers (**E**) are shown. Data are given as means ± SEM from three animals per age. p-value derived from Student's t-test is $^* p < 0.05$. Differences in morphology and distribution of Iba1$^+$ microglia between 6-month-old (**F**) and 24-month-old (**G**) mice. Scale bars indicate 20 µm in overview images and 7 µm in high magnification detail images. CC = corpus callsosum, CPu = caudatoputamen.

2.2. Detection of a Distinct Gene Expression Profile in Aged Cortical Microglia

As a next step, we addressed the transcriptional changes in aged cortical microglia. Therefore, frontal cortices from young and aged mice were dissected and microglia were isolated and stained for fluorescence activated cell sorting (FACS). Cd11b$^+$/Cd45^{low}-positive microglia were collected and RNA was isolated for cDNA microarrays (Figure 2A). Expression data were used for prediction of the biological processes (Figure 2B) and molecular functions (Figure 2C) of the top-regulated genes using the DAVID gene ontology (GO term) enrichment analysis. As shown in Figure 2B, immunological functions and cholesterol/steroid metabolic processes are predicted to be upregulated in aged cortical microglia. Activated molecular functions of aged microglia include ATP-binding, 2′-5′-oligoadenylate synthetase activity, double-stranded RNA binding and nucleotidyltransferase activity (Figure 2C). Data from cDNA microarray analysis revealed the upregulation of genes involved in immune responses including *Ifi204*, *Lilrb4*, *Arhgap15* and *Cd244*. Taken together, the data indicate activated immune responses and increased lipid metabolism in aged cortical microglia.

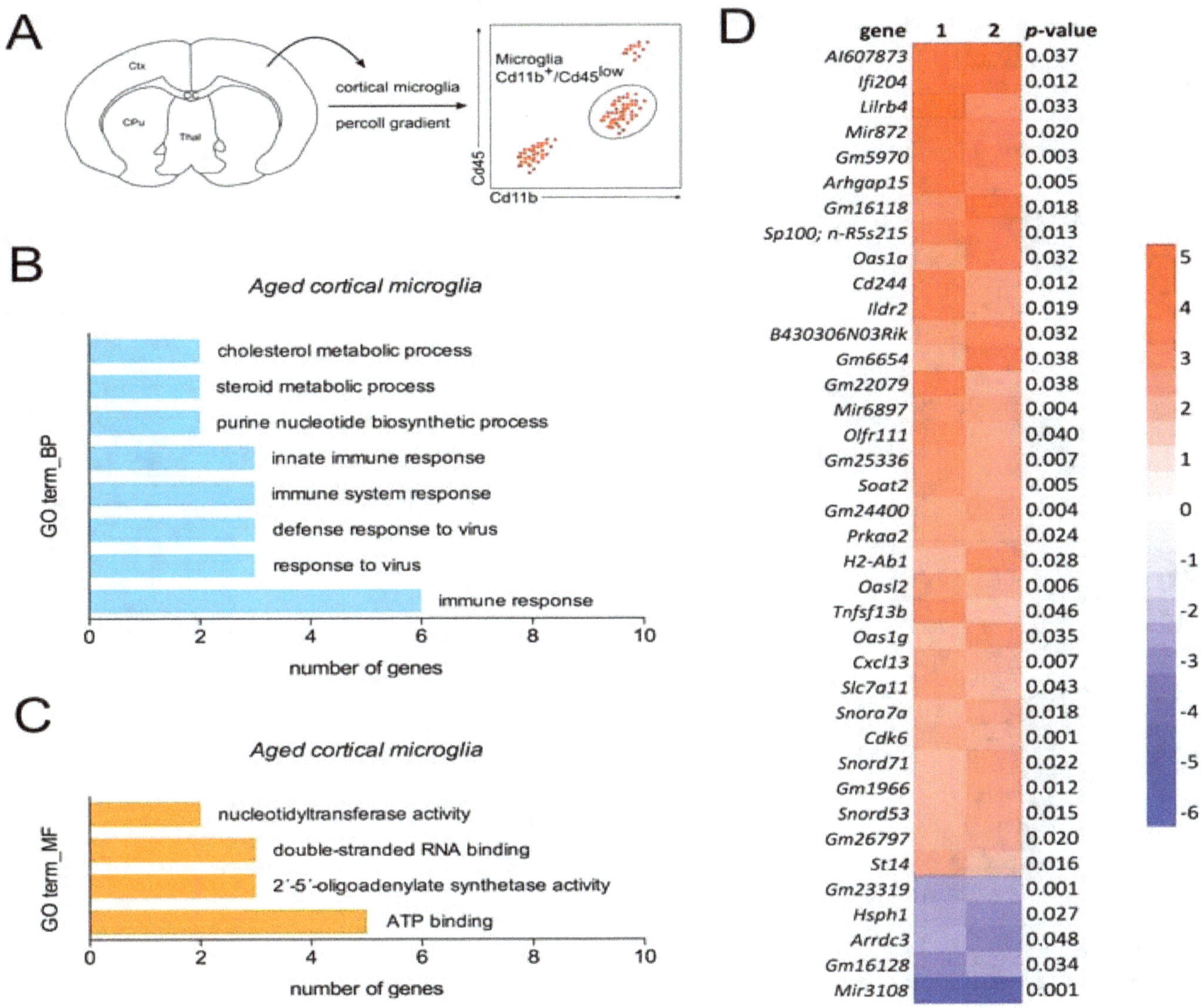

Figure 2. Gene expression pattern of aged cortical microglia. (**A**) Workflow scheme depicting microglia isolation and sorting strategy. (**B**,**C**) GO term enrichment analysis of biological processes (**B**) and molecular functions (**C**) as performed using DAVID Bioinformatics Resources 6.8. (**D**) Heatmap summarizing transcriptional changes in aged cortical microglia. Expression data from aged microglia are presented as $\log_2$-fold changes ($n = 2$) and compared to young (6-month-old) microglia. CC = corpus callosum, CPu = caudatoputamen, Ctx = cortex, Thal = thalamus.

2.3. Increased Expression of Cd206 and Cd36 in Aged Cortical Microglia

Using flow cytometry, the expression of microglia activation markers Cd206, Cd36 and Cd86 was determined. Cortical microglia were isolated using the percoll gradient method and subsequently stained against F4/80 as a microglia marker in combination with either Cd206, Cd36 or Cd86. Flow cytometry revealed that total numbers of F4/80$^+$ cortical microglia were significantly reduced in aged mice (Figure 3A,B), which confirms microglia quantifications depicted in Figure 1E. Moreover, we observed significant increases in Cd206$^+$ (Figure 3A,C), as well as Cd36$^+$ (Figure 3A,D) microglia. As given in Figure 3E, quantifications of F4/80$^+$/Cd86$^+$ microglia revealed that the percentages of Cd86^{high} microglia increase in the frontal cortices of aged mice; however, this increase did not reach statistical significance ($p = 0.069$). The results presented here demonstrate that aged cortical microglia display an activation pattern characterized by increased expression of M1-like as well as M2-like microglia activation markers. Based on the percentages of marker-positive microglia, it is highly likely that distinct cortical microglia subsets with specialized functions exist in aged mice. It further remains to be established to what extent these subsets contribute to anti-inflammatory and restorative functions in the aged cerebral cortex.

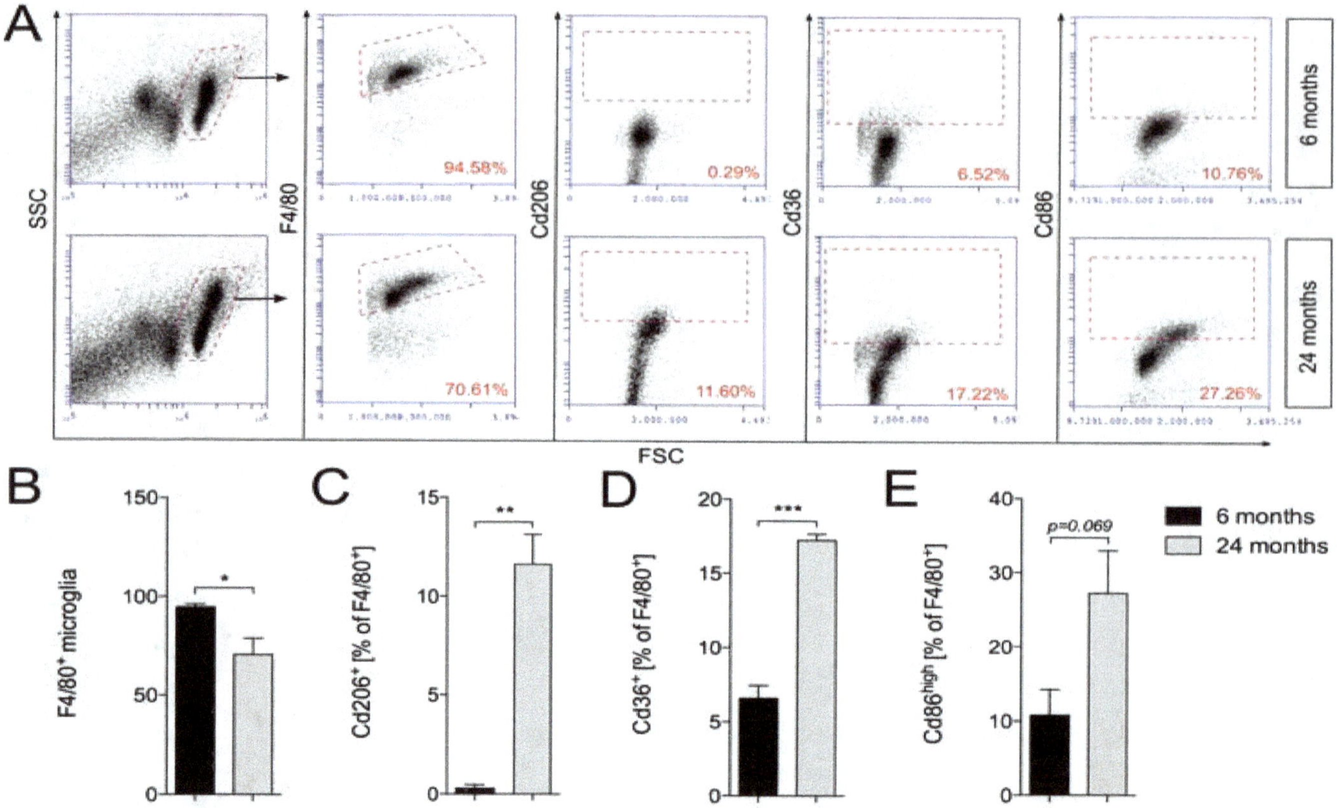

Figure 3. Expression of Cd206, Cd36 and Cd86 in F4/80$^+$ cortical microglia. (**A**) Gating strategy and representative dot plots of Cd206$^+$, Cd36$^+$ and Cd86^{high} cortical microglia from young (6 months) and aged (24 months) mice. Quantification of (**B**) F4/80$^+$, (**C**) Cd206$^+$, (**D**) Cd36$^+$ and (**E**) Cd86^{high} microglia. Data are given as percentages of F4/80$^+$ microglia $\pm$ SEM from three animals per age. p-values derived from student's t-test are * $p < 0.05$, ** $p < 0.01$ and *** $p < 0.001$.

3. Discussion

In the present study, we demonstrate that aging is associated with distinct changes in cortical microglia. We describe that numbers of cortical microglia significantly decreased in 24-month-old male mice and that the remaining microglia in aged mice showed slight morphological changes, as well as an uneven distribution pattern. This observation is in congruence with a recent report showing that microglia numbers decreased in the nigrostriatal system and cortices of 18-month- and 24-month-old mice, respectively [19]. However, a different mouse strain was used in the present study, thus resulting in the necessity of ruling out differences in age-dependent changes of microglia numbers between mouse strains. Morphological changes of aged microglia, including retracted processes and reduced process branching, have also been reported in aged human neocortex samples [20], indicating functional changes described during aging [21]. However, morphological changes of microglia do not necessarily reflect their functional states and, thus, analysis of microglial gene expression has been widely used to gain insights into their functional changes during aging and in several disease models [17,18]. In order to understand the impact of aging on cortical microglia, we have isolated aged (24-month-old) Cd11b$^+$/Cd45^{low} microglia and analyzed their gene expression profiles compared to young (6-month-old) microglia. Using cDNA microarray analysis, we demonstrated the upregulation of immune function related genes, including *Ifi204*, *Lilrb4*, *Arhgap15* and *Cd244*, and DAVID gene ontology (GO term) enrichment analysis further predicted the activation of innate immune responses in aged cortical microglia. However, detailed analysis of recent reports addressing the function of the above-mentioned genes suggests an immunoregulatory and/or anti-inflammatory phenotype of aged cortical microglia. However, the molecular functions of most of the observed upregulated genes are not understood in microglia and, thus, the prediction of potential microglia functions in the aged cerebral cortex can only be made based on recent reports addressing the role of these genes in other cell types. For instance, *Ifi204* expression has been described to increase in macrophages to inhibit proliferation and foster their differentiation [22]. Moreover, macrophage autophagy activation and IFN-β (interferon-β) release after bacterial infections has been linked to *Ifi204* expression [23]. Interestingly, the type I interferon IFN-β has been reported to limit CNS damage by abrogating chronic cytokine release. This functional feature of IFN-β might further explain its therapeutic potential in chronic autoimmune CNS pathologies such as multiple sclerosis [24]. The myeloid inhibitory receptor Lilrb4 (leukocyte immunoglobulin-like receptor b4), also referred to as Ilt3 (immunoglobulin-like transcript 3), Lir-5 (immunoglobulin-like receptor 5) or Cd85k, is a member of the leukocyte immunoglobulin-like receptor family (LILRs/LIRs), and represents an important mediator of immune tolerance [25]. Although the functions of LILRB4 in microglia are unknown and, thus, remain elusive, *Lilrb4*-deficiency has been demonstrated to result in increased Nf-κB (nuclear factor κB) signaling in atherosclerotic plaque-associated macrophages [26] and exaggerated LPS-induced cytokine/chemokine release from neutrophils [27]. In the CNS, increased expression of *Lilrb4* has been described in $Cd11c^+$ microglia, which are believed to counteract amyloid deposition by increased amyloid β-uptake and degradation in a mouse model for AD [28]. Another interesting upregulated gene in aged cortical microglia is the Rho GTPase activating protein 15 (*Arhgap15*), which serves as a potent inhibitor of Rac1 (rac family small GTPase 1) [29]. The small GTPase Rac1 has been implicated in Nox2 (NADPH oxidase 2 or $gp91^{phox}$)-mediated generation of reactive oxygen species (ROS) in microglia [30]. Notably, ROS generation via the Rac1-Nox2 axis has been demonstrated to be responsible for microglia-mediated neurotoxicity associated by Tnfα release and Nf-κB activation [31]. The SLAM (signaling lymphocytic activation molecule) receptor Cd244 was described to be essential in inhibiting the LPS-induced release of proinflammatory cytokines from splenic dendritic cells [32]. However, these functions in microglia have not been analyzed, so far. Taken together, the functional properties of the above-mentioned upregulated genes suggest a distinct phenotype of aged cortical microglia associated with regulation/inhibition of innate immune functions and anti-inflammatory and neuroprotective functions. This notion is further supported by increased surface expression of Cd206, also known as mannose receptor 1 (Mrc1) in aged cortical microglia. Cd206/Mrc1 expression was reported to be increased in alternatively activated microglia facilitating neuroprotective effects [33,34]. Furthermore, we provide evidence that the number of $Cd36^+$ microglia was significantly increased in frontal cortices of aged mice. Recently, increased expression of the scavenger receptor Cd36 in microglia was linked to triggering receptor expressed on myeloid cells 2 (Trem2)-mediated alleviations of AD symptoms by enhanced uptake of Aβ and abrogation of memory loss [35]. Moreover, lack of Cd36 exacerbated injury in cerebral ischemia models associated with reduced engulfment of apoptotic neurons and enhanced Nf-κB signaling [36,37]. It remains elusive how microglia might promote neuroprotection in the aged brain, but expression and release of neuroprotective factors is likely to be one major mechanism. Release of insulin like growth factor 1 (Igf1) from microglia has recently been shown to be essential for survival of cortical layer V neurons during postnatal development [38] and could also be a candidate in the aged cerebral cortex. However, sophisticated proteome-based studies are necessary to understand which microglia-derived factors contribute to neuroprotective effects.

It has been described that microglia in different brain regions show distinct expression patterns of immunoregulatory markers, suggesting the existence of a huge immunological diversity between microglia from different functional CNS regions [39]. In the present study, we clearly demonstrate that cortical microglia in aged mice show a distinct activation profile, which is characterized by immunoregulatory and anti-inflammatory functions. These results suggest that aged microglia might support neuron survival rather than promoting detrimental effects on cortical neuron populations. However, upregulation of Cd86 further indicates M1-like microglia activation in aged mice suggesting a microglia activation phenotype fostering neurodegeneration. It remains to be established to what extent different functional microglia subsets are present in the aged murine cerebral cortex, and whether these cortical microglia phenotypes are region-specific or can be detected in other functional systems of the aged CNS. Finally, data from aged mice need to be compared with recently published reports addressing age-dependent changes in aged human microglia [40,41]. Together, the results presented here further broaden our understanding of age-dependent changes in cortical microglia functions and activation states, and indicate that aging alone—without any additional inflammatory trigger—does not necessarily result in a pro-inflammatory microglia activation.

4. Materials and Methods

4.1. Animals

All animal experiments in this study were approved by the Federal Ministry for Nature, Environment and Consumer's Protection of the federal state of Baden-Württemberg (X-15/01A (9 February 2015), X-15/06A (1 December 2015), G-15/111 (3 December 2015)) and were conducted in accordance with the respective national, federal and institutional regulations. 6-month- and 24-month-old male C57BL/6JRj mice used for cortical microglia isolations (flow cytometry and RNA isolation) and immunohistochemistry were obtained from Janvier (Le Genest Saint Isle, France).

4.2. Microglia Isolation

Mice were deeply anesthetized by intraperitoneal injections of Ketamin (75 mg/kg)/Rompun (5.8 mg/kg) and transcardially perfused with ice-cold phosphate buffer solution (PBS). Brains were dissected and meninges were removed on absorbent paper. Brains were collected in cold buffer (1× HBSS (Hanks' balanced salt solution) containing 1% BSA (bovine serum albumin) and 1 mM EDTA (ethylenediaminetetraacetic acid)), homogenized using a glass homogenizer and filtered through 75 µm cell strainers (Falcon). Samples were centrifuged 12 min at 300× *g* and 10 °C. For density gradient centrifugation, the pellet was resuspended in 5 mL 37% Percoll (P1644, Sigma Aldrich, St. Louis, MO, USA) in PBS, underlayed with 4 mL 70% Percoll and overlayed with 4 mL 30% Percoll in a 15 mL Falcon Tube (Corning, New York, NY, USA). Gradients were centrifuged for 40 min, 600× *g*, 10 °C, without breaks. Finally, the cell layer was collected from the 70% and 37% interface and transferred to PBS containing 1% FCS and centrifuged for 5 min, 200× *g*, 4 °C.

4.3. Flow Cytometry

Cells were stained with primary antibodies directed against Cd11b (1:20, 53-0112-82, eBiosciene, Thermo Fisher Scientific, Waltham, MA, USA), Cd206 (5 µL, FAB2535C, R&D Systems, Minneapolis, MN, USA), Cd36 (5 µL, MCA2748A647, AbD Serotech, BIO-Rad, Puchheim, Germany), Cd45 (1:20, 17-0451-82, eBiosciene), Cd86 (5 µL, MCA2463PE, AbD Serotech) and F4/80 (5 µL, MCA497A488, AbD Serotech) at 4 °C for 15 min. Fc (fragment crystallizable region) receptor blocking (TrueStain fcX, 101319, Biolegend, San Diego, CA, USA) was used to avoid unspecific antibody binding. Cells were washed and analyzed using the BD Accuri C6 flow cytometer (BD, Heidelberg, Germany).

4.4. Histology and Immunohistochemistry

Anesthetized mice were transcardially perfused using PBS followed by 4% paraformaldehyde (PFA). Brains were extracted and post-fixed in 4% PFA overnight. Free-floating 50 µm vibratome (Leica, Wetzlar, Germany) sections were incubated overnight with anti-IBA1 (1:1000, 019-19741, Wako, Japan). Alexa Flour 488-conjugated secondary antibodies (Cell Signaling Technology, Danvers, MA, USA) were used at 1:200 for 2 h at room temperature. Nuclei were counterstained using 4′6-diamidino-2-phenylindole (DAPI, Roche, Basel, Switzerland) and sections were mounted on glass cover slips. Imaging was performed using the Leica TCS SP8 confocal laser scanning microscope (Leica, Wetzlar, Germany) and LAS AF image analysis software (Leica, Wetzlar, Germany). For DAB (3,3′-diaminobenzidine) staining, peroxidase-conjugated secondary antibodies (Dianova, Hamburg, Germany) were used. Images were captured using A Zeiss AxioImager I (Zeiss, Göttingen, Germany) and the Stereoinvestigator Software 8.0 (MicroBrightField, Magdeburg, Germany).

4.5. Determination of Cortical Thickness and Cortical Microglia Numbers

Cortical thicknesses and microglia numbers were determined after immunohistochemical stainings (Iba1) of 50 μm coronal vibratome sections. After image acquisition using a Zeiss AxioImager I (Zeiss, Göttingen, Germany) and the Stereoinvestigator Software 8.0 (MicroBrightField, Magdeburg, Germany). Four serial sections were opened with ImageJ (National Institutes of Health, Bethesda, MD, USA), and the cortical thicknesses were analyzed after setting the scale for pixel/micron conversation using the ImageJ-integrated measurement function. Means were calculated from four serial sections, and cortical thicknesses are given in μm. Cortical microglia numbers were obtained using the automatic cell counting function of the ImageJ toolbox. Four serial sections were used and $Iba1^+$ microglia were determined in a 0.67 mm^2 rectangle. Microglia numbers were calculated for 1 mm^2 and means from four sections per animals were plotted.

4.6. cDNA Microarray

Total RNA was extracted from $Cd11b^+/Cd45^{low}$ microglia after sorting with BD Cell Sorter FACS Aria Fusion or BD Cell Sorter FACS Aria III using the Picopure RNA extraction kit (Life technologies, Carlsbad, CA, USA) according to the manufacturer's instructions. Cortices of three mice were pooled to obtain sufficient numbers of $Cd11b^+/Cd45^{low}$ microglia for RNA isolation. RNA quality was controlled using RNA pico chips on a Bioanalyzer 2100 (Agilent, Santa Clara, CA, USA). 2 ng total RNA was labeled using the GeneChip WT Pico Reagent kit (catalog number 902623, Thermo Fisher Scientific, Waltham, MA, USA) and hybridized to Affymetrix Mouse Transcriptome Array, MTA 1.0 (Affymetrix, Inc., Santa Clara, CA, USA). In this procedure, first strand cDNA was synthesized with a combination of a Poly-dT and random primers containing a 5′-adaptor sequence. A 3′-adaptor was added to the single-stranded cDNA followed by low-cycle PCR amplification. Next, the cDNA was used as a template for in vitro transcription (IVT), which produces amplified amounts of antisense mRNA (cRNA). The cRNA was then used as input for a second round of first-strand cDNA synthesis, producing single-stranded sense cDNA. Finally, the cDNA was fragmented using uracil-DNA glycosylase (UDG) and end-labeled with biotin and terminal deoxynucleotidyl transferase (TdT). The labeled targets were hybridized to GeneChip MTA 1.0 cartridge arrays, which were stained on a GeneChip Fluidics Station 450 and scanned on a GeneChip scanner 3000 7G (Thermo Fisher Scientific, Waltham, MA, USA).

4.7. Statistics

Data are given as means $\pm$ standard error of the mean (SEM). Two-group analysis (young vs. aged) was performed using Student's t-tests. All statistical analyses were performed using GraphPad Prism 6 (GraphPad Software Inc., La Jolla, CA, USA) and p-values < 0.05 were considered as being statistically significant. To determine differential expression of genes in young and aged cortical microglia, the two-sample Bayesian t-test [42] was used.

Acknowledgments: The authors thank Ludmila Butenko for her excellent technical support. The work was funded by grants from the Deutsche Forschungsgemeinschaft (DFG, SP 1555/2-1). Funds from the University of Rostock were received to cover the costs of publishing in open access.

Author Contributions: Björn Spittau and Tanja Zöller conceived and designed the experiments; Tanja Zöller, Abdelraheim Attaai and Phani Sankar Potru performed the experiments; Tanja Zöller and Björn Spittau analyzed the data; Björn Spittau, Phani Sankar Potru and Tamara Ruß wrote the paper.

References

1. McHugh, D.; Gil, J. Senescence and aging: Causes, consequences, and therapeutic avenues. *J. Cell Biol.* **2018**, *217*, 65–77. [CrossRef] [PubMed]
2. Molteni, M.; Rossetti, C. Neurodegenerative diseases: The immunological perspective. *J. Neuroimmunol.* **2017**, *313*, 109–115. [CrossRef] [PubMed]
3. Kierdorf, K.; Erny, D.; Goldmann, T.; Sander, V.; Schulz, C.; Perdiguero, E.G.; Wieghofer, P.; Heinrich, A.; Riemke, P.; Hölscher, C.; et al. Microglia emerge from erythromyeloid precursors via Pu.1- and Irf8-dependent pathways. *Nat. Neurosci.* **2013**, *16*, 273–280. [CrossRef] [PubMed]
4. Greter, M.; Lelios, I.; Pelczar, P.; Hoeffel, G.; Price, J.; Leboeuf, M.; Kündig, T.M.; Frei, K.; Ginhoux, F.; Merad, M.; et al. Stroma-derived interleukin-34 controls the development and maintenance of Langerhans cells and the maintenance of microglia. *Immunity* **2012**, *37*, 1050–1060. [CrossRef] [PubMed]
5. Ginhoux, F.; Greter, M.; Leboeuf, M.; Nandi, S.; See, P.; Gokhan, S.; Mehler, M.F.; Conway, S.J.; Ng, L.G.; Stanley, E.R.; et al. Fate mapping analysis reveals that adult microglia derive from primitive macrophages. *Science* **2010**, *330*, 841–845. [CrossRef] [PubMed]
6. Bennett, M.L.; Bennett, F.C.; Liddelow, S.A.; Ajami, B.; Zamanian, J.L.; Fernhoff, N.B.; Mulinyawe, S.B.; Bohlen, C.J.; Adil, A.; Tucker, A.; et al. New tools for studying microglia in the mouse and human CNS. *Proc. Natl. Acad. Sci. USA* **2016**, *113*, E1738–E1746. [CrossRef] [PubMed]
7. Butovsky, O.; Jedrychowski, M.P.; Moore, C.S.; Cialic, R.; Lanser, A.J.; Gabriely, G.; Koeglsperger, T.; Dake, B.; Wu, P.M.; Doykan, C.E.; et al. Identification of a unique TGF-β-dependent molecular and functional signature in microglia. *Nat. Neurosci.* **2014**, *17*, 131–143. [CrossRef] [PubMed]
8. Askew, K.; Li, K.; Olmos-Alonso, A.; Garcia-Moreno, F.; Liang, Y.; Richardson, P.; Tipton, T.; Chapman, M.A.; Riecken, K.; Beccari, S.; et al. Coupled Proliferation and Apoptosis Maintain the Rapid Turnover of Microglia in the Adult Brain. *Cell Rep.* **2017**, *18*, 391–405. [CrossRef] [PubMed]
9. Ajami, B.; Bennett, J.L.; Krieger, C.; Tetzlaff, W.; Rossi, F.M.V. Local self-renewal can sustain CNS microglia maintenance and function throughout adult life. *Nat. Neurosci.* **2007**, *10*, 1538–1543. [CrossRef] [PubMed]
10. Goldmann, T.; Wieghofer, P.; Jordão, M.J.C.; Prutek, F.; Hagemeyer, N.; Frenzel, K.; Amann, L.; Staszewski, O.; Kierdorf, K.; Krueger, M.; et al. Origin, fate and dynamics of macrophages at central nervous system interfaces. *Nat. Immunol.* **2016**, *17*, 797–805. [CrossRef] [PubMed]
11. Spittau, B. Aging Microglia-Phenotypes, Functions and Implications for Age-Related Neurodegenerative Diseases. *Front. Aging Neurosci.* **2017**, *9*, 194. [CrossRef] [PubMed]
12. Raj, D.D.A.; Jaarsma, D.; Holtman, I.R.; Olah, M.; Ferreira, F.M.; Schaafsma, W.; Brouwer, N.; Meijer, M.M.; de Waard, M.C.; van der Pluijm, I.; et al. Priming of microglia in a DNA-repair deficient model of accelerated aging. *Neurobiol. Aging* **2014**. [CrossRef] [PubMed]
13. Raj, D.D.A.; Moser, J.; van der Pol, S.M.A.; van Os, R.P.; Holtman, I.R.; Brouwer, N.; Oeseburg, H.; Schaafsma, W.; Wesseling, E.M.; den Dunnen, W.; et al. Enhanced microglial pro-inflammatory response to lipopolysaccharide correlates with brain infiltration and blood-brain barrier dysregulation in a mouse model of telomere shortening. *Aging Cell* **2015**, *14*, 1003–1013. [CrossRef] [PubMed]
14. Sierra, A.; Gottfried-Blackmore, A.C.; McEwen, B.S.; Bulloch, K. Microglia derived from aging mice exhibit an altered inflammatory profile. *Glia* **2007**, *55*, 412–424. [CrossRef] [PubMed]
15. Facci, L.; Barbierato, M.; Marinelli, C.; Argentini, C.; Skaper, S.D.; Giusti, P. Toll-like receptors 2, -3 and -4 prime microglia but not astrocytes across central nervous system regions for ATP-dependent interleukin-1β release. *Sci. Rep.* **2014**, *4*, 6824. [CrossRef] [PubMed]
16. Fonken, L.K.; Frank, M.G.; Kitt, M.M.; D'Angelo, H.M.; Norden, D.M.; Weber, M.D.; Barrientos, R.M.; Godbout, J.P.; Watkins, L.R.; Maier, S.F. The Alarmin HMGB1 Mediates Age-Induced Neuroinflammatory Priming. *J. Neurosci.* **2016**, *36*, 7946–7956. [CrossRef] [PubMed]
17. Holtman, I.R.; Raj, D.D.; Miller, J.A.; Schaafsma, W.; Yin, Z.; Brouwer, N.; Wes, P.D.; Möller, T.; Orre, M.; Kamphuis, W.; et al. Induction of a common microglia gene expression signature by aging and neurodegenerative conditions: A co-expression meta-analysis. *Acta Neuropathol. Commun.* **2015**, *3*, 31. [CrossRef] [PubMed]
18. Hickman, S.E.; Kingery, N.D.; Ohsumi, T.K.; Borowsky, M.L.; Wang, L.-C.; Means, T.K.; El Khoury, J. The microglial sensome revealed by direct RNA sequencing. *Nat. Neurosci.* **2013**, *16*, 1896–1905. [CrossRef] [PubMed]

19. Sharaf, A.; Krieglstein, K.; Spittau, B. Distribution of microglia in the postnatal murine nigrostriatal system. *Cell Tissue Res.* **2013**, *351*, 373–382. [CrossRef] [PubMed]
20. Davies, D.S.; Ma, J.; Jegathees, T.; Goldsbury, C. Microglia show altered morphology and reduced arborization in human brain during aging and Alzheimer's disease. *Brain Pathol.* **2017**, *27*, 795–808. [CrossRef] [PubMed]
21. Koellhoffer, E.C.; McCullough, L.D.; Ritzel, R.M. Old Maids: Aging and Its Impact on Microglia Function. *Int. J. Mol. Sci.* **2017**, *18*. [CrossRef] [PubMed]
22. Dauffy, J.; Mouchiroud, G.; Bourette, R.P. The interferon-inducible gene, *Ifi204*, is transcriptionally activated in response to M-CSF, and its expression favors macrophage differentiation in myeloid progenitor cells. *J. Leukoc. Biol.* **2006**, *79*, 173–183. [CrossRef] [PubMed]
23. Chunfa, L.; Xin, S.; Qiang, L.; Sreevatsan, S.; Yang, L.; Zhao, D.; Zhou, X. The Central Role of IFI204 in IFN-β Release and Autophagy Activation during *Mycobacterium bovis* Infection. *Front. Cell. Infect. Microbiol.* **2017**, *7*, 169. [CrossRef] [PubMed]
24. Blank, T.; Prinz, M. Type I interferon pathway in CNS homeostasis and neurological disorders. *Glia* **2017**, *65*, 1397–1406. [CrossRef] [PubMed]
25. Cheng, H.; Mohammed, F.; Nam, G.; Chen, Y.; Qi, J.; Garner, L.I.; Allen, R.L.; Yan, J.; Willcox, B.E.; Gao, G.F. Crystal structure of leukocyte Ig-like receptor LILRB4 (ILT3/LIR-5/CD85k): A myeloid inhibitory receptor involved in immune tolerance. *J. Biol. Chem.* **2011**, *286*, 18013–18025. [CrossRef] [PubMed]
26. Jiang, Z.; Qin, J.-J.; Zhang, Y.; Cheng, W.-L.; Ji, Y.-X.; Gong, F.-H.; Zhu, X.-Y.; Zhang, Y.; She, Z.-G.; Huang, Z.; et al. LILRB4 deficiency aggravates the development of atherosclerosis and plaque instability by increasing the macrophage inflammatory response via NF-κB signaling. *Clin. Sci.* **2017**. [CrossRef] [PubMed]
27. Zhou, J.S.; Friend, D.S.; Lee, D.M.; Li, L.; Austen, K.F.; Katz, H.R. gp49B1 deficiency is associated with increases in cytokine and chemokine production and severity of proliferative synovitis induced by anti-type II collagen mAb. *Eur. J. Immunol.* **2005**, *35*, 1530–1538. [CrossRef] [PubMed]
28. Kamphuis, W.; Kooijman, L.; Schetters, S.; Orre, M.; Hol, E.M. Transcriptional profiling of CD11c-positive microglia accumulating around amyloid plaques in a mouse model for Alzheimer's disease. *Biochim. Biophys. Acta* **2016**, *1862*, 1847–1860. [CrossRef] [PubMed]
29. Zamboni, V.; Armentano, M.; Sarò, G.; Ciraolo, E.; Ghigo, A.; Germena, G.; Umbach, A.; Valnegri, P.; Passafaro, M.; Carabelli, V.; et al. Disruption of ArhGAP15 results in hyperactive Rac1, affects the architecture and function of hippocampal inhibitory neurons and causes cognitive deficits. *Sci. Rep.* **2016**, *6*, 34877. [CrossRef] [PubMed]
30. Bedard, K.; Krause, K.-H. The NOX family of ROS-generating NADPH oxidases: Physiology and pathophysiology. *Physiol. Rev.* **2007**, *87*, 245–313. [CrossRef] [PubMed]
31. Li, Q.; Spencer, N.Y.; Pantazis, N.J.; Engelhardt, J.F. Alsin and SOD1(G93A) proteins regulate endosomal reactive oxygen species production by glial cells and proinflammatory pathways responsible for neurotoxicity. *J. Biol. Chem.* **2011**, *286*, 40151–40162. [CrossRef] [PubMed]
32. Georgoudaki, A.-M.; Khodabandeh, S.; Puiac, S.; Persson, C.M.; Larsson, M.K.; Lind, M.; Hammarfjord, O.; Nabatti, T.H.; Wallin, R.P.A.; Yrlid, U.; et al. CD244 is expressed on dendritic cells and regulates their functions. *Immunol. Cell Biol.* **2015**, *93*, 581–590. [CrossRef] [PubMed]
33. Porrini, V.; Lanzillotta, A.; Branca, C.; Benarese, M.; Parrella, E.; Lorenzini, L.; Calzà, L.; Flaibani, R.; Spano, P.F.; Imbimbo, B.P.; et al. CHF5074 (CSP-1103) induces microglia alternative activation in plaque-free Tg2576 mice and primary glial cultures exposed to beta-amyloid. *Neuroscience* **2015**, *302*, 112–120. [CrossRef] [PubMed]
34. Xiao, Q.; Yu, W.; Tian, Q.; Fu, X.; Wang, X.; Gu, M.; Lü, Y. Chitinase1 contributed to a potential protection via microglia polarization and Aβ oligomer reduction in D-galactose and aluminum-induced rat model with cognitive impairments. *Neuroscience* **2017**, *355*, 61–70. [CrossRef] [PubMed]
35. Kim, S.-M.; Mun, B.-R.; Lee, S.-J.; Joh, Y.; Lee, H.-Y.; Ji, K.-Y.; Choi, H.-R.; Lee, E.-H.; Kim, E.-M.; Jang, J.-H.; et al. TREM2 promotes Aβ phagocytosis by upregulating C/EBPα-dependent CD36 expression in microglia. *Sci. Rep.* **2017**, *7*, 11118. [CrossRef] [PubMed]
36. Li, F.; Faustino, J.; Woo, M.-S.; Derugin, N.; Vexler, Z.S. Lack of the scavenger receptor CD36 alters microglial phenotypes after neonatal stroke. *J. Neurochem.* **2015**, *135*, 445–452. [CrossRef] [PubMed]
37. Woo, M.-S.; Wang, X.; Faustino, J.V.; Derugin, N.; Wendland, M.F.; Zhou, P.; Iadecola, C.; Vexler, Z.S. Genetic deletion of CD36 enhances injury after acute neonatal stroke. *Ann. Neurol.* **2012**, *72*, 961–970. [CrossRef] [PubMed]

38. Ueno, M.; Fujita, Y.; Tanaka, T.; Nakamura, Y.; Kikuta, J.; Ishii, M.; Yamashita, T. Layer V cortical neurons require microglial support for survival during postnatal development. *Nat. Neurosci.* **2013**, *16*, 543–551. [CrossRef] [PubMed]
39. De Haas, A.H.; Boddeke, H.W.G.M.; Biber, K. Region-specific expression of immunoregulatory proteins on microglia in the healthy CNS. *Glia* **2008**, *56*, 888–894. [CrossRef] [PubMed]
40. Olah, M.; Patrick, E.; Villani, A.-C.; Xu, J.; White, C.C.; Ryan, K.J.; Piehowski, P.; Kapasi, A.; Nejad, P.; Cimpean, M.; et al. A transcriptomic atlas of aged human microglia. *Nat. Commun.* **2018**, *9*, 539. [CrossRef] [PubMed]
41. Mrdjen, D.; Pavlovic, A.; Hartmann, F.J.; Schreiner, B.; Utz, S.G.; Leung, B.P.; Lelios, I.; Heppner, F.L.; Kipnis, J.; Merkler, D.; et al. High-Dimensional Single-Cell Mapping of Central Nervous System Immune Cells Reveals Distinct Myeloid Subsets in Health, Aging, and Disease. *Immunity* **2018**. [CrossRef] [PubMed]
42. Fox, R.J.; Dimmic, M.W. A two-sample Bayesian *t*-test for microarray data. *BMC Bioinform.* **2006**, *7*, 126. [CrossRef] [PubMed]

15

Who is Classified as Untestable on Brief Cognitive Screens in an Acute Stroke Setting?

Emma Elliott *, Bogna A. Drozdowska, Martin Taylor-Rowan, Robert C. Shaw, Gillian Cuthbertson and Terence J. Quinn

Institute of Cardiovascular and Medical Sciences, University of Glasgow, New Lister Building, Glasgow Royal Infirmary, Glasgow G31 2ER, UK
* Correspondence: e.elliott.2@research.gla.ac.uk

Abstract: Full completion of cognitive screening tests can be problematic in the context of a stroke. Our aim was to examine the completion of various brief cognitive screens and explore reasons for untestability. Data were collected from consecutive stroke admissions (May 2016–August 2018). The cognitive assessment was attempted during the first week of admission. Patients were classified as partially untestable (≥1 test item was incomplete) and fully untestable (where assessment was not attempted, and/or no questions answered). We assessed univariate and multivariate associations of test completion with: age (years), sex, stroke severity (National Institutes of Health Stroke Scale (NIHSS)), stroke classification, pre-morbid disability (modified Rankin Scale (mRS)), previous stroke and previous dementia diagnosis. Of 703 patients admitted (mean age: 69.4), 119 (17%) were classified as fully untestable and 58 (8%) were partially untestable. The 4A-test had 100% completion and the clock-draw task had the lowest completion (533/703, 76%). Independent associations with fully untestable status had a higher NIHSS score (odds ratio (OR): 1.18, 95% CI: 1.11–1.26), higher pre-morbid mRS (OR: 1.28, 95% CI: 1.02–1.60) and pre-stroke dementia (OR: 3.35, 95% CI: 1.53–7.32). Overall, a quarter of patients were classified as untestable on the cognitive assessment, with test incompletion related to stroke and non-stroke factors. Clinicians and researchers would benefit from guidance on how to make the best use of incomplete test data.

Keywords: feasibility; cognitive screening instruments; cognition; stroke

---

1. Introduction

Cognitive screening following a stroke is recommended in international clinical guidelines [1,2] and routinely performed in acute stroke settings in many countries. However, completion of a cognitive test battery in a medically unwell person with recent neurological insult is challenging. Previous research has demonstrated that around 20% of stroke patients cannot fully complete many of the cognitive screening tests commonly used in stroke practice, for example the Montreal Cognitive Assessment (MoCA) [3] and the Mini-Mental State Examination (MMSE) [4]. Test non-completion is reported in both acute stroke [5] and rehabilitation settings [6] (Table 1). However, published data appear conflicting and other centres have reported that a lengthy neuropsychological battery can be performed in the acute setting [7].

Table 1. Previous studies addressing feasibility of cognitive assessments post-stroke.

Study	Test	Number of Patients	Inclusion Criteria Relevant to Feasibility	Time Point	Completion Rate
			Setting: Acute		
Alderman et al. [8] (CA)	Battery of 8 tests	27	Mild strokes and TIAs	≤24 h	96%
Collas 2016 [9] (CA)	OCS	155	No relevant exclusions	5 days (mean)	89%
Horstmann et al. [10]	MoCA	842	IS and ICH. No relevant exclusions	2 days (median)	81%
Pasi et al. [5]	MoCA	137	IS and ICH. No relevant exclusions	5–9 days	83%
Pendlebury et al. [11]	AMT MMSE	1097	No relevant exclusions	4 days (median)	76% partially testable 69% fully testable
Van Zandvoort et al. [7]	1.5-h NPB	57	IS only, no previous stroke, maximum age 80, mRS 2–4, no psychiatric history or comorbidity that could influence cognitive functioning	4–22 days	75%
			Setting: Sub-Acute/Rehabilitation		
Barnay et al. [12]	CASP MMSE MoCA	44	All aphasic patients	42 ± 22 days	CASP 82% MMSE 64% MoCA 70%
Benaim et al. [6]	CASP MMSE MoCA	50	Non-aphasic patients only	40 ± 17 days	CASP 100% MMSE 100% MoCA 94%
Cumming et al. [13]	MoCA	220	IS and ICH. No relevant exclusions	3 months	Mild stroke 87% Moderate stroke 79% Severe stroke 67%
Kwa et al. [14]	CAMCOG	129	IS only	≥3 months	88%
Mancuso et al. [15]	OCS MMSE	325	No previous stroke, able to consent themselves, no previous psychiatric/neurological disease	33.9 ± 41.8 days	Fully untestable: MMSE 2%, OCS 1% Highest incompletion for individual OCS tasks: trails 28/325 (9%)
Lees et al. [16]	ACE-III MMSE MoCA	51	No relevant exclusions	36 days (median)	ACE-III 27% MMSE 43% MoCA 39%

Abbreviations: Abbreviated Mental Test (AMT); Addenbrooke's Cognitive Examination III (ACE-III); Cambridge Cognition Examination (CAMCOG); Cognitive assessment scale for stroke patients (CASP); conference abstract (CA); ischaemic stroke (IS); intracerebral haemorrhage (ICH); Mini-Mental State Examination (MMSE); Montreal Cognitive Assessment (MoCA); neuropsychological battery (NPB); Oxford Cognitive Screen (OCS); transient ischaemic attack (TIA); modified Rankin Scale (mRS).

Feasibility of completing a cognitive assessment is multifactorial; some aspects may relate to the stroke (extent of damage, presence of aphasia, limb weakness) and others may relate to the nature of the testing (timing and length of assessment, complexity). Looking at the patient characteristics and approaches to assessment can explain the apparently contradictory findings in the literature. Patients included in studies of cognitive tests are often not representative of a typical stroke unit. For example, studies may favour the inclusion of those with minor strokes, no (or little) pre-stroke disability and those who are able to provide informed consent, whilst patients with severe aphasia or an existing diagnosis of dementia are often excluded [17]. This selection bias will underestimate the true incidence of untestable patients.

An incomplete cognitive test has clinical implications. Inexperienced assessors may erroneously ascribe an incomplete test to cognitive impairment, when in the context of stroke, non-completion may relate to physical impairments. Ultimately, test non-completion could risk false positive and false negative diagnosis of cognitive problems with attendant harm. An understanding of the extent of test non-completion and knowledge of factors relating to untestability could potentially avoid this. The issue of test incompletion also complicates stroke research and audit. Often patients with incomplete assessments are excluded from analyses (since a total score cannot be calculated). This practice biases results, underestimates levels of cognitive impairment and could also lead to erroneous results [11]. Various approaches to incorporate incomplete tests have been proposed but there is no consensus on the best method [16].

There are different ways to address these feasibility issues, but the approach taken will depend on the aspect of feasibility of greatest relevance. For example, one may decide to choose a test specifically designed for a stroke (e.g., Oxford Cognitive Screen (OCS) [18]). This approach recognises that many traditional cognitive tests were designed for memory clinic populations and are not suited to the specific challenges encountered in acute stroke settings. Stroke specific, multi-domain tests are described and may be less biased by physical, communication and visuospatial impairments. Another approach may be to choose a shorter cognitive screen. This approach may be particularly suited to the acute medical setting where clinicians have limited time and other investigations may be prioritised in the first few days. Shorter tests may also be attractive to patients as there will be a reduced test burden. Short cognitive screens have been largely ignored in research conducted in the stroke setting. Stroke care is continuously evolving and differs internationally, but there is currently a paucity of feasibility research on cognitive tests in an acute, National Health Service (NHS) context. Our research aimed to meet these two gaps.

Our primary aim was to describe the test completion (feasibility) of some of the shortest cognitive screens (deliverable in under five min) in an unselected group admitted to our hyper-acute stroke unit. Our secondary aims were to explore reasons for assessors giving a patient a label of being untestable and to describe factors associated with being untestable.

2. Methods

We conducted an observational, cross-sectional study, using routinely collected data from an urban UK, teaching hospital. This was approved by the West of Scotland Research Ethics Committee (ws/16/0001) on 4 February 2016. We followed Standards of Reporting of Neurological Disorders (STROND) guidance [19] for the design, conduct and reporting of the study.

2.1. Setting and Population

We collected anonymised, routine, clinical data from consecutive admissions to our hyper-acute stroke unit (HASU). The unit admits all suspected stroke and transient ischaemic attack (TIA) patients with no exclusions in relation to age, disability or comorbidity. The unit offers level two (high dependency) clinical care and only patients requiring multi-organ support would be admitted to a higher-level care facility. Recruitment occurred during four timepoints: May 2016–February 2017; April–June 2017; October–December 2017; and July–August 2018. For the purposes of this study, we made no exclusions around stroke severity or stroke-related impairments. Written informed consent was not required for assessment.

2.2. Clinical and Demographic Assessment

Clinical and demographic data were collected for each patient by five trained researchers (four postgraduate students in psychology/neuroscience and one undergraduate medical student). Data collected were a mix of prospective assessment and retrospective derivation from medical case notes. Stroke severity was determined by the National Institutes of Health Stroke Scale (NIHSS) [20] on admission. Medical history, including any pre-stroke diagnosis of dementia, was recorded using medical notes and primary care summary data. Pre-stroke functioning was established using the modified Rankin Scale (mRS) [21–23]. Bamford stroke classification was completed for both ischaemic and haemorrhagic patients.

2.3. Cognitive Assessment

The cognitive assessment consisted of 13 questions, covering 8 different cognitive screening tests: the 10-point Abbreviated mental test score (AMTS) [24] and its shorter version AMT-4 [25], General Practitioner Assessment of Cognition (GPCOG) (patient section) [26], Mini-Cog [27], six item cognitive impairment test (6-CIT) [28], National Institute Neurological Disorders S-Canadian Stroke Network (NINDS-CSN) 5-min MoCA [29], abbreviated MoCA [30], and the 4 'A's Test (4AT) (Available online: www.the4AT.com) (Table 2). Each of these individual tests can be administered in under 5 min (and so suitable for use in acute clinical practice). They cover a variety of cognitive domains and have some supporting validation work in primary and geriatric care [31].

Table 2. Short cognitive tests ordered by number of items.

Test Name	Number of Items		Questions	Maximum Score	% of Assessments We Could Score in Full
Mini-Cog [27]	2	1	3-word delayed recall	5	75%
		2	Clock draw (numbers, hands)		
Abbreviated MoCA [30]	2	1	5-word delayed recall	8	75%
		2	Clock draw (face, numbers, hands)		
4-AMT [25]	4	1	Age	4	81%
		2	Year		
		3	Place		
		4	Date of birth		
4AT (Available online: www.the4AT.com)	5	1	Alertness	12	100%
		2	Age		
		3	Current year		
		4	Place		
		5	Date of birth		
		6	Months backwards		
6-CIT [28]	6	1	Time	28	78%
		2	Month		
		3	Yearl		
		4	Count backwards from 20		
		5	5-part delayed recall		
		6	Months backwards		
GPCOG [26]	7	1	Date	9	75%
		2	Month		
		3	Year		
		4	Date of birth		
		5	5-part delayed recall		
		6	Clock draw (numbers, hands)		
		7	News item		
NINDS-CSN 5 min MoCA [29]	7	1	Date	12	79%
		2	Month		
		3	Year		
		4	Day		
		5	Place		
		6	City		
		7	5-word delayed recall		
		8	Fluency (letter F)		
10-AMT [24]	10	1	Age	10	79%
		2	Time		
		3	Year		
		4	Place		
		5	Two-person recognition		
		6	Date of birth		
		7	Year of WW1		
		8	Current prime minister		
		9	Count backwards from 20		
		10	3-part delayed recall		

Abbreviations: Abbreviated mental test (AMT); General Practitioner Assessment of Cognition (GPCOG); Montreal Cognitive Assessment (MoCA); National Institute of Neurological disorders and stroke and the Canadian stroke network (NINDS-CSN); Six item cognitive impairment test (6-CIT).

Assessment was attempted during the first week of admission. Patients were only approached once for assessment, unless the patient requested for the assessment to be done at a later time-point, the assessment was interrupted by another clinical investigation (e.g., scan) or if the patient requested the assessment to be done over two sessions. Patients were not approached at all (and categorised fully untestable) if the parent clinical team reported that the patient was too unwell to undergo assessment or if the assessor felt that any form of direct testing would not be possible. In these patients, who could not be directly assessed, we checked if a cognitive assessment was documented by the parent clinical team since admission.

2.4. *Defining the Test Completion Outcomes*

Patients were classified as fully untestable when no part of the assessment was attempted (decision made by researcher in consultation with parent clinical team) and/or when no questions were answered when testing was attempted. Partially untestable was defined when at least one item in a test could not be completed or was not attempted (decided by either the patient, parent clinical team or researcher). A list of potential categories was created by the authors based on clinical experience, previous literature and initial scoping of free text responses. The free text reasons documented for each patient classified as untestable by the individual assessor were later collated into categories (e.g., aphasia and dysarthria both captured under speech problems) by the lead author (E.Elliott) with discussion with the stroke consultant (T.Quinn). Where more than one reason was listed, we chose the primary factor deemed to have the greatest impact on assessment (e.g., a patient documented as both acutely confused and dysarthric was categorised under confusion). Cases where a test item was attempted but poorly completed, for example, a patient with limb weakness who attempted the clock-draw with their weak or non-dominant hand, were classed as testable.

2.5. *Statistical Analysis*

We described patients as fully or partially untestable using the definitions above. We looked at the completion rate of each question in our assessment and then calculated completion rates for the different tests. Patients who ended up with a non-stroke diagnosis were kept in the analyses as we were interested in the feasibility of tests within all patients admitted with a suspected stroke and we retained admission NIHSS for these patients where it was completed.

We assessed univariable and multivariable associations with outcomes of interest using logistic regression. Variables were chosen based on previous literature [10,11] and plausible associations with feasibility. The following 12 covariates were used in both univariate and multivariate analyses: age (years), sex, NIHSS, Bamford stroke classification (TIA, partial anterior circulation stroke—PACS, total anterior circulation stroke—TACS, posterior circulation stroke—POCS, lacunar stroke—LACS, non-stroke (used as reference group)), pre-morbid mRS, presence of intracerebral haemorrhage (ICH), previous diagnosis of dementia and previous TIA/stroke. We did not include delirium in the model since our only measure was the 4AT scale and all untestable patients would have ended up with a label of delirium. Associations were described as odds ratios (OR) with corresponding 95% confidence intervals. We used the rule of 10 outcome events per predictor variable to determine the number of covariates we could include in the model and so required 120 "cases" for the model.

Analyses were run twice to account for how partially untestable patients are treated differently in the literature; in the first analysis they were treated as testable and in the second treated as untestable (grouped with the fully untestable patients). All data analyses were performed using the statistical software package SPSS (version 25 IBM, Armonk, NY, USA).

3. Results

The full sample included 703 patients (mean age 69.4 ± 13.7, 382 (54%) males, median NIHSS 2 (interquartile range, IQR 1–5)) (Table 3 for full patient characteristics). Of these, 119 (17%) were classified as fully untestable on all tests. Reasons for fully untestable fell under eight categories but for more than half of the group this was due to neurological deterioration (e.g., patients who were unresponsive, very unwell, palliative) (62/119, 54%). A further 58 (8%) patients in the full sample were separately classified as partially untestable (did not attempt ≥1 question); reasons fell under nine categories, with limb weakness 15 (26%) and speech problems 13 (22%) being most prevalent (full breakdown of reasons detailed in Figure 1). A large proportion of patients in the fully untestable group (n = 50, 42%) had a TACS, compared to only 3 (5%) in the partially untestable group.

Table 3. Characteristics of the sample.

Characteristics	Full Sample (n = 703)	Partially Untestable (n = 58)	Fully Untestable (n = 119)
Sex (male)	382 (54%)	27 (47%)	59 (50%)
Age mean (SD)	69.4 (13.7) Missing data (n = 2)	76.6 (9.7)	76.8 (12.5) Missing data (n = 2)
IS ICH TIA Non-stroke	429 IS 22 ICH 137 TIA 109 N/S Missing data (n = 6)	42 IS 4 ICH 5 TIA 7 N/S	85 IS 8 ICH 11 TIA 13 N/S Missing data (n = 2)
Bamford classification (IS and ICH)	66 TACS 174 PACS 100 POCS 111 LACS Missing data (n = 6)	3 TACS 25 PACS 12 POCS 6 LACS	50 TACS 31 PACS 8 POCS 4 LACS Missing data (n = 2)
NIHSS median (IQR)	2 (1–5) Missing data (n = 15)	4 (3–7) Missing data (n = 1)	8 (4–16) Missing data (n = 2)
Pre-morbid mRS median (IQR)	1 (0–3) Missing data (n = 5)	2 (0–3)	3 (0–3) Missing data (n = 1)
Previous stroke (IS/ICH) or TIA (yes)	218 (31%)	20 (34%)	36 (30%)
Previous diagnosis of dementia (yes)	61 (9%)	8 (14%)	30 (25%)

Abbreviations: ischaemic stroke (IS); interquartile range (IQR); intracerebral haemorrhage (ICH); lacunar stroke (LACS); modified Rankin Scale (mRS); National Institute for Health Stroke Scale (NIHSS); non-stroke (N/S); partial anterior circulation stroke (PACS); posterior circulation stroke (POCS); transient ischaemic attack (TIA); total anterior circulation stroke (TACS).

Patients who ended up with a non-stroke diagnosis (n = 109) were a diverse group (diagnoses included migraine, subarachnoid haemorrhage and vasovagal events). Of these, 20 (18%) were untestable in some way. Only 12 patients (2%) of the full sample declined the cognitive assessment; three declined the full assessment and nine declined certain questions. Characteristics: 7 (58%) males, mean age of 74.3 (SD = 13.9), median NIHSS of 3 (IQR 2–5), diagnoses: 1 non-stroke, 3 TIAs, 3 PACS, 3 POCS and 2 LACS.

We looked at the completion of each individual question within our full cognitive assessment (Table S1). Clock-draw had the lowest completion rate (533/703 (76%)), whilst age had the highest (583/703 (83%)). For 25/58 (43%) patients in the partially untestable group, clock-draw was the only task that they did not attempt. The completion rate of each individual test is given in Table 2; the 4AT was the only test which could be scored in full for all patients.

In the univariate analyses: higher age, TACS, ICH, higher NIHSS, higher pre-morbid mRS and a previous diagnosis of dementia were associated with being untestable, whilst a lacunar stroke was associated with being testable (Table 4). In the first multivariable regression analysis ($n = 680$), independent associations with fully untestable status were: higher NIHSS score (OR: 1.18, 95% CI: 1.11–1.26), higher pre-morbid mRS (OR: 1.28, 95% CI: 1.02–1.60) and pre-stroke dementia (OR: 3.35, 95% CI: 1.53–7.32). A lacunar stroke classification was associated with being testable (OR: 0.19, 95% CI: 0.06–0.65). In the second analysis (where the partially untestable group was combined with the fully untestable), the above variables remained significant. In addition, the following associations were found for being untestable: older age (OR: 1.04, 95% CI: 1.02–1.06) and presence of ICH (OR: 3.44, 95% CI: 1.13–10.44); whilst a TIA classification was associated with being testable (OR: 0.45, 95% CI: 0.20–0.997) (Table 4).

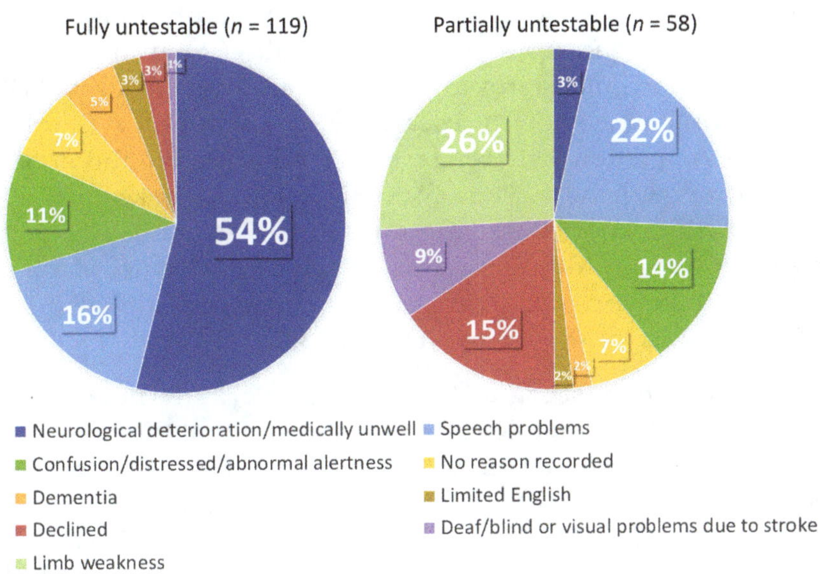

Figure 1. Reasons for fully/partially untestable.

Table 4. Feasibility associations.

Variables	Univariate for Fully Untestable	Multivariate (Partially Treated as Testable)	Multivariate (Partially Treated as Untestable)
	OR (95% CI)	**OR (95% CI)**	**OR (95% CI)**
Age (years)	**1.06 (1.04–1.08)**	1.02 (1.00–1.04)	**1.04 (1.02–1.06)**
Sex (male)	0.80 (0.54–1.18)	1.32 (0.77–2.26)	0.97 (0.62–1.51)
Stroke classification (non-stroke used as reference group):			
TACS	**23.08 (10.29–51.76)**	2.96 (0.98–8.93)	1.47 (0.50–4.34)
PACS	1.60 (0.80–3.22)	0.73 (0.32–1.65)	0.92 (0.46–1.83)
LACS	**0.28 (0.08–0.88)**	**0.19 (0.06–0.65)**	**0.26 (0.10–0.64)**
POCS	0.64 (0.25–1.62)	0.39 (0.14–1.12)	0.73 (0.33–1.61)
TIA	0.65 (0.28–1.50)	0.55 (0.21–1.40)	**0.45 (0.20–1.00 *)**
ICH	**2.96 (1.21–7.23)**	2.48 (0.72–8.59)	**3.44 (1.13–10.44)**
NIHSS	**1.30 (1.23–1.36)**	**1.18 (1.11–1.26)**	**1.23 (1.14–1.31)**
Pre-morbid mRS	**1.64 (1.41–1.91)**	**1.28 (1.02–1.60)**	**1.24 (1.03–1.50)**
Pre-stroke diagnosis of dementia	**6.01 (3.47–10.42)**	**3.35 (1.53–7.32)**	**2.74 (1.32–5.70)**
Previous stroke (IS, ICH) or TIA	0.96 (0.62–1.47)	0.82 (0.45–1.48)	0.91 (0.56–1.49)

* 0.997. Bold: significant associations. Abbreviations: intracerebral haemorrhage (ICH); ischaemic stroke (IS); lacunar stroke (LACS); modified Rankin Scale (mRS); National Institute for Health Stroke Scale (NIHSS); partial anterior circulation stroke (PACS); posterior circulation stroke (POCS); total anterior circulation stroke (TACS); transient ischemic attack (TIA).

4. Discussion

In an unselected sample of 703 patients admitted to our HASU, a quarter were classified as partially or fully untestable on brief cognitive screening tests. In those patients classified as partially untestable, the clock-draw was the most problematic, so tests including this item had the lowest completion rate. The 4AT was the only test which could be scored in full for all patients as it includes a score for being untestable. Factors associated with being fully untestable were previous diagnosis of dementia, higher pre-morbid mRS and higher NIHSS on admission, whilst a diagnosis of lacunar stroke was associated with being testable.

4.1. Research in Context

Our findings are generally in keeping with the limited literature on test feasibility. The associations of non-completion with stroke severity and dementia have face validity and the reasons given for a label of untestable were similar to those described in previous studies (for example limb weakness [5,11,16], aphasia [5,10,11], pre-morbid functional status [5] and reduced consciousness [11]), although reporting reasons for cognitive test non-completion in research is the exception rather than the norm. These findings highlight that non-completion is driven by both stroke specific and non-stroke related factors. Our finding that the clock-draw was the most problematic test is also in keeping with previous research findings for a stroke population; Lees et al. [16] found the lowest rates of completion on test items that required copying or drawing. Although tasks which assess visuospatial abilities, such as the clock-drawing test, can be challenging for stroke patients, they provide useful information on a key cognitive domain and can predict longer-term outcomes [32].

We decided to focus on the shortest cognitive tests available, in the hopes that they would be more practical for both the patient and clinician. Our results showed that the rates of completion for these short tests were similar to the completion rates for longer multi-domain cognitive tests previously studied (MoCA, MMSE). This should not be interpreted as meaning that the shortest tests are just as likely to be incomplete as more detailed tests. We did not include or directly compare longer tests with our short screens and our unselected population is not comparable with the patients tested in previous studies. There is a concern that shorter cognitive tests are inferior to longer, more detailed tests. Previous work has suggested that there is a trade-off between duration of administration and diagnostic accuracy [33] in the context of dementia. A focus on length of assessment alone (number of questions, administration time) is perhaps too simplistic, and test content is likely to be more important. For example, a long test could assess one area of cognition in depth yet neglect other domains.

4.2. Strengths and Weaknesses of the Research

A major strength of our study is that we had access to an unbiased, real-world sample, including patients who are often excluded from research (for example those with severe aphasia and dementia). While using clinical data have these benefits, we also have to acknowledge that due to the 'messy reality' of acute clinical practice, data are often missing. Our approach allowed us to retrospectively derive missing data from various sources including inpatient medical records, primary care data and consultation with the parent clinical team. Retrospective scoring can increase some inaccuracy, for example, calculating NIHSS based on the symptoms documented in medical case notes, rather than carrying it out directly with the patient.

There were some potentially interesting aspects of feasibility/applicability where we did not record data. We did not record the total number of patients who had limb weakness from their stroke and attempted the clock-draw using their weak or non-dominant hand (classed as testable). Data on this subgroup would be useful as many will lose points or score zero for poorly completed drawing tasks. We also did not record if an assessment had to be completed over two sessions or if any part of the assessment was interrupted.

Although we operationalised our concept of partially and fully untestable there is still subjectivity in the interpretation. It is essentially a judgement call by the clinician whether patients with aphasia, limb weakness and visual problems can complete a task (if the patient does not decline themselves). The same patient could therefore be classified differently purely based on who assessed them. This is particularly relevant in our study, where differing assessors performed the cognitive testing. This could be considered both a strength and weakness as it provides further real-world validity (some people might be better at encouraging patients to complete an assessment than others).

Finally, a limitation of determining feasibility of different questions and their resulting tests is the order in which the questions are asked. We acknowledge asking questions in the same order for each patient introduces some bias and is an issue because some patients will struggle to focus for longer periods of time or are easily fatigued.

4.3. Recommendations for Future Research and Practice

The strict administration and scoring criteria required for cognitive tests can be problematic for the stroke setting. Clinicians and researchers can therefore expect to encounter a number of stroke patients that will be untestable on certain tasks, or patients who are testable, but their stroke-related impairments result in a misleading test score. While in clinical practice an assessment can be put into context, in research it is more important that a-priori rules are set for dealing with incomplete tests. The importance of doing this is highlighted by the fact our analyses showed different results depending on how partially untestable patients were classified. Numerous approaches exist to deal with missing data [16], but to maximise the utility of the data collected, we recommend, where possible, that researchers make full use of incomplete participant data, rather than applying a complete-case analysis approach.

Tests which incorporate scoring for untestable patients, such as the 4AT, are helpful. Although the 4AT is primarily a delirium screen, the same approach could be applied to general cognitive tests. Guidance documents exist for scoring other stroke scales such as the NIHSS in patients who are comatose, confused, etc., so these types of resources could be made available for challenging cases in cognitive assessment.

Test completion rates are just one measure of feasibility. Feasibility covers a range of factors relating to the patient, assessor and the ward setting (Figure 2), so future research studies should include data addressing these other perspectives. To date, there has been little data published on the clinician's experience of cognitive assessment, environmental factors affecting assessment on the ward (noise, space, interruptions) and practical aspects, such as how assessors have misinterpreted administration/scoring instructions. With the increased use of computerised versions of cognitive tests in the future, feasibility issues from the assessor's side are likely to improve; for example, automatic scoring saves time and reduces scoring errors and subjectivity. Future research should also make use of routinely collected clinical data, such as that collected by the Sentinel Stroke National Audit Programme (SSNAP) and the Scottish stroke care audit in the United Kingdom. One could argue that any study using a researcher to administer a scale, rather than a clinical member of staff, is not truly addressing broader feasibility and implementation issues.

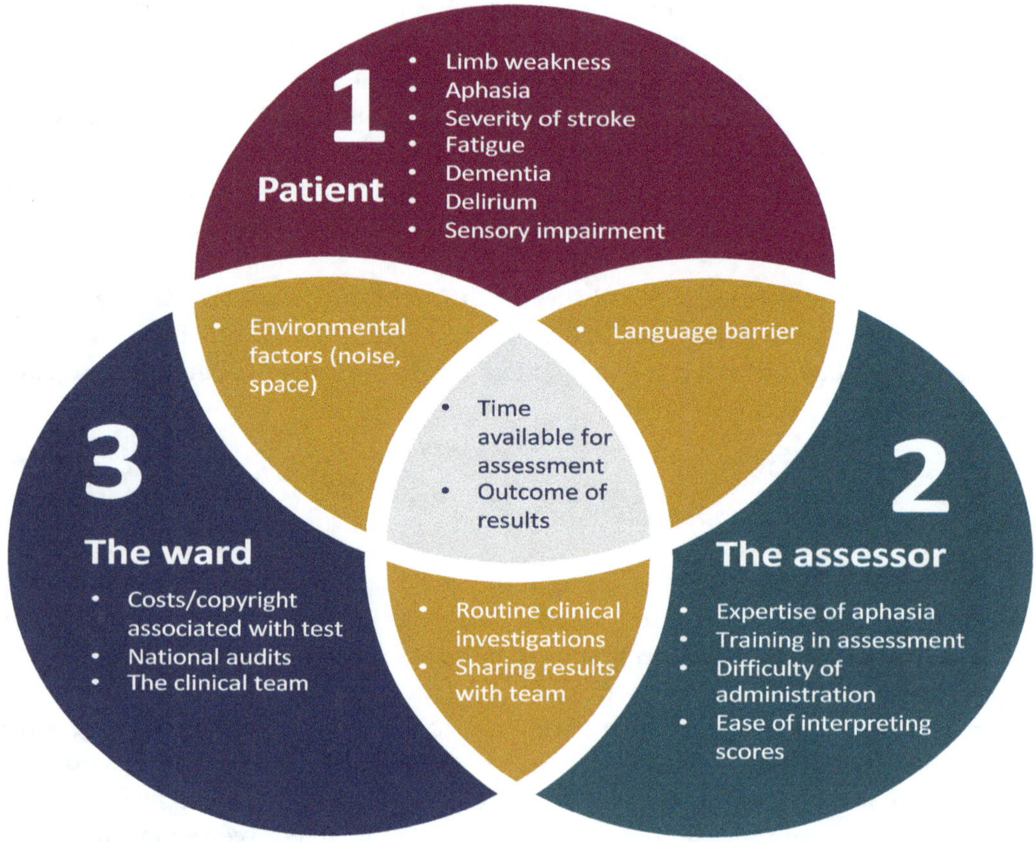

Figure 2. Factors affecting feasibility of cognitive assessment in acute stroke. Factors listed are illustrative but not exhaustive.

5. Conclusions

In a real-world sample, a quarter of patients in our HASU were classified as fully or partially untestable on brief cognitive screening tests. Clinicians and researchers should make a-priori plans on how to address incomplete assessments. Feasibility is a multi-faceted term, and factors from both clinician and patient point of view should be considered.

Author Contributions: Conceptualisation, T.J.Q.; data collection, E.E., B.A.D., M.T.-R., R.C.S., G.C.; formal Analysis, E.E.; writing-original draft, E.E.; writing-reviewing & editing, all authors; supervision, T.J.Q.

References

1. Quinn, T.J.; Elliott, E.; Langhorne, P. Cognitive and Mood Assessment Tools for Use in Stroke. *Stroke* **2018**, *49*, 483–490. [CrossRef] [PubMed]
2. Intercollegiate Stroke Working Party. *National Clinical Guideline for Stroke*, 5th ed.; Royal College of Physicians: London, UK, 2016.
3. Nasreddine, Z.S.; Phillips, N.A.; Bedirian, V.; Charbonneau, S.; Whitehead, V.; Collin, I.; Cummings, J.L.; Chertkow, H. The Montreal Cognitive Assessment, MoCA: A brief screening tool for mild cognitive impairment. *J. Am. Geriatr. Soc.* **2005**, *53*, 695–699. [CrossRef] [PubMed]
4. Folstein, M.F.; Folstein, S.E.; McHugh, P.R. "Mini-mental state". A practical method for grading the cognitive state of patients for the clinician. *J. Psychiatr Res.* **1975**, *12*, 189–198. [CrossRef]
5. Pasi, M.; Salvadori, E.; Poggesi, A.; Inzitari, D.; Pantoni, L. Factors predicting the Montreal cognitive assessment (MoCA) applicability and performances in a stroke unit. *J. Neurol* **2013**, *260*, 1518–1526. [CrossRef] [PubMed]

6. Benaim, C.; Barnay, J.L.; Wauquiez, G.; Bonnin-Koang, H.Y.; Anquetil, C.; Perennou, D.; Piscicelli, C.; Lucas-Pineau, B.; Muja, L.; le Stunff, E.; et al. The Cognitive Assessment scale for Stroke Patients (CASP) vs. MMSE and MoCA in non-aphasic hemispheric stroke patients. *Ann. Phys. Rehabil. Med.* **2015**, *58*, 78–85. [CrossRef] [PubMed]
7. van Zandvoort, M.J.E.; Kessels, R.P.C.; Nys, G.M.S.; de Haan, E.H.F.; Kappelle, L.J. Early neuropsychological evaluation in patients with ischaemic stroke provides valid information. *Clin. Neurol. Neurosurg.* **2005**, *107*, 385–392. [CrossRef]
8. Alderman, S.; Vahidy, F.; Bursaw, A.; Savitz, S. Abstract TP337: Feasibility of Cognitive Testing in Patients with Acute Ischemic Stroke. *Stroke* **2013**, *44*, ATP337. [CrossRef]
9. Collas, D. Detecting Cognitive Impairment in Acute Stroke Using the Oxford Cognitive Screen: Characteristics of Left and Right Hemisphere Strokes, with More Severe Impairment in AF Strokes (P1.190). *Neurology* **2016**, *86*, P1.190.
10. Horstmann, S.; Rizos, T.; Rauch, G.; Arden, C.; Veltkamp, R. Feasibility of the Montreal Cognitive Assessment in acute stroke patients. *Eur. J. Neurol.* **2014**, *21*, 1387–1393. [CrossRef]
11. Pendlebury, S.T.; Klaus, S.P.; Thomson, R.J.; Mehta, Z.; Wharton, R.M.; Rothwell, P.M. Methodological Factors in Determining Risk of Dementia After Transient Ischemic Attack and Stroke: (III) Applicability of Cognitive Tests. *Stroke* **2015**, *46*, 3067–3073. [CrossRef]
12. Barnay, J.L.; Wauquiez, G.; Bonnin-Koang, H.Y.; Anquetil, C.; Perennou, D.; Piscicelli, C.; Lucas-Pineau, B.; Muja, L.; le Stunff, E.; de Boissezon, X.; et al. Feasibility of the cognitive assessment scale for stroke patients (CASP) vs. MMSE and MoCA in aphasic left hemispheric stroke patients. *Ann. Phys. Rehabil. Med.* **2014**, *57*, 422–435. [CrossRef]
13. Cumming, T.B.; Bernhardt, J.; Linden, T. The montreal cognitive assessment: Short cognitive evaluation in a large stroke trial. *Stroke* **2011**, *42*, 2642–2644. [CrossRef]
14. Kwa, V.I.H.; Limburg, M.; Voogel, A.J.; Teunisse, S.; Derix, M.M.A.; Hijdra, A. Feasibility of cognitive screening of patients with ischaemic stroke using the CAMCOG A hospital-based study. *J. Neurol.* **1996**, *243*, 405–409. [CrossRef]
15. Mancuso, M.; Demeyere, N.; Abbruzzese, L.; Damora, A.; Varalta, V.; Pirrotta, F.; Antonucci, G.; Matano, A.; Caputo, M.; Caruso, M.G.; et al. Using the Oxford Cognitive Screen to Detect Cognitive Impairment in Stroke Patients: A Comparison with the Mini-Mental State Examination. *Front. Neurol.* **2018**, *9*, 101. [CrossRef]
16. Lees, R.A.; Hendry Ba, K.; Broomfield, N.; Stott, D.; Larner, A.J.; Quinn, T.J. Cognitive assessment in stroke: Feasibility and test properties using differing approaches to scoring of incomplete items. *Int. J. Geriatr. Psychiatry* **2017**, *32*, 1072–1078. [CrossRef]
17. Pendlebury, S.T.; Chen, P.J.; Bull, L.; Silver, L.; Mehta, Z.; Rothwell, P.M. Methodological factors in determining rates of dementia in transient ischemic attack and stroke: (I) impact of baseline selection bias. *Stroke* **2015**, *46*, 641–646. [CrossRef]
18. Demeyere, N.; Riddoch, M.J.; Slavkova, E.D.; Bickerton, W.L.; Humphreys, G.W. The Oxford Cognitive Screen (OCS): Validation of a stroke-specific short cognitive screening tool. *Psychol. Assess.* **2015**, *27*, 883–894. [CrossRef]
19. Bennett, D.A.; Brayne, C.; Feigin, V.L.; Barker-Collo, S.; Brainin, M.; Davis, D.; Gallo, V.; Jette, N.; Karch, A.; Kurtzke, J.F.; et al. Development of the standards of reporting of neurological disorders (STROND) checklist: A guideline for the reporting of incidence and prevalence studies in neuroepidemiology. *Eur. J. Epidemiol.* **2015**, *30*, 569–576. [CrossRef]
20. Brott, T.; Adams, H.P., Jr.; Olinger, C.P.; Marler, J.R.; Barsan, W.G.; Biller, J.; Spilker, J.; Holleran, R.; Eberle, R.; Hertzberg, V.; et al. Measurements of acute cerebral infarction: A clinical examination scale. *Stroke* **1989**, *20*, 864–870. [CrossRef]
21. Rankin, J. Cerebral vascular accidents in patients over the age of 60. I. General considerations. *Scott. Med. J.* **1957**, *2*, 127–136. [CrossRef]
22. van Swieten, J.C.; Koudstaal, P.J.; Visser, M.C.; Schouten, H.J.; van Gijn, J. Interobserver agreement for the assessment of handicap in stroke patients. *Stroke* **1988**, *19*, 604–607. [CrossRef]
23. Fearon, P.; McArthur, K.S.; Garrity, K.; Graham, L.J.; McGroarty, G.; Vincent, S.; Quinn, T.J. Prestroke modified rankin stroke scale has moderate interobserver reliability and validity in an acute stroke setting. *Stroke* **2012**, *43*, 3184–3188. [CrossRef]

24. Hodkinson, H.M. Evaluation of a mental test score for assessment of mental impairment in the elderly. *Age Ageing* **1972**, *1*, 233–238. [CrossRef]
25. Swain, D.G.; Nightingale, P.G. Evaluation of a shortened version of the Abbreviated Mental Test in a series of elderly patients. *Clin. Rehabil.* **1997**, *11*, 243–248. [CrossRef]
26. Brodaty, H.; Pond, D.; Kemp, N.M.; Luscombe, G.; Harding, L.; Berman, K.; Huppert, F.A. The GPCOG: A new screening test for dementia designed for general practice. *J. Am. Geriatr. Soc.* **2002**, *50*, 530–534. [CrossRef]
27. Borson, S.; Scanlan, J.M.; Chen, P.; Ganguli, M. The Mini-Cog as a screen for dementia: Validation in a population-based sample. *J. Am. Geriatr. Soc.* **2003**, *51*, 1451–1454. [CrossRef]
28. Brooke, P.; Bullock, R. Validation of a 6 item cognitive impairment test with a view to primary care usage. *Int. J. Geriatr. Psychiatry* **1999**, *14*, 936–940. [CrossRef]
29. Hachinski, V.; Iadecola, C.; Petersen, R.C.; Breteler, M.M.; Nyenhuis, D.L.; Black, S.E.; Powers, W.J.; DeCarli, C.; Merino, J.G.; Kalaria, R.N.; et al. National Institute of Neurological Disorders and Stroke-Canadian Stroke Network vascular cognitive impairment harmonization standards. *Stroke* **2006**, *37*, 2220–2241. [CrossRef]
30. Panenková, E.; Kopecek, M.; Lukavsky, J. Item analysis and possibility to abbreviate the Montreal Cognitive Assessment. *Ceska Slov. Psychiatr.* **2016**, *112*, 63–69.
31. Ismail, Z.; Rajji, T.K.; Shulman, K.I. Brief cognitive screening instruments: An update. *Int. J. Geriatr. Psychiatry* **2010**, *25*, 111–120. [CrossRef]
32. Champod, A.S.; Gubitz, G.J.; Phillips, S.J.; Christian, C.; Reidy, Y.; Radu, L.M.; Darvesh, S.; Reid, J.M.; Kintzel, F.; Eskes, G.A. Clock Drawing Test in acute stroke and its relationship with long-term functional and cognitive outcomes. *Clin. Neuropsychol.* **2019**, *33*, 817–830. [CrossRef] [PubMed]
33. Larner, A.J. Speed versus accuracy in cognitive assessment when using CSIs. *Prog. Neurol. Psychiatry* **2015**, *19*, 21–24. [CrossRef]

Permissions

All chapters in this book were first published by MDPI; hereby published with permission under the Creative Commons Attribution License or equivalent. Every chapter published in this book has been scrutinized by our experts. Their significance has been extensively debated. The topics covered herein carry significant findings which will fuel the growth of the discipline. They may even be implemented as practical applications or may be referred to as a beginning point for another development.

The contributors of this book come from diverse backgrounds, making this book a truly international effort. This book will bring forth new frontiers with its revolutionizing research information and detailed analysis of the nascent developments around the world.

We would like to thank all the contributing authors for lending their expertise to make the book truly unique. They have played a crucial role in the development of this book. Without their invaluable contributions this book wouldn't have been possible. They have made vital efforts to compile up to date information on the varied aspects of this subject to make this book a valuable addition to the collection of many professionals and students.

This book was conceptualized with the vision of imparting up-to-date information and advanced data in this field. To ensure the same, a matchless editorial board was set up. Every individual on the board went through rigorous rounds of assessment to prove their worth. After which they invested a large part of their time researching and compiling the most relevant data for our readers.

The editorial board has been involved in producing this book since its inception. They have spent rigorous hours researching and exploring the diverse topics which have resulted in the successful publishing of this book. They have passed on their knowledge of decades through this book. To expedite this challenging task, the publisher supported the team at every step. A small team of assistant editors was also appointed to further simplify the editing procedure and attain best results for the readers.

Apart from the editorial board, the designing team has also invested a significant amount of their time in understanding the subject and creating the most relevant covers. They scrutinized every image to scout for the most suitable representation of the subject and create an appropriate cover for the book.

The publishing team has been an ardent support to the editorial, designing and production team. Their endless efforts to recruit the best for this project, has resulted in the accomplishment of this book. They are a veteran in the field of academics and their pool of knowledge is as vast as their experience in printing. Their expertise and guidance has proved useful at every step. Their uncompromising quality standards have made this book an exceptional effort. Their encouragement from time to time has been an inspiration for everyone.

The publisher and the editorial board hope that this book will prove to be a valuable piece of knowledge for researchers, students, practitioners and scholars across the globe.

List of Contributors

Sunghee Kim, Kwisoon Choe and Kyoungsook Lee
Department of Nursing, Chung-Ang University, Dongjak-gu, Seoul 06974, Korea

Edyta Socha, Piotr Kośliński, Marcin Koba and Marcin Gackowski
Department of Toxicology and Bromatology, Faculty of Pharmacy, Collegium Medicum of Nicolaus Copernicus University, 85-067 Bydgoszcz, Poland

Katarzyna Mądra-Gackowska and Kornelia Kędziora-Kornatowska
Department of Geriatrics, Faculty of Health Sciences, Collegium Medicum of Nicolaus Copernicus University, 85-067 Bydgoszcz, Poland

Emilia Daghir-Wojtkowiak
Department of Biopharmaceutics and Pharmacodynamics, Medical University of Gdańsk, 80-210 Gdańsk, Poland

Michelle A. Erickson and William A. Banks
VA Puget Sound Healthcare System, Geriatric Research Education and Clinical Center, Seattle, WA 98108, USA
Division of Gerontology and Geriatric Medicine, Department of Medicine, University of Washington, Seattle, WA 98104, USA

Troy A. A. Harkness
Department of Anatomy and Cell Biology, University of Saskatchewan, Saskatoon, SK S7N 5E5, Canada

Mikhail V. Trostnikov, Natalia V. Roshina and Stepan V. Boldyrev
Institute of Molecular Genetics of RAS, Kurchatov Sq. 2, 123182 Moscow, Russia
Vavilov Institute of General Genetics, Russian Academy of Sciences, Gubkin 3, 119991 Moscow, Russia

Ekaterina R. Veselkina, Andrey A. Zhuikov and Elena G. Pasyukova
Institute of Molecular Genetics of RAS, Kurchatov Sq. 2, 123182 Moscow, Russia

Anna V. Krementsova
Institute of Molecular Genetics of RAS, Kurchatov Sq. 2, 123182 Moscow, Russia
Emmanuel Institute of Biochemical Physics, Russian Academy of Sciences, Kosygin St. 4, 119334 Moscow, Russia

Avital Sternin
Brain and Mind Institute, Department of Psychology, University of Western Ontario, London, ON N6A 3K7, Canada

Alistair Burns
Division of Neuroscience & Experimental Psychology, Manchester Institute for Collaborative Research on Ageing, School of Social Sciences, University of Manchester, Manchester M13 9PL, UK

Adrian M. Owen
Brain and Mind Institute, Department of Psychology, University of Western Ontario, London, ON N6A 3K7, Canada
Department of Physiology and Pharmacology, University of Western Ontario, London, ON N6A 3K7, Canada

Consolacion Garcia-Contreras, Laura Torres-Rovira and Susana Astiz
Comparative Physiology Group, SGIT-INIA, 28040 Madrid, Spain

Antonio Gonzalez-Bulnes
Comparative Physiology Group, SGIT-INIA, 28040 Madrid, Spain
Faculty of Veterinary Sciences, Universidad Complutense de Madrid, 28040 Madrid, Spain

Marta Vazquez-Gomez and Beatriz Isabel
Faculty of Veterinary Sciences, Universidad Complutense de Madrid, 28040 Madrid, Spain

Jorge Gonzalez
Micros Veterinaria, Campus de Vegazana, 24007 Leon, Spain

Esteban Porrini
Institute of Biomedical Technology (ITB), Universidad de La Laguna, 38200 Tenerife, Spain

Magali Gonzalez-Colaço
Central Unit of Clinical Research and Clinical Assays (UCICEC), Universitary Hospital of Canary Island, 28010 Tenerife, Spain

Hartmut Lehfeld
Department of Psychiatry and Psychotherapy, Paracelsus Medical University, 90419 Nuremberg, Germany

Mark Stemmler
Institute of Psychology, University of Erlangen-Nuremberg, 91052 Erlangen, Germany

Daniela Vieira, João Durães, Beatriz Santiago, Diana Duro, Marisa Lima and Miguel Tábuas-Pereira
Neurology Department, Centro Hospitalar e Universitário de Coimbra, 3000-045 Coimbra, Portugal

Maria João Leitão
Neurology Department, Centro Hospitalar e Universitário de Coimbra, 3000-045 Coimbra, Portugal
Center for Neuroscience and Cell Biology, University of Coimbra, 3000-070 Coimbra, Portugal

Inês Baldeiras and Isabel Santana
Neurology Department, Centro Hospitalar e Universitário de Coimbra, 3000-045 Coimbra, Portugal
Faculty of Medicine, University of Coimbra, 3000-070 Coimbra, Portugal
Center for Neuroscience and Cell Biology, University of Coimbra, 3000-070 Coimbra, Portugal

Magdalena Krajewska-Włodarczyk
Department of Rheumatology, Municipal Hospital in Olsztyn, 10-900 Olsztyn, Poland
Department of Internal Medicine, School of Medicine, Collegium Medicum, University ofWarmia and Mazury, 10-900 Olsztyn, Poland
Department of Pathophysiology, School of Medicine, Collegium Medicum, University of Warmia and Mazury, 10-900 Olsztyn, Poland

Adam Osowski
Department of Pathophysiology, School of Medicine, Collegium Medicum, University of Warmia and Mazury, 10-900 Olsztyn, Poland

Agnieszka Owczarczyk-Saczonek and Waldemar Placek
Department of Dermatology, Sexually Transmitted Diseases and Clinical Immunology, School of Medicine, Collegium Medicum, University of Warmia and Mazury, 10-900 Olsztyn, Poland

Joanna Wojtkiewicz
Department of Pathophysiology, School of Medicine, Collegium Medicum, University of Warmia and Mazury, 10-900 Olsztyn, Poland
Laboratory for Regenerative Medicine, School of Medicine, Collegium Medicum, University of Warmia and Mazury, 10-900 Olsztyn, Poland

Jiz-Yuh Wang
Graduate Institute of Medicine, College of Medicine, Kaohsiung Medical University, Kaohsiung 80708, Taiwan
Department of Medical Research, Kaohsiung Medical University Hospital, Kaohsiung 80708, Taiwan

Chen-Yen Lin
Graduate Institute of Medicine, College of Medicine, Kaohsiung Medical University, Kaohsiung 80708, Taiwan

Chiou-Lian Lai
Department of Neurology, Faculty of Medicine, College of Medicine, Kaohsiung Medical University, Kaohsiung 80708, Taiwan
Department of Neurology, Kaohsiung Medical University Hospital, Kaohsiung 80756, Taiwan

Ching-Tien Lee
Department of Nursing, Hsin-Sheng College of Medical Care and Management, Taoyuan 32544, Taiwan

Catherine Pennington
ReMemBr Group, University of Bristol, Bristol Brain Centre, Southmead Hospital, Southmead Road, BS10 5NB Bristol, UK
Centre for Dementia Prevention, University of Edinburgh, 9A Bioquarter, 9 Little France Road, Edinburgh EH16 4UX, UK

Harriet Ball and Marta Swirski
ReMemBr Group, University of Bristol, Bristol Brain Centre, Southmead Hospital, Southmead Road, BS10 5NB Bristol, UK

Rónán O'Caoimh
Centre for Gerontology and Rehabilitation, University College Cork, St Finbarr's Hospital, Douglas road, T12 XH60 Cork City, Ireland
Department of Geriatric Medicine, Mercy University Hospital, Grenville Place, T12 WE28 Cork City, Ireland

D. William Molloy
Centre for Gerontology and Rehabilitation, University College Cork, St Finbarr's Hospital, Douglas road, T12 XH60 Cork City, Ireland

Tanja Zöller
Institute for Anatomy and Cell Biology, Department of Molecular Embryology, Faculty of Medicine, University of Freiburg, Freiburg 79104, Germany

Björn Spittau
Institute for Anatomy and Cell Biology, Department of Molecular Embryology, Faculty of Medicine, University of Freiburg, Freiburg 79104, Germany
Institute of Anatomy, University of Rostock, Rostock 18057, Germany

Abdelraheim Attaai
Institute for Anatomy and Cell Biology, Department of Molecular Embryology, Faculty of Medicine, University of Freiburg, Freiburg 79104, Germany
Faculty of Biology, University of Freiburg, Freiburg 79104, Germany
Department of Anatomy and Histology, Faculty of Veterinary Medicine, Assiut University, Assiut 71526, Egypt

Phani Sankar Potru and Tamara Ruß
Institute of Anatomy, University of Rostock, Rostock 18057, Germany
Emma Elliott, Bogna A. Drozdowska, Martin Taylor-Rowan, Robert C. Shaw, Gillian Cuthbertson and Terence J. Quinn
Institute of Cardiovascular and Medical Sciences, University of Glasgow, New Lister Building, Glasgow Royal Infirmary, Glasgow G31 2ER, UK

Index

www.ingramcontent.com/pod-product-compliance
Lightning Source LLC
LaVergne TN
LVHW081013210926
848485LV00004B/848
* 9 7 8 1 6 3 9 2 7 5 8 0 9 *